UNEQUAL HEALTH

The scandal o

Danny Dorling

First published in Great Britain in 2013 by

The Policy Press
University of Bristol
Fourth Floor
Beacon House
Queen's Road
Bristol BS8 1QU
UK
t: +44 (0)117 331 4054
f: +44 (0)117 331 4093
tpp-info@bristol.ac.uk
www.policypress.co.uk

North America office:
The Policy Press
c/o The University of Chicago Press
1427 East 60th Street
Chicago, IL 60637, USA
t: +1 773 702 7700
f: +1 773-702-9756
e:sales@press.uchicago.edu
www.press.uchicago.edu

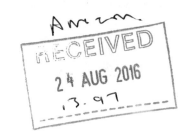

British Library Cataloguing in Publication Data
A catalogue record for this book is available from the British Library.

Library of Congress Cataloging-in-Publication Data
A catalog record for this book has been requested.

ISBN 978 1 44730 513 2 paperback
ISBN 978 1 44730 514 9 hardcover

Cover design by The Policy Press
Front cover: images kindly supplied by members of www.stockxchang.com
Printed and bound in Great Britain by Hobbs, Southampton
The Policy Press uses environmentally responsible print partners.

For Robbie, Izzy and Sol

Contents

Section V: Global inequality

Section VI: Thinking, drawing and counting

Section VII: Changing demographics and ageing populations

Sources of extracts

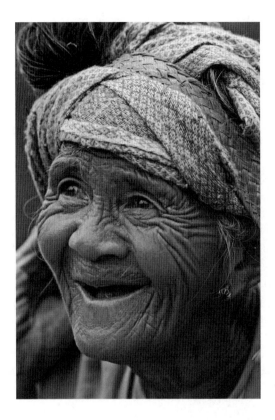

The following research centres, journals, publishers, newspapers, activists and websites all generously gave permission for previously published work to be included here; many thanks to all.

Section I: The long view

1: Figure 1.3 from www.mydavidcameron.com/posters/cam-nhs1

2: Figure 2.5 from Duncan Rickelton; Figure 2.7 from www.bbc.co.uk

3: Dorling, D., Mitchell, R., Shaw, M., Orford, S. and Davey Smith. G. (2000) 'The ghost of Christmas past: health effects of poverty in London in 1896 and 1991', *British Medical Journal*, vol 321, no 7276, December, pp 1547-51; and Dorling, D., Mitchell, R., Orford, S., Shaw, M. and Davey Smith, G. (2005) 'Inequalities and Christmas yet to come', *British Medical Journal*, vol 331, p 1409.

4: Dorling, D. (2006) 'Infant mortality and social progress in Britain, 1905–2005', in E. Garrett, C. Galley, N. Shelton and R. Woods (eds) *Infant mortality*, Aldershot: Ashgate, chapter 11.

5: Shaw, M. and Dorling, D. (2004) 'Who cares in England and Wales? The Positive Care Law: cross-sectional study', *Journal of General Practice*, vol 54, pp 899-903.

Section II: The liberal record

6: Figure 6.2 from a photograph by John Giles/Press Association.

7: Shaw, M., Davey Smith, G. and Dorling, D. (2005) 'Health inequalities and New Labour: how the promises compare with real progress', *British Medical Journal*, vol 330, pp 1016-21.

8: Dorling, D. (2007) 'Health', in J. Crudas *et al* (eds) *Closer to equality? Assessing New Labour's record on equality after 10 years in government*, London: Compass.

9: Dorling, D. (2007) 'Social harm and social policy in Britain', in Roberts, R. and McMahon, W. (eds) *Social justice and criminal justice*, London: Centre for Crime and Justice Studies, chapter 10.

10: Thomas, B., Dorling, D. and Davey Smith, G. (2010) 'Inequalities in premature mortality in Britain: observational study from 1921 to 2007', *British Medical Journal*, 23 July.

Section III: Medicine and politics

11: Figure 11.1 was redrawn from an original produced by the Association of Physicians.

12: Shaw, M., Mitchell, R. and Dorling, D. (2000) 'Time for a smoke: one cigarette is equivalent to 11 minutes of life expectancy', *British Medical Journal*, vol 320, p 53.

13: McCloskey, B., Macfarlane, A., Heyman, B., Dorling, D. *et al* (2002) 'Letter: Select Committee's report used parliamentary privilege unacceptably', *British Medical Journal*, vol 324, p 1584.

14: Shaw, M., Dorling, D., Mitchell, R. and Davey Smith, G. (2005) 'Labour's "Black Report" moment', *British Medical Journal*, vol 331, p 575.

15: Dorling, D. (2007) 'Guest Editorial: The real Mental Health Bill', *Journal of Public Mental Health*, vol 6, no 3, pp 6-13.

16: McCartney, G., Collins, C. and Dorling, D. (2010) 'Observation: Would action on health inequalities have saved New Labour?', *British Medical Journal*, 23 June, vol 340, p 1388.

17: Dorling, D. and Thomas, B. (2011) 'Mapping inequalities in Britain', *Sociology Review*, vol 21, no 1, pp 15-19.

18: Hennig, B.D. and Dorling, D. (2012) 'In focus: London's political landscapes', *Political Insight*, vol 3, no 1, p 38.

Section IV: Despair and joy

19: Figure 19.1 was redrawn from the original by Sebastian Kraemer; Figure 19.2 was redrawn from the original graphic in Norton-Taylor, R. (2012) 'Arms sales rise during downturn to more than $400bn, report reveals', *The Guardian*, London, 29 February.

20: Dorling, D. and Gunnell, D. (2003) 'Suicide: the spatial and social components of despair in Britain 1980-2000', *Transactions of the Institute of British Geographers*, vol 28, no 4, pp 442-60.

21: Shaw, M., Dorling, D. and Davey Smith, G. (2002) 'Editorial: Mortality and political climate: how suicide rates have risen during periods of Conservative government, 1901-2000', *Journal of Epidemiology and Community Health*, vol 56, no 10, pp 722-7.

22: Dorling, D. and Barford, A. (2009) 'The inequality hypothesis: thesis, antithesis, and a synthesis', *Health & Place*, vol 15, no 4, pp 1166-9.

23: Dorling, D. (2011) *Housing and identity: How place makes race*, Better Housing Briefing 17, London: Race Equality Foundation.

24: Dorling, D. (2011) 'Border controls? Here's a long line of reasons to relax', *The Guardian*, 8 November.

25: Dorling, D. (2011) 'Poor kids', Interview with Kerry O'Brien, Four Corners, Australian Broadcasting Corporation, 3 October, online transcript.

Section V: Global inequality

26: Figures 26.1 and 26.2 are reproduced as a public domain work prepared by an officer or employee of the US Government as part of that person's official duties.

27: Dorling, D. and Barford, A. (2011) 'How do the other four-fifths live?', *New Internationalist*, vol 442, p 51.

28: Dorling, D., Shaw, M. and Davey Smith, G. (2006) 'HIV and global health: global inequality of life expectancy due to AIDS', *British Medical Journal*, vol 32, pp 662-4.

29: Barford, A. Dorling, D., Davey Smith, G. and Shaw, M. (2006) 'Editorial: Women's life expectancy', *British Medical Journal*, vol 332, pp 1095-6.

30: Rigby, J.E. and Dorling, D. (2007) 'Mortality in relation to sex in the affluent world', *Journal of Epidemiology and Community Health*, vol 61, no 2, pp 159-64.

31: Dorling, D. (2007) 'Anamorphosis: the geography of physicians, and mortality', *International Journal of Epidemiology*, vol 36, no 4, pp 745-50.

32: Dorling, D., Mitchell, R. and Pearce, J. (2007) 'The global impact of income inequality on health by age: an observational study', *British Medical Journal*, vol 335, pp 873-5.

33: Dorling, D. and Coles, P. (2009) 'Featured graphic: wars, massacres, and atrocities of the 20th century', *Environment and Planning A*, vol 41, no 8, pp 1779-80.

34: Barford, A., Dorling, D. and Pickett, K. (2010) 'Re-evaluating self-evaluation. A commentary on Jen, Jones, and Johnston', *Social Science & Medicine*, vol 70, pp 496-7.

35: Hennig, B.D. and Dorling, D. (2011) 'In focus: America's debt to the world', *Political Insight*, vol 2, no 3, p 34.

Section VI: Thinking, drawing and counting

36: Figure 36.2 was redrawn from a graph originally produced by the National Institute of Economic and Social Research.

37: Dorling, D. (2007) 'Worldmapper: the human anatomy of a small planet', *PLoS Medicine*, vol 4, no 1, pp 13-18.

38: Dorling, D. (2009) 'Using statistics to describe and explore data', *Key methods in geography*, London: Sage Publications, chapter 21.

39: Tunstall, H., Mitchell, R., Dorling, D., Gibbs, J. and Platt, S. (2012) 'Socio-demographic diversity and unexplained variation in death rates among the most deprived areas in Britain', *Journal of Public Health*, vol 34, no 2, pp 296–304.

40: Dorling, D. (2012) 'What if it were not the custard cream that did for them? Review of disease maps: epidemics on the ground by Tom Koch', *International Journal of Epidemiology*, vol 41, no 2, pp 572-3.

Section VII: Changing demographics and ageing populations

41: Figure 41.1: image reproduced from *The Guardian*.

42: Ballas, D. and Dorling, D. (2007) 'Measuring the impact of major life events upon happiness', *International Journal of Epidemiology*, vol 36, no 6, pp 1244-52.

43: Dorling, D. (2011) 'Roads, casualties and public health: the open sewers of the 21st century', Publication of PACTS 21st Westminster Lecture, London: Parliamentary Advisory Council for Transport Safety (PACTS).

44: Pearce, J. and Dorling, D. (2009) 'Tackling global health inequalities: closing the health gap in a generation', *Environment and Planning A, Commentary*, vol 41, pp 1-6.

45: Dorling, D. (2011) 'How will we care for the centenarians of the future?', *The Guardian*, 23 May.

46: Dorling, D. (2011) 'We're all ... just little bits of history repeating, Part 1: History, Part 2: Future', *Significance Magazine* website, 13 June.

47: Dorling, D. and Hennig, B.D. (2011) 'In focus: global population shifts', *Political Insight*, vol 2, no 2, p 34.

48: Figure 48.1 was reproduced from an original article, in turn attributed to Thinkstock.

Foreword

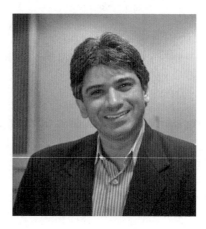

When Danny Dorling asked me to write a foreword to his forthcoming book, which, he informed me, was a collection of his prior articles on the subject of health inequalities, as well as some new chapters, I readily agreed. It was an absolute honour to present an opening to the two decades of passionate and engaging scholarship by Danny Dorling on the subject of health inequalities. Subsequently, when I received the draft it consisted of 48 chapters, nine of them new, grouped into seven sections. Even though I have followed Danny Dorling's previous work over the years, I had underestimated the size and substance of his contributions to the field of health inequalities until I saw them under one cover. Put simply, the whole was handsomely more than the sum of its parts and makes the reading (and re-reading) of the 48 chapters worthwhile. The scope of the scholarly work presented here, alongside some very interesting perspective pieces on a variety of issues that on a first glance appears highly eclectic, makes it a considerable challenge to write a short foreword in a manner that does justice to this magnificent collection.

Unequal health, with its bold subheading, *The scandal of our times*, has two central messages. First, the levels of inequalities in health that we currently observe in the UK (and everywhere else) are unprecedented and among the largest even when viewed from a historical perspective. And, second, these increasing health inequalities are largely a reflection of the ever-increasing inequalities in income and wealth that have been a characteristic feature of the recent trajectory of economic growth and development. In situating the narrative of health inequalities within the deeply polarising nature of people's socioeconomic circumstances, *Unequal health* reminds us – both in terms of substance and style – of *The health of nations: Why inequality is harmful to your health* by Ichiro Kawachi and Bruce Kennedy, and the more recent *The spirit level: Why greater equality makes societies stronger* by Richard Wilkinson and Kate Pickett. What distinguishes *Unequal health* at the same time is a uniquely historical and geographical perspective that Danny Dorling brings to our understanding of health inequalities. I also could not help going back to re-read Danny Dorling's *Injustice:*

Why social inequality persists, after reading *Unequal health*, and the two together make one of the most compelling arguments to view health and social inequalities as a singular, and not two separate, issues.

Turning to specifics, in what remains one of my all-time favourite articles on the subject of health and social inequalities, and which is retained in this collection as Chapter 3, Danny Dorling, along with his collaborators, show how place-variation in measures of poverty and affluence constructed in 1896 independently predicted the place-variation in mortality rates in London as measured a century later. The basic message that current health inequalities match the 19th-century patterns of wealth inequalities could conceivably generate a nonchalant reaction that social inequalities have always been and will always remain with us. So what's the big deal? Indeed, in light of the progress that every country (and possibly every population group) in the world has made with regard to health, especially as measured through standard measures of mortality, and life expectancy, an indifferent view to the existence of health inequalities might even appear justified. I encounter this view ever so often in my conversations with my economist colleagues who feel that epidemiologists (and let's say all non-economist health researchers) appear to be disproportionally inclined to focus on society's collective failures with regard to improving public health, ignoring the remarkable gains we have made.

However, as Danny Dorling shows directly or indirectly through several papers grouped in Section I, the view of secular improvements is only partial. In what is the most comprehensive account of historical trends of infant mortality in Britain, he shows that at the turn of the 20th century in England and Wales one in six babies died in their first year of life; a hundred years later less than one in 186 babies died before reaching their first birthday; round one to the cheerfully disposed economists. However, as is painstakingly pointed out, the inequalities in infant mortality rate between wealthy and deprived areas, during the same time, increased sixfold in the UK; in 2001 more than six infants were dying in the most deprived places for every one dying in the least deprived, and the corresponding figure for 1901 was 2.5 to 1. Importantly, as Danny Dorling shows, these inequalities were entirely modifiable, since considerable progress in reduction of inequalities (not just secular improvements) had occurred in the first half of the 20th century only to be reversed later towards the last quarter of the 20th century and increasing into the first decade of the 21st century.

In Sections II and III, Danny Dorling presents to readers (especially those unfamiliar with the UK context) a collection of papers that together argue the interconnections between polity, economy and health. These interconnections are explored using current issues, making it extremely timely and facilitating a wider interest, in particular in those matters related to the logic of privatisation of the UK's National Health Service and evaluating the dismal record in particular of the New Labour government in the first decade of the 21st century in narrowing health inequalities despite it being a core objective when the party came into power in the late 1990s. The life expectancy gap between the worst and the best local authorities in the UK increased from about nine years to 13 years during the time New Labour was in power. To support his core argument, Danny Dorling pinpoints much of the blame on New Labour not doing enough to control increases in income and wealth inequalities in the UK.

Professor Dorling's frameworks of discussion in Sections II and III are reflective of Rudolph Virchow's declaration that 'Medicine is a social science, and politics is nothing else but medicine on a large scale'. But as with all of Danny Dorling's writings, these large frameworks are presented with clear data and insightful observations. On the latter, Danny Dorling drives home the point about the connections between polity and health in a telling observation on the amount of wordage that was devoted in an email sent from the central administration in his University to two announcements – the death of a cleaner, and the appointment of a bureaucrat to the senior management of the University; the latter got over 10 times the wordage, suggesting the implicit (or explicit) value that people place on these individuals which in turn is contingent on their position in the social hierarchy of our societies. The narrative and tenor of the chapters presented in the first two sections are extended and applied to aspects of well being, mental health and life satisfaction, including suicide, in Section IV, with one of the most telling examples being the linking of suicide rates to periods of Conservative government during the 20th century.

While much in the papers presented in this collection are issues drawn from the experiences of the UK, Section V explores similar themes drawn from more international experiences. In particular, in concordance with the theme of the collection, among others, Danny Dorling shows that high-income inequalities are closely associated with higher mortality in both poor and rich nations and especially during young adulthood. His attempt to also address some of the critiques of the income inequality thesis, as proposed by Richard Wilkinson, will be of particular interest to readers who follow this literature. His insight with regard to distinguishing between objectives and subjective measures of health, as well as the need to recognise this distinction within the context of between and within countries, is particularly informative.

Section VI showcases the means that Danny Dorling has used to convey substantive points. The creative geographer in Danny is evident in the essays that are both pedagogical as well as model applications of cartograms for understanding health inequalities. In particular, the take-home message here is a hard one given the conditioning of our brains to expect a particular representation when we see a world map, but one that Danny Dorling continues to work doggedly to get across, that is that the geographical representation of any health phenomenon using the conventional Mercatorian projection (the map that we are most familiar, but which substantially distorts the size to retain the shape) can be seriously misleading (also see www.worldmapper.org for an extensive collection of maps where the focus is on the subject of interest rather than the shape of the country).

In the set of chapters presented in the final section, Danny identifies emerging issues that have not received very much attention, at least in mainstream epidemiology. In particular his essay on linking the issue of road casualties in contemporary times to the issue of open sewers in the late 19th century is a classic application of the principles of formal graphical presentation, and of historical understanding, to contemporary problems.

We might, and perhaps should, continue to debate and discuss the precise point at which we should start caring about inequalities that afflict modern societies. At the same time, the collective writings presented in *Unequal health* make a compelling case that it is time to seriously discuss this in academic as well as public domains. As of 29 June 2012, the phrase 'health inequalities' returns over half a million writings in Google Scholar. If current trends in income and wealth inequalities continue, one can only expect health inequalities to further increase and mirror this trend. With this collection, Professor Dorling has laid an exemplary foundation for future generations of researchers to engage in a science that is strongly rooted in the ideas of fairness and social justice.

S. V. Subramanian, PhD
Professor of Population Health and Geography
Harvard University
3 July 2012

Acknowledgements

This book is, in effect, a follow-up to an earlier edited collection, *Fair play: A reader on social justice*. Unlike that earlier book, over 30,000 words here are new, and so a little more help was needed! Alison Shaw at The Policy Press oversaw the project and was very encouraging and engaged in the work at all stages. Alongside her I am grateful to Jo Morton who saw the book through production, to Dawn Rushen for patient copyediting, to Laura Vickers and Rebecca Tomlinson who checked all the copyright clearances, and to Dave Worth who typeset the complex text.

As with *Fair play*, Vassiliki (Vicky) Yiagopoulou helped select the images used at the start of each chapter and Paul Coles again patiently redrew all the figures and set all the tables ready for typesetting. Bronwen and David Dorling again read through all the material early on and again wondered what they had done so wrong that their son could produce so many simple errors in such a small number of words.

I am especially grateful to S.V. Subramanian for agreeing to write the Foreword.

I had a little more help this time because so much of the material here is new. George Davey Smith provided extremely useful criticism of an earlier version of some of this new writing; Sebastian Kraemer commented and added his usual very kind and constructive suggestions. I am also grateful for a great many suggestions from the students undertaking the Master's course in Social and Spatial Inequalities in Sheffield in spring 2012 who got to read and comment on all the early drafts: Eleanor Carter, Anika Forde, Thomas Fowler, Alice Gaskell, Nicholas Hood, Katie James, Katherine Littlewood, Christina Mak, Laura Simpkins, Amy Sweet, William Titmuss and Amber Wilson.

I have some more specific thanks. I am grateful to Peter Pearson for the George Orwell quote used in Chapter 1; for helping to produce Chapter 3 thanks were originally (and are still) due to Kevin Holohan for his digitising work, Nichola Tooke for her historical research and Jonathan Tooby for his photographic advice. Special thanks also to Michael Thrasher of the University of Plymouth for data used in Chapter 18, and for Chapter 23 I remain extremely grateful to Kat Nower, Tracey Bignall and Jabeer Butt of the Race Equality Foundation for advice on restructuring, and to Fiona Harris who copyedited the original.

I am also still in debt to Sarah Blandy of the School of Law, University of Leeds, for her comments on the legality of the right-to-sell, and to Ricky Joseph of the Centre on Household Assets and Savings Management at the University of Birmingham, who gave me advice on the latest research on 'race' and wealth inequalities emerging from the US and comparable work being planned for the UK. For Chapter 29 Charles Pattie and Eilidh Garrett gave very helpful comments on an earlier version of the typescript. For helping with Chapter 37, I remain grateful to my colleagues Graham Allsopp, Anna Barford, Ben Wheeler and John Pritchard at the University of Sheffield and to Mark Newman at the University of Michigan for their collaboration with this work, and Simon Brooker of the London School of Hygiene and Tropical Medicine for his helpful comments on an earlier draft. For Chapter 38 Chris Keylock very kindly suggested some of the examples used. And for Chapter 42 I would still like to thank the editor and three anonymous referees for their invaluable comments on an earlier draft of this article and John Lynch for his editorial pruning and guidance. Tom Hennell and Kat Smith were also very kind in discussing the latest evidence on possible reductions in inequalities in health in the UK as I was checking these proofs. That leaves a lot of other anonymous reviewers and less anonymous editors, production assistants and colleagues not properly thanked, but this list gives an idea for a few chapters of how much help I have had in creating what follows.

Finally, thanks to my wife Alison Dorling, for tolerating my obsession with getting everything down on paper in multiple formats before my time is up (so much to write, so few years in a lifetime) and to our children, Robbie, Izzy and Sol, for tempering the obsession.

All the suggestions and errors made below remain my sole responsibility, although if I can find a way of blaming them on someone else....

SECTION I
The long view

1

Unequal health: why a scandal, and why now?

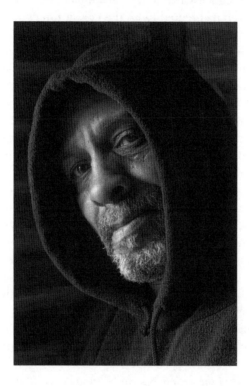

Inequalities in the health status of social groups have been observable for *at least* two millennia. For example, during the Roman occupation of Britain, variations in diet between the Romans and those they ruled resulted in the skeletons of poorer groups being stunted. And it was not just that the poor ate less well – the amount of labour demanded of different social groups varied, which contributed to the skeletons of those deemed to be inferior being further stunted.

Living under the tyranny of an occupation not only reduces the number of both necessities and luxuries people have in life, it also damages self-resolve and self-respect, although these are hard to measure, especially in archaeological records. Poorer people, for example, could be identified as those with fewer grave furnishings. And examination of dental remains has revealed that those with fewer possessions at the time of death suffered more from disease during life (Griffin *et al*, 2011). From this you may conclude that great health inequality has always been with us, but that is simply not true – the extent of inequalities has varied greatly over time.

The archaeological remains discussed here came from a Roman cemetery discovered in 1925 in Baldock, Hertfordshire (in Roman times Baldock was a settlement on the Icknield Way). Today Baldock is a tiny market town, sandwiched between the Great North Road and the A1 motorway. Among its claims to fame is that from 1936 onwards, the writer George Orwell lived nearby. Orwell wrote widely on issues that often touched on self-resolve and self-respect. He lived in Baldock because the rent was cheap; it was cheap because of the state of the housing there at the time – Orwell regularly had to fix a leaking cesspit. But just a decade ago the very home that Orwell had rented (with the cesspit long gone) was on the market for £395,000, and many young locals have recently had to leave the area because house prices have become so high (Clark, 2003).

During the 1930s, before moving to Baldock, Orwell travelled through northern England. He collected stories that were subsequently published in his 1937 book, *The road to Wigan Pier*, stories about the scandal of the inequalities he saw, of how dire the situation in many northern towns was and how bleak appeared the outlook. We later learned that during the years Orwell was travelling, inequalities in health across Britain had been falling through to the late 1930s and then through the 1950s, all the way to the 1970s. Orwell may well have had a less bleak outlook had he known what was to come, but he might not have written so well had he been more complacent and not so shocked by what he was living through.

During the 1970s, when falls in inequalities in health between different areas of Britain came to an end, it was possibly a sign that complacency had risen.[1] In hindsight we can see that it was partly because of what people like Orwell wrote in the 1930s and 1940s that the outlook had brightened, with acts of great selfishness more often curtailed between the 1930s and late 1970s than before or after. Lessons from the past are often lost, however, and it is when warnings are forgotten that inequalities are allowed to rise again, often in very similar form in similar places. Some features of British society today remain eerily reminiscent of Orwell's descriptions of the 1930s:

> *Nevertheless, in spite of the frightful extent of unemployment, it is a fact that poverty – extreme poverty – is less in evidence in the industrial North than it is in London. Everything is poorer and shabbier, there are fewer motor-cars and fewer well-dressed people; but also there are fewer people who are obviously destitute. Even in a town the size of Liverpool or Manchester you are struck by the fewness of the beggars. London is a sort of whirlpool which draws derelict people towards it, and it is so vast that life there is solitary and anonymous.* (Orwell, 1937 [1986], p 73)

Today, as cars are now much more a necessity than a luxury, there are many times more of them, even in the poorest of areas of the North, although outside of London lack of access to a car still differentiates the very worst-off places from those just badly off. In contrast, to be 'well-dressed' has for centuries been a necessity to securing basic respect and self-esteem.

---

[1] See Table 10.2 on p 134 in Chapter 10, which shows the trend in geographical inequalities in premature mortality falling from around 1921 to 1950, falling again from around 1963 to 1973, and then rising.

Seeing past scandals in the present

The writer Stephen Armstrong recently retraced Orwell's steps on the 75th anniversary of his journey north. He set out from London, aware that within London the 'sort of whirlpool' still exists, although many living in the richest parts of the capital are still often almost oblivious to it.[2] The affluent today, as in the 1930s, are similarly far too often unaware of how many people have had no work for many years, but unlike in the 1930s, it is now the young who are being hit the hardest:

> *August 2011 figures from the Office for National Statistics showed more than 20 per cent of 16–24 year olds were unemployed and 100,000 had been on the dole for two years or more. Earlier in the year, the first full comparison of numbers from local authorities showed that men and women in Manchester, Liverpool and Blackburn die ten years younger than men and women living in Kensington and Chelsea.* (Armstrong, 2012, pp 9-10)

Inequalities in income both create inequalities in wealth and reduce the overall level of health and the quality of life of the population as a whole. Figure 1.1(a) and (b) demonstrate this using the latest data for every country for which comparable figures on the income share of the top 1 per cent have been published. Each circle in the graph represents a country, with the circle area drawn in proportion to the country's population.

Any population that has suffered more insults, both physical and mental, will record poorer health and, ultimately, more premature mortality. And living in a regime of great income inequality is just one of many factors contributing to such insults that can reduce life expectancy. The more the richest 1 per cent take as their share of total income, the less there is for the rest. However, many insults contribute to national life expectancy averages, not simply the adverse effects of income inequality. One of the simplest to measure the effects now of is smoking.

Even in quite equitable countries, if, for example, people smoked more than average in the past, such as in Denmark, life expectancy today would be lower. As smoking rates among younger Danes are much lower, we should expect to see life expectancy rise there more rapidly than in places where a different kind of redistribution than simply less smoking is required. Other harder to quantify insults, such as the physiological harms that come from suffering racism, are similarly known to have independent adverse effects on health. Although all these separate insults matter, in affluent countries one appears to matter the most – inequality in income, which often correlates highly with the other insults. For example, the poor smoke more, and poorer members of minority ethnic groups are easier targets for racists.

---

[2] Chapter 39 records the whirlpool effect of migration in and out of London; this is the damping of mortality figures there among the poor, as so many are spun out before dying early elsewhere, although even poorer Londoners tend to be healthier due to migration selection.

Figure 1.1: LIfe expectancy (2009) of all people versus income share of the best-off 1% (latest year), all countries with recent 'top income' data

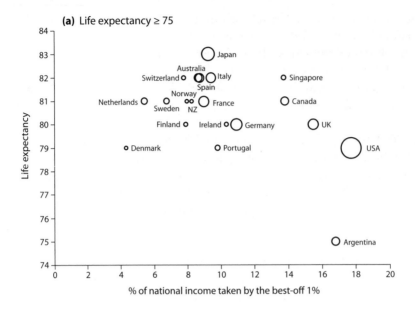

(a) Life expectancy ≥ 75

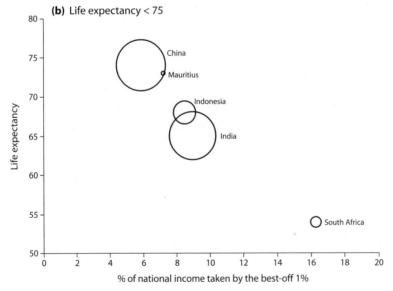

(b) Life expectancy < 75

Note: Circle area is proportional to the population in 2010.
The inequality data used is from the Paris School's World Top Income database: http://g-mond.parisschool ofeconomics.eu/topincomes/ (excluding Tanzania, where only data to 1970 were included).

Source: Life expectancy and population figures from WHO data: http://apps.who.int/ghodata?vid= 710#income (Australian statisticians dispute the WHO figure for life expectancy shown here).

Figure 1.1 is split into two halves, differentiating richer and poorer countries. In richer countries today life expectancy is above 75 years, while it is generally below that in poorer nations. However, where income inequalities are very high, individual income is reduced further for the great majority (99 per cent) of the population. During the 1930s the countries in the top half of Figure 1.1(a) experienced life expectancy rates more like those in the bottom half of Figure 1.1(b) because, in general, the populations were poorer, and also because fewer treatments for disease existed, particularly for its prevention through vaccination.

One great change between the 1930s and the 2010s is that while people today in an affluent area such as Kensington and Chelsea mostly live long lives and rarely experience poverty, they should now find it harder to avoid learning that they are part of the problem of inequality, as far more information on inequality and its harms is now available. During the 1930s many still believed that premature mortality, especially of infants, was an act of god rather than a tragedy that was almost entirely preventable, although others had begun to think differently. Now in rich countries we most often count the costs of health inequalities in terms of years lost at the end of life rather than lives lost at their very start.

Later on in his revision of Orwell's *The road to Wigan Pier*, Armstrong quotes figures from Michael Marmot's 2010 official independent review of health inequalities (Marmot, 2010), which claimed: '*... if everyone in England had the same death rates as the most advantaged, people who are currently dying young thanks to health inequalities would, in total, have enjoyed between 1.3 and 2.5 million extra years of life. They would, in addition, have had a further 2.8 million years free of limiting illness or disability*' (Armstrong, 2012, p 214).

Within Britain the scandal of our times is not that inequalities in health are now wider than they were in the 1920s or 1930s[3]; it is that we allowed them to become this wide knowing all we know today that was not known in the 1930s. Today almost everyone lives longer, on average, but the gaps between the expected length of life, according to where you live and your access to wealth, have grown to be the greatest recorded for a century, and the quality of life of those living shorter lives is now deteriorating as living standards fall in both absolute and relative terms. Meanwhile, income and wealth inequalities are continuing to rise, again uniquely today, given the depth of the 2008 economic crash this is found no matter whether those economic inequalities are measured in absolute or relative terms.

The outbreaks of mass poverty in the 1920s and 1930s were not planned. Neither was the beginning of reparation particularly well planned. In the decades before the Second World War in the UK (and not until that war in the US) inequalities in income, wealth and health began to fall greatly. In contrast, since the late 1970s, inequalities in income, health and wealth have all been rising as measured between different parts of Britain, and these rises are no longer the shock reaction to recent economic turmoil. Between 1979 and 2010 not enough work was done in any year

---

[3] See Chapter 25 and the text around Figure 48.2, p 452, in Chapter 48, for data, discussion and illustration of the effects of the recent trends that have led to inequalities becoming wider.

to curtail the rise of inequality. By 2012 the situation had become so dire that Liam Donaldson, former Chief Medical Officer for England, directly accused the new Coalition government of 2010 of showing disregard for people's lives in comparison with the New Labour government that had come before. In short, the Coalition government, in the decisions it took, may have '… *contributed to a rise in deaths in the year after the flu pandemic, according to the former chief medical officer Sir Liam Donaldson. In a new paper, Donaldson, who led the fight against the flu pandemic in 2009 but stepped down when the coalition took power in May 2010, says the change of government response was the key difference between the two years and criticizes the "laissez-faire" attitude of Andrew Lansley's Department of Health'* (Boseley, 2012).

The scandal of our times

During the two years from May 2010 to May 2012 it was often suggested that Andrew Lansley had become the most hated Secretary of State for Health that Britain had ever had. Even a normally Conservative-biased newspaper ran the following headline on Lansley's attempts to privatise the NHS: *'The firm that hijacked the NHS: MoS [Mail on Sunday] investigation reveals extraordinary extent of international management consultant's role in Lansley's health reforms'* (*Mail on Sunday*, 13 February 2012). David Cameron sacked him as Secretary of State in September 2012.

It is not impossible that we will soon be recording actual rises in mortality rates for particular groups in particular parts of Britain if the trends both to privatise healthcare and to allow inequality and poverty to rise continue (Pollock et al, 2012). The last time actual rises in mortality occurred was against the general background of social improvement experienced between the two world wars, at a time when unemployment rates were historically high and rising and in the aftermath of a global financial crash (Davey Smith and Marmot, 1991).

The position of the UK shown in Table 1.1 (the table of statistics that are plotted in Figure 1.1) is poor. The table is sorted by life expectancy and includes every country for which comparable income inequality data on the top 1 per cent are available. There are often reasons why the relationship between inequality and early mortality is not neater. In Denmark people live shorter lives because smoking rates in the 1980s were higher than in the UK, although those rates have since plummeted. In Singapore people live longer, on average, despite higher inequality, because of a system of deporting some of the poorest people and because some of those in the poorest groups of guest workers abort their babies to avoid the threat of deportation.[4] If such reasons are accounted for, then the correlation between tolerating extreme inequality within a country and poorer overall health becomes even stronger.

As income and wealth inequalities rise, so too do health inequalities. By May 2010 it had become apparent that men and women had a combined average life expectancy of 74.3 years in Glasgow compared to 88.7 in the Royal Borough of Kensington and Chelsea (2007–09 data; see Figure 41.3, on p 381 of Chapter 41). Therefore the

---

[4] See Chapter 36 for the estimates of the number of people directly and indirectly affected.

gap between an affluent enclave of London and economically run-down Glasgow exceeded 14 years, a 19 per cent difference. It is necessary to go back to the recession of the 1880s to find a greater gap between areas. At that time life expectancy was 46 years in Bristol compared to 36 years in Liverpool, a 10-year absolute, and (then) 28 per cent relative difference between the two ports (Szreter and Mooney, 1998, table 1). By May 2012, as recorded later in this volume in Chapter 41, that gap between

Table 1.1: Income inequality and life expectancy, all countries with data, 2009

Country	Year of latest available income inequality data	Top 1% richest people's share of all income (%)	Life expectancy in years 2009	Population estimate 2010 (millions)
Japan	2005	9.20	83	126.6
Switzerland	1995	7.76	82	7.6
Australia	2008	8.59	82	22.3
Spain	2008	8.61	82	46.1
Italy	2009	9.38	82	60.6
Singapore	2009	13.7	82	5.1
Netherlands	1999	5.38	81	16.6
Sweden	2009	6.72	81	9.4
Norway	2008	7.94	81	4.9
New Zealand	2009	8.22	81	4.4
France	2006	8.94	81	62.8
Canada	2007	13.78	81	34.0
Finland	2002	7.86	80	5.4
Ireland	2000	10.30	80	4.5
Germany	1998	10.88	80	82.3
United Kingdom	2007	15.45	80	62.0
Denmark	2005	4.29	79	5.6
Portugal	2005	9.77	79	10.7
United States	2008	17.67	79	310.4
Argentina	2004	16.75	75	40.4
China	2003	5.87	74	1348.9
Mauritius	2008	7.20	73	1.3
Indonesia	2004	8.46	68	239.9
India	1999	8.95	65	1224.6
South Africa	2007	16.25	54	50.1

Note: Table is sorted by life expectancy.
The inequality data used is from the Paris School's World Top Income database: http://g-mond.parisschool
ofeconomics.eu/topincomes/ (excluding Tanzania, where only data to 1970 were included).

Source: Life expectancy and population figures from WHO data: http://apps.who.int/ghodata?vid=
710#income (Australian statisticians dispute the WHO figure for life expectancy shown
here).

areas had widened yet again, but inequalities between social classes as measured by children's survival chances had suddenly narrowed.[5]

Sometimes it can feel as though the geography of inequality in Britain is stuck in a kind of rut, but we must remember just how much worse off in absolute terms people were when the great-great-grandparents of today's students were children. Szreter and Mooney show that in the registration district of Liverpool (as opposed to the whole city), life expectancy in the 1880s was only 29 years, some 19 years lower than the 48 years recorded then in the affluent Clifton district of Bristol. Similarly, in Glasgow in earlier years life expectancies as low as in Liverpool were recorded, only 27 years around 1840. Infant mortality was key to determining these low overall ages, dragging average life expectancies down as so many died in the first year of life. Manchester's life expectancy for 1801 to 1850 was possibly the lowest ever recorded in a large city that was not wiped out as a result; it was calculated at 25.3 years, which affected a population of 235,000 people in 1841.

Inequalities in health in Britain are the scandal of our times today because you have to travel back to these Victorian statistics to last find life expectancy gaps between places greater than today, even though the overall levels of health were then much worse. But what of the time before the Victorians?

The higher social status of groups in an area has not always been reflected in better health there. More than a century before Manchester first recorded such low life expectancies, in the decades running up to 1700, *'major and minor aristocracy experienced similar life expectancy and infant mortality to the overall population.... As Johansson (1999) has suggested, it took knowledge to convert wealth into health'* (Davey Smith, 2007, p 221, relying in turn on Johansson, 1999). This apparent equality of health was hypothesised to be due to the higher number of people the wealthy came into contact with, and the fact that at that time they knew much less about the causes of ill health. The scandal then was not inequality but ignorance.

Why economic inequality harms health

The general explanation that living under conditions of high social inequality is detrimental to health (Wilkinson, 1999) is not yet easily supported by a simple biological model, but this does not make it a bad explanation, just a relatively new one. Critics of the theory that inequality 'of itself' is detrimental to health relied on older and hence possibly less reliable data than that used here (Davey Smith, 2007, figure 7, relying in turn on Lynch *et al*, 2001).

In 2012 a biological model was proposed for why rank inequality might have an effect on health in primates (Tung *et al*, 2012). However, within the same month

---

[5] See Figure 41.3 on p 381 of Chapter 41, for trends by area, and Figure 44.1 on p 432 of Chapter 44, for trends by social class. Note that it is possible that, in very recent years, just prior to publication of this book, geographical inequalities in health by area may have narrowed in a similar way to those seen by class in Figure 44.1. The 2011 Census reveals that there were fewer people living in Kensington and Chelsea than had been thought to live there, so life expectancy in this very affluent borough will not be as high as was believed to be the case prior to summer 2012.

a review was then published which suggested no evidence among primates that rank was adversely related to increased risk of coronary artery disease (Petticrew and Davey Smith, 2012). And then, at almost exactly the same time again, an article was published suggesting that stress caused by increased rank differentiation was the probable explanation for rising obesity in particular societies (Pickett and Wilkinson, 2012).

A biological explanation for why income inequality harms health could be summarised as 'stress causes raised steroid levels which cause weight gain'. A social explanation might be 'in more unequal countries advertisers are less curtailed from advertising fatty foods'. The argument over precisely how high inequality causes poorer health will continue for some time. In relatively poorer areas people die earlier, and countries with higher inequality are home to more people who are relatively poor. But there is much more to why inequality 'of itself' is harmful to good health than simply increasing poverty.

One way in which high economic inequality harms health is that it pushes medical practitioners away from those most in need. Figure 1.2 shows a rough inverse relation between the proportion of the population who have health needs in different parts of the country and the proportion who are qualified working-age medical doctors but who are not working in medicine. Medical doctors are more likely to be found in areas of better health, not because it is there that they make more people better, but because it is there that more prefer to live and work. This is in preference to living and working where people's health is worse and the areas are poorer. (Chapter 5 includes figures that show this is the case for all those doctors working in medicine.) The exceptions to the rule, Gwent, Carmarthenshire and Torfaen, are places where relatively high numbers of doctors moved to, working at something but not as practising medical doctors. Only 0.06 per cent of Torfaen's population are qualified medical doctors working in medicine, which is less than the numbers of the working-age population who were qualified but not working as medical doctors in that district!

In more equitable countries there are fewer inequalities in health between areas, and doctors tend not to avoid serving areas with greater health problems simply because there are fewer such obviously needy areas. In more unequal countries physicians tend to live and work further away from those who are in need of their care.[6] What may be less well appreciated is that more qualified physicians in more unequal countries may be choosing not to actually work as physicians. In more unequal countries do more young people choose to study medicine because of the high incomes doctors receive rather than because they actually want to help people get better?

What Figure 1.2 shows is that the proportion of qualified medical practitioners who are in employment but who are not working as doctors is inversely related to the proportion of the population reporting health needs. In general the more people who are ill in a city or county within Britain, the smaller the proportion of doctors

---

[6] Chapter 5, this volume, shows that qualified physicians working as practising physicians tend to be found in greatest numbers where people are least ill (see Figure 5.3, p 75).

who will be working there, but even smaller is the proportion of qualified doctors not working in medicine but still living and working there.

When health inequalities are high and there are large variations between areas, doctors appear not to want to live in areas with high health needs. This is even more the case for groups labelled 'other health professionals' (not including doctors, nurses and dentists). Most other health professionals, such as osteopaths and psychologists, work in private practice and so tend to gravitate to where people have more money and are less sick.

Figure 1.2: Qualified physicians not working in medicine versus health needs, 2001, Britain

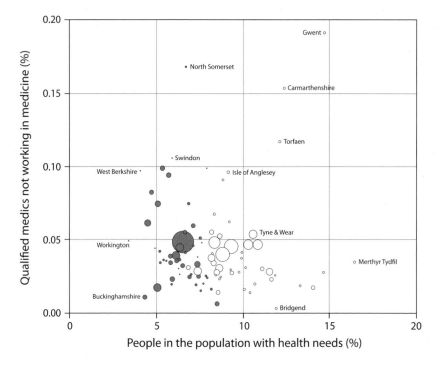

Note: Each circle is an area of Britain, county or major city. Areas in the South of England are coloured darker and the area of each circle is drawn in proportion to its population. Selected circles are named.

Source: Same data as used in Shaw, M. and Dorling, D. (2004) 'Who cares in England and Wales? The Positive Care Law: cross-sectional study', *Journal of General Practice*, vol 54, pp 899-903 www.dannydorling.org/?page_id=1475

When it comes to keeping away from the sick, dentists tend to live even further away from those in greatest need. In fact, nurses are the only group of health professionals to be found in slightly higher numbers in areas where there are greater health needs (Shaw and Dorling, 2004). More dentists in poorer areas would not help prevent many premature deaths, but they could relieve a great deal of suffering instead of, for example, carrying out cosmetic whitening in richer areas.

The chapters that follow in this first section concern, first, the more distant history of health inequalities by considering epidemics, pandemics and in particular, cholera (Chapter 2), then the persistence of the geography of poverty (Chapter 3); next is a chapter that considers how the greatest reductions in infant mortality have been achieved (Chapter 4). The section ends by considering the continued strength of the inverse care law in health (Chapter 5). These four chapters have been placed together to try to provide a general introduction to the subject of unequal health, but what we know is always changing. Despite the natural tendency of health researchers to concentrate on what is worse at any one time, there are always pointers to how things might be improved, and sometimes signs of hope.

Why cooperation helps us all

As the draft of this chapter was being finished a study was released that strengthened the case for greater equality improving performance and well-being. The study suggested that an argument could be made, even among people at the most highly paid end of the income structure, for how greater equality brings greater benefits (Bucciol and Piovesan, 2012). And this information reached me via a bank! The Economic Research Division of the Federal Reserve Bank of St Louis disseminated the paper through their support of the Research Papers in Economics website. The blog TrackBack (2012) has neatly summarised the findings of the paper, which was a study of footballers:

> *Pay dispersion has an overall negative impact on team performance … doubling pay dispersion [as measured by the Theil index] decreases by 6% the probability of winning a match. This is a big effect. The authors estimate that if a team changes from everyone being paid the same wage of €600k pa (the average in their sample) to a superstar earning €1.5m pa and everyone else in the team getting €510k, the chances of the team winning a game falls by 20 percentage points. That's almost as big an effect as having to play every game away from home. This adverse effect comes because pay dispersion worsens individuals' performance….*

This quote about Italian Series A football league clubs was then followed by page after page of further analysis, not by the authors, but by apparently statistically addicted football fans adding comments online.[7] Fun though such musings are, and also potentially informative, the problems of most people are not how best to maximise the number of goals 11 very cosseted young men might score depending on how much they are paid. The problems of most people in Britain and similar

---

[7] The authors of the paper were two Italians, one a Professor of Econometrics with a degree partly in statistics who works at the University of Verona, the other now an Economics Research Fellow at Harvard Business School in the US.

places are how to live healthily and happily in a society that is becoming more and more financially and socially divided with each year that passes, as our health service is increasingly privatised (see Figure 1.3) and our media are slow to appreciate what we are in great danger of returning to.

Figure 1.3: An example of airbrushing and what non-misleading advertising would look like.

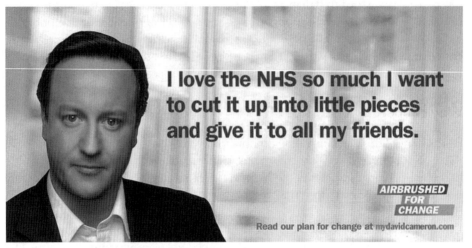

see colour version in plate section

Source: http://www.mydavidcameron.com/posters/cam-nhs1

References

Armstrong, S. (2012) *The road to Wigan Pier revisited*, London: Constable.

Boseley, S. (2012) 'Government laxity on flu led to more deaths, says report', *The Guardian*, 16 April (www.guardian.co.uk/society/2012/apr/16/flu-deaths-government-failure).

Bucciol, A. and Piovesan, M. (2012) *Pay dispersion and work performance*, Harvard Business School Working Paper 12-075, Boston, MA: Harvard Business School (www.hbs.edu/research/pdf/12-075.pdf).

Clark, R. (2003) 'At the gates of Animal Farm', *Daily Telegraph*, 24 September (www.netcharles.com/orwell/articles/col-afgates.htm).

Davey Smith, G. (2007) 'Boyd Orr lecture: Life-course approaches to inequalities in adult chronic disease risk', *Proceedings of the Nutrition Society*, vol 66, pp 216-36.

Davey Smith, G. and Marmot, M. (1991) 'Trends in mortality in Britain 1920-1986', *Annals of Nutrition and Metabolism*, vol 25 (supplement 1), pp 53-63.

Griffin, R., Pitts, M., Smith, R. and Brook, A. (2011) 'Inequality at late Roman Baldock, UK: the impact of social factors upon health and diet', *Journal of Anthropological Research*, vol 67, no 4, pp 533-56.

Johansson, S.R. (1999) *Death and the doctors: Medicine and elite mortality in Britain from 1500 to 1800*, Working Paper Series No 7, Cambridge: Cambridge Group for the History of Population and Social Structure.

Lynch, J., Davey Smith, G., Hillemeier, M., Shaw, M., Raghunathan, T. and Kaplan, G. (2001) 'Income inequality, the psychosocial environment, and health: comparisons of wealthy nations', *The Lancet*, vol 358, pp 194-200.

Marmot, M. (2010) *Fair society, healthy lives: The Marmot review*, London: The Marmot Review.

Orwell, G. (1937 [1986]) *The road to Wigan Pier*, London: Penguin. [Also freely available to read at http://gutenberg.net.au/ebooks02/0200391.txt]

Petticrew, M. and Davey Smith, G. (2012) 'The monkey puzzle: a systematic review of studies of stress, social hierarchies, and heart disease in monkeys', *PLOS One*, vol 7, no 3: e27939, doi:10.1371/journal.pone.0027939.

Pickett, K. and Wilkinson, R. (2012) 'Income inequality and psychosocial pathways to obesity', *Proceedings of the British Academy*, vol 174, chapter 10.]

Pollock,. M., Price, D. *et al* (2012) 'How the Health and Social Care Bill 2011 would end entitlement to comprehensive health care in England', *The Lancet*, vol 379, no 9814, pp 387-9.

Shaw, M. and Dorling, D. (2004) 'Who cares in England and Wales? The Positive Care Law: cross-sectional study', *Journal of General Practice*, vol 54, pp 899-903

Szreter, S. and Mooney, G. (1998) 'Urbanization, mortality, and the standard of living debate: new estimates of the expectation of life at birth in nineteenth-century British cities', *Economic History Review*, vol 51, no 1, pp 84-112

TrackBack (2012) 'Robin Van Persie and the cost of inequality', Stumbling and Mumbling blog, 15 March (http://stumblingandmumbling.typepad.com/stumbling_and_mumbling/2012/03/robin-van-persie-the-cost-of-inequality.html).

Tung, J., Barreiroa, L.B., Johnson, Z.P., Hansen, K.D., Michopoulos, V., Toufexis, D., Michelini, K., Wilson, M.E. and Gilad, Y. (2012) 'Social environment is associated with gene regulatory variation in the rhesus macaque immune system', *PNAS Early Edition* (www.pnas.org/lookup/suppl/doi:10.1073/pnas.1202734109/-/DCSupplementl), pp 1-6.

Wilkinson, G. (1999) 'Health, hierarchy, and social anxiety', *Annals of the New York Academy of Sciences*, vol 896, pp 48–63.

2

The long view: from 1817 to 2012

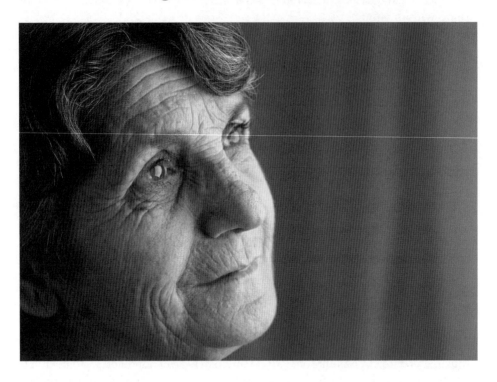

And he that was never yet connected with his poorer neighbour, by deeds of charity or love, may one day find, when it is too late, that he is connected with him by a bond which may bring them both, at once, to a common grave. (Budd, 1931)

When you take the long view, the recent past looks so much better than the distant past. For example, maps of disease in the 19th century concentrated, above all else, on cholera (Hamlin, 2009). There were so many outbreaks and so many of them were mapped that, if you have lived much of your life in Britain or similar places, you could, if morbidly inclined, chart your own personal biography through the plotting of some of the most painful and tragic epidemics that caused so many premature deaths in the not too distant past.

Cholera arrived in Britain in 1831, and about 30,000 people died during 1832. It had been endemic in India and was reported, from an outbreak there in Bengal (in 1817), to be spreading outwards and northwards through Russia and west across Europe (Davey Smith, 2002). The arrival of cholera occurred within a few years of the doubling of the numbers of warehouses in cities such as Manchester, cities that were exporting goods to places like India. Cholera slowly came back with the ships, from port to port, country to country, and first broke out in Britain about 14 years after its initial 1817 identification as a potential pandemic disease.

Approximately 1,325 people were known to have contracted cholera in Manchester in 1832. Just over half of them died. Whenever and wherever it hit, the shock of dealing with the immediate tragedy and its aftermath led local physicians to try to explain what was occurring. In Manchester in 1833 Dr Henry Gaulter mapped the progress of cholera through the city. He followed cartographic conventions first set down in Germany (Koch, 2011). Germany, being nearer Russia, was the first more affluent nation to be struck by the disease.

On street plans of Manchester Dr Gaulter drew black dots at addresses where victims had died. This would become a common way of mapping death in Britain in later epidemics (see Busteed and Hindle, 2010). But he also mapped each street, dwelling by dwelling, both within Manchester and out to nearby Warrington (see Figure 2.1). He suggested theory after theory as to what might be causing and spreading cholera. Later on in his book he suggested that:

> *The truth is that in the greater part of Manchester there are no sewers at all, and that where they do exist they are so small and badly constructed that instead of contributing to the purification of the town, they become themselves nuisances of the worst description.…* *The contrast between the localities which the rich and poor inhabit, exhibits perhaps the most striking example of the substantial advantages, as far as health is concerned, which affluence can bestow.…* (Gaulter, 1833, pp 118-19; see Figure 2.8 on p 35 in the annex at the end of this chapter for the full quotation)

Dr Gaulter went on to suggest that it was the very poorest who suffered most from cholera, people who had just arrived in the city and who were living in the most crowded of lodging houses or those who had recently lost or had failed to gain factory employment:

> *Of the whole number of Manchester cases very few indeed were employed by the factories at all [due to] the general comfort and cleanliness of these establishments.* (Gaulter, 1833, pp 119-20)

Unlike in later decades, securing a factory job in the 1830s was a great achievement, a step up for the desperate. However, the extent to which cholera was most constrained to those who were so desperate is now more contested than the consensus reached during the Victorian era. It is possible that cholera deaths were more constrained to a particular group of people because it was more dangerous to that group and it was not such a risk to those who were better off, but fear of cholera helped in speeding up general social improvement as the better-off were led to believe they were at even greater risk than they actually were.

Disease at the population level and the structure of human society are always closely linked. It might not be so foolish to claim that cholera was turned into a pandemic disease by the colonisation of the subcontinent that under British rule

Figure 2.1: The localities of cholera, Manchester, 1832

see colour version in plate section

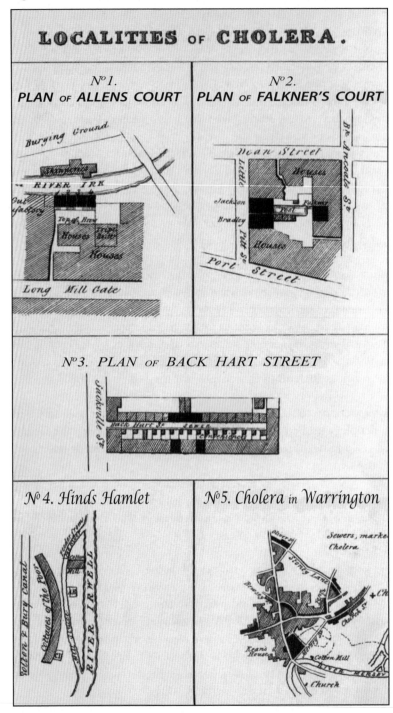

Source: Gaulter (1833, frontispiece)

(www.archive.org/stream/originandprogre00gaulgoog#page/n10/mode/2up)

came to be called India. It was not that there was a utopian order to society in the Indian subcontinent prior to British rule – there was no harmonious pre-existing Indian social structure. However, what there was, in the form of established customs, systems of agriculture, industry and services, came to be so severely disrupted by colonisation as to heap further poverty most forcibly on those who were already the poorest and most marginalised. Local elites were often co-opted by the colonisers. All this was a precursor to pandemic.

Once local elites began to work for foreign masters, those who were already poor in India became further impoverished through those actions necessary to sustain colonisation. Local textile industries were decimated to create a market for British cotton goods. It was partly as a result of this that social stability in India was reduced under British rule. Before the British came there had been despotism, suffering and hunger, but only one major famine recorded every century or so.

From Medinipur to Manchester[1]

Under British rule there was famine in 1770 in Bengal, in 1783 in Bihar, Bengal and Punjab, followed by famines in 1787, 1790, 1803 and 1813 (Davies, 2000). Famines continued throughout the 19th century and up until independence. But those early 18th-century famines, and the more general trials of living under occupation, were possibly enough to harass the population sufficiently to provide a ready pool of weakened victims and a fall in general living standards that made the people ripe for the harbouring, mutation, strengthening and spreading of diseases already present but as yet uncommon. Colonisation also meant more travel between the lands of the colonisers and the colonised, and that in turn meant more scope to spread disease.

The colonisation of India and the destruction of its textile industry provided a much increased market for US-grown cotton, much of which was spun in Manchester and thereabouts. In the short term it brought profit to Manchester, and the first factories were clean. In the medium term competition between producers meant that conditions in the factories deteriorated, and trade to India in the end brought back the cholera its colonial initiation had helped to stoke. The number of cotton mills peaked in Manchester in 1853 at 108 (Manchester City Council, 2012). At around that peak, and partly because of the peaking, one of the most deadly outbreaks of cholera engulfed Britain.

Today we hardly ever think of what a major disease outbreak is like, how it alters much more than the lives of those who are infected and killed, how it changes people's views on the world, how it can elicit great despair but also galvanise others to act, to graph, to map and to measure – and to advocate things they had always wished for, practices which might not necessarily immediately alleviate suffering from (and lessen the risk of) cholera, but policies which might improve underlying

---

[1] Medinipur is in Bengal; it was also the centre of revolts and dissent long before Manchester took the role of being the place that first inspired modern communism.

social conditions and be less opposed due to the fear of cholera – turning a crisis into an opportunity.

To begin to see this story and to try to get a feel for times past, you could look back at what happened just a few generations ago where you live. I grew up in Oxford. If I search for old maps of Oxford what I often find are maps of cholera. Oxford suffered outbreaks of cholera in 1832, 1849 and 1854. In the first half of the 19th century it was almost impossible to know why. Almost every conceivable theory had been proposed.

In Oxford another doctor called Henry, this time Henry Wentworth Acland, plotted cases of cholera on city maps. He also noted that the number of times the sound of thunder supposedly unaccompanied by lightning was heard in the city in the three outbreak years was 2, 8 and 4 respectively (Acland, 1856, p 62). He contrasted that with the figures for many other years. Thunder occurring without lightning was then seen as just another of many hundreds of possible causes of the cholera outbreaks.

It is hard to imagine the diligence with which people recorded every conceivable cause in the search for an understanding of terrifying diseases such as cholera, a disease which was as terrifying to the rich as it was to the poor. In Russia an earlier epidemic had killed over 100 nobles. And an outbreak could easily result in rioting and panic. A menacing, fleeing and simultaneously very poor population does not make a good workforce, or, necessarily, a particularly loyal body of subjects. So the rich feared cholera for many reasons, in addition to their fear of contracting the disease itself.

More useful than tabulating lightning and thunder were Dr Acland's actual maps of cholera spreading through Oxford. These plotted contours for altitude and showed, in 1854, that the higher up people lived, the less likely they were to die of the disease. Maps can be very useful, but it is also very easy to see patterns in maps, patterns that may be more imagined than real.

Under the High Level Bridge

When I was 18 I moved to Newcastle upon Tyne and stayed there for 10 years. When the 1854 cholera outbreak struck that city the cases were most densely clustered just north of the Tyne. South of the Tyne in the town of Gateshead they were a little more spread out. In Gateshead, if you look at the map in Figure 2.2, you might imagine a cluster to be found just to the west of the High Level Bridge. Look down to your left next time you travel north on the East Coast main line as you begin to cross the Tyne.

If you could actually see 28 dots below you – to your left from the train window, or on the 1854 map – having seen the apparent cluster of cases, you might have been tempted to search for a possible cause. You could, for example, have found the source of water drunk by people there and have claimed that that was the reason. Had it been from the pump of a well you could even have removed the pump handle. Alternatively you could have stepped back a little and looked at the physical and social contours of Gateshead. Physically this is what you might find:

That the town of Gateshead, separated from that of Newcastle by the river Tyne only, is mainly situated on a steep slope ascending from that river, in some places with great abruptness, and at the southern extremity of the borough reaching a height of 500 feet; that the great bulk of the town lies at a very considerable elevation, the lowest thoroughfares,

Figure 2.2: Cholera in Gateshead in 1845 (cases)

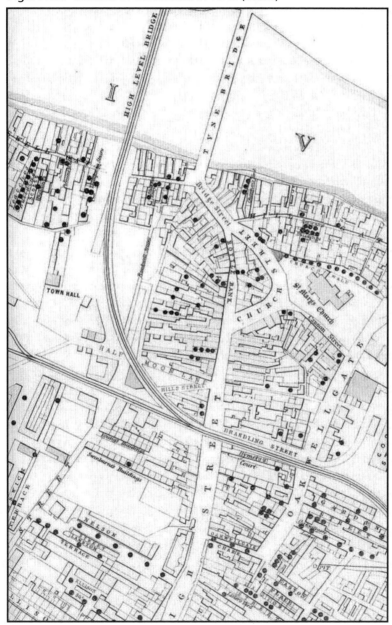

Source: www.genuki.org.uk/big/eng/NBL/Cholera/Mp2.html

those immediately along the verge of the river, being from 4 to 5 feet above spring tide high water. (Royal Commission, 1854, part 4, introduction)

When the Royal Commission carried out their thorough study of Newcastle, Tynemouth and Gateshead, rather than produce a huge plethora of possibilities, including thunder without lightning, or identify a particular pump (or well) as the problem, they came to a much broader conclusion. It was announced that it was the sanitary conditions of the population at large that were amiss:

That the poorer classes of Gateshead are not only exceedingly ill lodged, but also much overcrowded in their lodgings; that it is an habitual thing for an entire family to live, sleep, cook, eat and wash, &c.; in a single room; the corners of single rooms thus occupied being occasionally further sub-let to other families or lodgers. (Royal Commission, 1854, part 114)

The notion of cholera coming from the poorer classes, often seen as the 'dangerous classes' – and therefore alleviation being required to prevent its spread to the better-off – grew in importance with respect to the implementation of preventative initiatives as the 19th century progressed. Cholera may actually not have been particularly strongly socially patterned (Davey Smith, 2012), but the perception that it was, was important for social reform as the 'dangerous classes' became seen as the sink for sustaining the disease, and so it was felt that improving their living conditions would improve the general good. Scientific 'truth' may thus have been constructed on a potential misunderstanding, but a socially useful one (Young, 1977).

The upper classes were drawn to live in cities (country life could be tedious and not especially profitable). The affluent often did not have separate water supplies, and came into close contact with their servants and others in crowded streets and homes. Cholera may well not have been a disease of poverty other than that the poor were housed more often in low-lying land where water was frequently stagnant and where sewage accumulated and the disease could be most easily transmitted.

What was highlighted during the 19th century, through the scare stories and then a particular subset of them, and what caused the high-profile stories, was what came to fit best into the consolidating narrative. 'Unsanitary surroundings' fitted best partly because it served wider social goals in an age of great social change and led to policy changes that were more widely beneficial: *'British sanitary systems became the universal mark of adequate public provision for health'* (Hamlin, 1998, p 2). As we move forward in time, and move from place to place, we often realise that what we thought was once true in one place may not have been so straightforward.

I moved from Newcastle to Bristol in 1996 and for a short time lived at Richmond Terrace, in Clifton. It is not that I am cursed (or necessarily obsessed) by my personal geographic history; the point I am trying to make here is that wherever you are in Britain and any other country rich enough to have records, if you take a little care to look, you will find that there will have been disease outbreaks all around you, especially a century-and-a-half ago.

Epidemic outbreaks were particularly acute during industrialisation and colonisation, at those times before we had learned to control disease a little, which in a circular way may well have been by sharing out resources a 'tad' more fairly, to improve sanitary conditions. Later would come more personalised treatment, vaccines and antibiotics, for other diseases. Before that came better public health, but often the public health improvement required a simple story to first be told. Here is part of the story of Dr William Budd, who settled in Bristol in 1842:

> *In 1847, as a general practitioner, he visited a patient with fever in Richmond Terrace, Clifton, a suburb of the city. He diagnosed the fever as typhoid and soon realized that there was a minor epidemic among the homes of Richmond Terrace; of 34 households, 13 experienced at least one case of fever. The only thing the 13 houses had in common was the use of a well; the 21 without fever had different water supplies. He hypothesized that the disease was being spread by water; and in 1849, when he became responsible for the water supplies in Bristol, he concluded that cholera was spread from person to person in similar fashion. In consequence the Bristol water supplies were improved.*
> (Moorhead, 2002, p 562)

Epidemiological imaginations

This story of the use of just one infected well is contagious. Dr Budd was far from the first to use it, and similar stories have been played out innumerable times since. It is a nice simple story, and it can – for a short time – circumvent questions of jerry-built homes, poverty wages and nasty social attitudes, to replace these with the tale of the heroic physician who removed the handle from the pump and saved the day. This is not to say that the jerry-building and people living in cellars (in their own and others' sewage) provide the answer to why cholera spread, as neither is simply the passage of the disease from India. What it is fair to say is that given all the confusion over a new disease, simple stories of a single infected water source are especially alluring.

In fact, even in the most famous case of all (of which more below), the 1854 Broad Street outbreak in Soho, London, investigated by Dr Snow, the pump in question may well not have been the source and, even if it were, its handle was removed too late to have had any great effect (see Figure 2.3). Dr Snow was the London-based Yorkshire doctor now viewed as one of the founding fathers of epidemiology for his work on the cholera epidemic of 1854, which convinced the authorities to remove the handle of a water pump on Broad Street:[2]

> *There is no doubt that the mortality was much diminished, as I said before, by the flight of the population, which commenced soon after the outbreak; but the attacks had*

---

[2] See Chapter 40, this volume, for more on the world's most famous pump handle remover, and a reproduction of Dr Snow's map (Figure 40.2, p 367) and further discussion of medical cartography.

so far diminished before the use of the water was stopped, that it is impossible to decide whether the well still contained the cholera poison in an active state, or whether, from some cause, the water had become free from it. The pump-well has been opened, and I was informed by Mr Farrell, the superintendent of the works, that there was no hole or crevice in the brickwork of the well, by which any impurity might enter; consequently in this respect the contamination of the water is not made out by the kind of physical evidence detailed in some of the instances previously related. I understand that the well is from twenty-eight to thirty feet in depth, and goes through the gravel to the surface of the clay beneath. (Snow, 1855)

Figure 2.3: Cholera outbreak in Golden Square, Broad Street, London, 1854

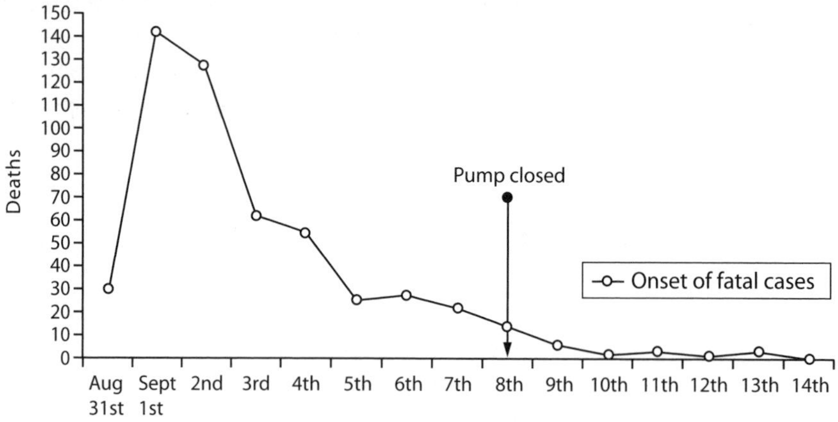

(668 deaths: onset date unknown)

Source: Davey Smith (2002, Figure 4)

We will, in all probability, never really know whether the well and its pump in Broad Street was the cause of the Soho outbreak, as all we have to go on are contemporary accounts, such as that from Reverend Henry Whitehead, a strong critic of Dr Snow at the time, who *'felt that an intensive inquiry would reveal the falsity of the Snow's hypothesis regarding the Broad Street pump'*, and he undertook such an inquiry. Then *'Slowly and I may add reluctantly [the conclusion was reached] that the use of water [from the Broad Street pump] was connected with the continuation of the outburst'* (Whitehead, 1855). Of course, failing to falsify a hypothesis does not mean it has been confirmed.

The fact that the outbreak declined long before the pump handle was removed casts doubt on Dr Snow's hypothesis. But the myth of how sure people then were that the cause was the pump in Broad Street is simply too strong a myth to kill. Look up the definition of 'human geography' in Wikipedia and, at least as of February 2012, you are greeted with Dr Snow's dot map of cholera in London in 1854, but no mention is made of the fact that no microscopic dirt was found in the well, nor that many cases of cholera found further away from the well were not drawn on the map, nor that it was a fishing exercise as simple as that you have just been encouraged to engage in above by looking at the map of Gateshead (see Figure 2.2). In fact:

> *As the tale of the Broad Street pump has been transformed into an anecdote resembling an urban legend, a recurring theme represents Snow as a clear-eyed modern thinker who saw the facts, and was opposed by defenders of ancient preconceived theories. But it misrepresents history, and does Snow an injustice, to imagine that he was not guided every bit as much by his own theory as his opponents were by theirs.* (Brody *et al*, 2000, p 68)

There is a chance that the myth of the medical map as a scientific tool of discovery will *not* simply be replaced by its being recognised as partly sustaining a self-promoting fraud, but that the earlier and other work on mapping cholera will come to be seen as key to changing hearts and minds in favour of public expenditure on public health for the common good, *and* on looking in general at how human beings are connected, not just within a city, but from as far as Bengal is from Manchester and as 1817 is from today. As the biographer of Dr Budd ended his short history of the doctor, he claimed Budd had added another task to the work of such general practitioners:

> *For the thinking general practitioner he added a fifth task – to study the interaction of human beings with themselves, with living organisms and within their shared environments. This is the task of human ecology.* (Moorhead, 2002, p 564)

Of course no one person adds a task on their own. More than a dozen years before Dr Budd knocked on that (later my?) door in Richmond Terrace, Clifton, Bristol, and more than 20 years before the Royal Commissioners in the North East of England suggested that it was the living conditions of the poor that were to blame, Dr Robert Baker, in *The Report to the Leeds Board of Health*, publishing quickly after those first large outbreaks in January 1833, wrote that:

> *We are of the opinion that the streets in which malignant cholera prevailed most severely, were those in which the drainage was most imperfect; and that the state of the general health of the inhabitants would be greatly improved, and the probability of a future visitation from such malignant epidemics diminished, by a general and efficient system of drainage, sewerage and paving, and the enforcement of better regulations as to the cleanliness of the streets.* (British Library, 2012)

An extract from Robert Baker's map is reproduced as Figure 2.4. In fact, it is not at all obvious from the map that cases of cholera were most concentrated in the poorest areas; in the fields just by the area labelled 'Little London' that lies on the northern edge of the map, then not a very poor area,[3] is the area where the buildings of the

---

[3] It is poorer now, but not the poorest part of Leeds; see Nick Davies (1998) for details.

University of Leeds were later erected. The School of Geography at the University of Leeds is now sited there and it overlooks a large cemetery. The cemetery land has been considerably raised up due to the volume of bodies from pandemics such as that shown in Figure 2.4. I mention this detail as I moved from being a lecturer in Bristol to next work as a professor right by that cemetery in the University of Leeds. Almost wherever you go in Britain you are never that far from previous sites of epidemic and pandemic concentration (the darkened homes in Figure 2.4).

Figure 2.4: Cholera in Leeds in 1832 (section of map)

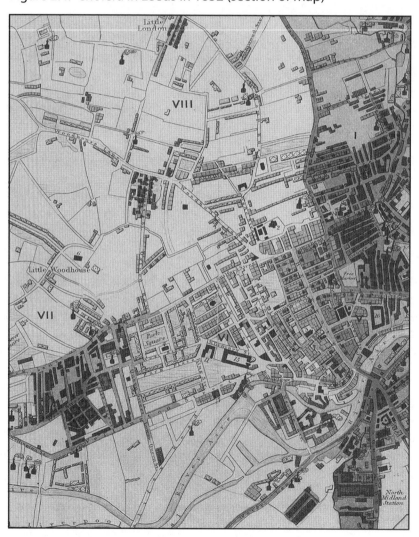

Note: Streets and homes where cholera struck are shaded black.

Source: www.bl.uk/learning/images/makeanimpact/publichealth/large12727.html

The ghosts of past times

At the time I moved to Leeds, in 2000, colleagues and I had published the paper that forms the basis of the next chapter, Chapter 3, 'The ghost of Christmas past' (Dorling *et al*, 2000). It has subsequently been recycled more than once, but it does show that geographical patterns are also recycled, even when very different populations move into an area and many of the old population leave. The paper suggested that the impact of inequalities, particularly of health, could span generations despite great population turnover. It drew on maps of London produced at the end of the 19th century and contrasted them with ones drawn on a very similar basis but taken from the census of 100 years later, in 1991.

The area of Little London (just north of Woodhouse Lane in Leeds) is today relatively poor, but 100 years ago it was almost certainly a little more affluent, and cholera was not that discriminatory. Public works did result in the worst of the slums being demolished and rebuilt with back-to-backs. These were then demolished and the area was rebuilt with modern council housing, which was in turn again, often shortly afterwards, demolished. All the time the housing of the affluent was improved, or newly built further out (to the north and west in Leeds), as also happened in many other British cities.

Despite huge improvements in public health, places that were poor in the past have often continued to be so, while affluent areas have similarly tended to stay affluent or have reverted to being affluent again because of the geographical advantages of their location. Overall health as measured in absolute terms may improve, but as infectious disease has been reduced, and as the rich come again to believe they could be immune to many of the troubles of the poor, relative gaps grow.

Chapter 4 (Dorling, 2006) shows how, as infant mortality became more rare in England and Wales, its association with poverty, rather than its links with chance epidemic or other factors based on medical, environmental and social conditions, strengthened. The annex to Chapter 3 (Dorling *et al*, 2005) shows how the longer someone lives both in poverty and in a poor area, the earlier they tend to die. And this outcome applies not only to past, but also present, generations. Chapter 5 shows that these divides have recently been rising and are typified by a growing North–South divide, all characterised by social polarisation of the population by poverty, wealth, and consequently, poor and good health (Dorling and Thomas, 2009).

Popular government discourse often appears to allege that inequalities in health and income have decreased over time as a consequence of policies and initiatives that politicians have put in place; although in average absolute terms, there has been great improvement, most of this recent improvement has been associated with the diminishing popularity of smoking from the 1950s to the 1970s as both knowledge and life chances in general improved. The claim that government today has been narrowing gaps stands contrary to the general lack of progress in narrowing made over recent times and contrasts sharply with the public health achievements that began to be made within Britain towards the end of the 19th century and that came to full fruition in the first 70 years of the 20th century.

In Britain, to next find health inequalities as great as those suffered at the end of the time of cholera we have to jump from Victorian times to the neo-Victorian era of Margaret Thatcher (1979 to 2012 onwards). Although gains have been made in public health since the 1970s, the benefits have been disproportionately felt by the affluent who, in turn, continue to marginalise the poor, so when governments talk about the strides made in diminishing health inequalities, they are largely speaking about an exclusive portion of the population, and perpetuating a discourse that is consistently separated from the life experiences of average people, of the majority of citizens, and especially of the most disadvantaged people within society.

We need to remember public health advocacy in the distant past to draw hope for the future, and to learn again from when, over a century ago, we were last confronted by rising inequality. Both economic and health inequalities have expanded over the last three decades. Despite increasing life expectancy overall, inequalities in life expectancy between the poorest and richest groups in society have widened. Furthermore, rising inequalities in life expectancy between areas are concurrent with rising economic inequalities that have emerged between different parts of Britain.

As yet, nowhere in Britain has seen a fall in life expectancy or an absolute increase in mortality rates for any group (the last recorded absolute falls were for people aged 25 and over between 1921 and 1940; see Davey Smith and Marmot, 1991, table 1).

Infant mortality rates (IMRs) remain highest today in areas in which they were highest a century ago. This is despite a recent dramatic reduction in overall IMRs that has corresponded with the increasing concentration of higher IMRs in the poorest regions. It is also important not to forget that in recent decades inequalities in health for adults have continuously risen despite all the government rhetoric and subsequent initiatives aimed at reducing health inequalities. The rhetoric began with Margaret Thatcher's commitment to *reduce* health inequalities by 25 per cent by the year 2000, a promise made in 1985; they *increased* by more than that target. Both Conservative and New Labour government policy has largely been symbolic and has failed to tackle the disparities in income and wealth that drive rising health inequalities as measured across society. Instead, more potent and redistributive policies are needed to initiate change and greater equality.

Although much of the rest of this book may seem pessimistic, there are, nonetheless, reasons for optimism. Unlike in the US, where in certain states and for certain groups living standards as reflected by life expectancy have fallen in absolute terms, there is as yet no such trend anywhere in the UK. In the US in some states infant mortality among the babies of black parents has been rising since 2007 (Census Bureau, 2012). Nowhere in the UK has infant mortality yet risen. Moreover, greater equality can be convincingly claimed to be beneficial for the health of wealthy and poorer people, and hence, the whole of society. The drink and drug intake of wealthy North Americans is partly so high, it is argued, because they live in such an unequal society. But when all poor health can be ascribed to apparent individual weakness and without such obvious motivators as cholera epidemics to bring the rich to their senses, it may be harder to sell redistributive policies today. A general

Figure 2.5: If pounds were pixels – one of many hundreds of images of dissent in 2012

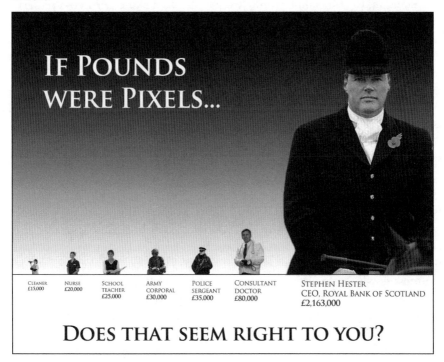

IF POUNDS WERE PIXELS...

| CLEANER £15,000 | NURSE £20,000 | SCHOOL TEACHER £25,000 | ARMY CORPORAL £30,000 | POLICE SERGEANT £35,000 | CONSULTANT DOCTOR £80,000 | STEPHEN HESTER CEO, ROYAL BANK OF SCOTLAND £2,163,000 |

DOES THAT SEEM RIGHT TO YOU?

see colour version in plate section

Note: Image created by Duncan Rickelton.

Source: http://zoom.it/yE58

and widespread rise in disgust with the rich (rather than envy) might be what we need next to help us most, both in the UK and the US (see Figure 2.5).

The beginnings and the ends

The following chapters, and much of the rest of this book, explore the beginnings and ends of life – how birth and death, although unifying events, are severely unequal as revealed by rates of infant mortality and ratios of premature death risk between the rich and poor. Birth and death are unifying in that when giving birth you have more in common with others giving birth than anyone else (regardless of class). The same is true of death.

The next section of this book begins by considering recent Coalition government reforms (Chapter 6). In the remainder of this section, the New Labour record on reducing health inequalities is placed in the context of rising geographical inequalities in health over the last century. Two core New Labour targets were to reduce the gap in infant mortality across social groups and to raise life expectancy within the most disadvantaged areas. The first target may be close to being attained, but the second is not. Detailed analysis of trends in area-based life expectancy show that life expectancy in the richest areas continued to rise faster than anywhere else in the UK as measured up to 2009 and beyond. Just like the men and pigs in George Orwell's animal farm, it has become hard to tell Conservatives and New Labour apart in the 21st century because of the effect of Thatcherism on both.

Although people are no longer the kinds of chattels they were in the 19th century and all, on average, live much longer, some live much longer than others. A note of caution has to be woven into the story of declining infant mortality over the 20th century. While it reduced dramatically over the period, and became more rare, its association with poverty, rather than chance, has been increasing, and this reflects the overall health divide. However, its association with poverty as indicated by social class has reduced in recent years.[4]

As far as we know, to date, the tactics of the 2000s for raising the living standards of the poorest people in Britain have failed to cut down health inequalities. It is possible that there may still be a delayed effect, and inequalities are now increasing largely because of harm done in the 1980s. Time will tell. Intriguingly, in the historical record, reductions in infant mortality have been coincident not with moments of rapidly rising income levels, but when GNP (gross national product) per capita has risen most slowly (in the late 1940s and early 1950s). Infant mortality should react much more quickly to current events, although it is also influenced by parents' past environments, especially the mother's (Subramanian et al, 2012). Health inequalities in the last hundred years were lowest when the lives of the rich and the poor were less different. This leads to calls for a 'stronger dose' of redistribution of wealth.

The ghost of Christmas past still looms large over Britain. Images of Victorian squalor (and vice) are readily brought to mind through the vivid works of Dickens, the author of that ghost. The 200th anniversary of Charles Dickens' birth was celebrated in early 2012, but how many policy makers would associate patterns of poverty from the Victorian era with the health outcomes of today? The next chapter in particular brings an historical lens to relationships between the spatial distribution of poverty and mortality in London. The analysis shows that for diseases related to deprivation in early life, contemporary mortality is better predicted by the distribution of poverty in 1896 than in 1991.

A great deal of the findings in the following chapters raise issues around the stability of 'poor places' over time and, again, sharpen the evidence for less miserly, more redistributive, fairer, policies, which, a cynic might suggest, includes motherhood and apple pie; but what is the alternative? Is it to suggest that if a person looks after him or herself, ensures that his or her water source and air is clean, then '… *it is to his complete protection from their influence that the rich man is indebted for his immunity from cholera quite as much if not more, than to any remarkable freedom from the agency of the predisposing causes, which his wealth confers. The contrast between the localities which the rich and poor inhabit, exhibits perhaps the most striking example of the substantial advantages,*

---

[4] See Figure 44.1 and footnote 2 on p 432 in Chapter 44 for declines in class inequalities in infant mortality recorded in 2009 and 2010. The falls are coincident with the increased numbers of children being taken into care following the death of 'Baby P' on 3 August 2007 and the subsequent investigation into his death.

as far as health is concerned, which affluence can bestow …' (Gaulter, 1833, p 118). (See Figure 2.8 in the annex to this chapter on p 35.)

Conclusion

Monuments were erected around Britain to remember those who died of cholera in the 19th century and to serve as a warning for what might return if we do not continue to learn the lessons of the past (see Figure 2.6). The cholera epidemics were brought under significant control long before Robert Koch's theses on germ theory were published in 1876.

It is not medical science that could most improve health and well-being today but, as before, a better understanding of how we all influence each other. Another way of looking at arguments for the redistribution of income and wealth is that

Figure 2.6: Sheffield cholera monument

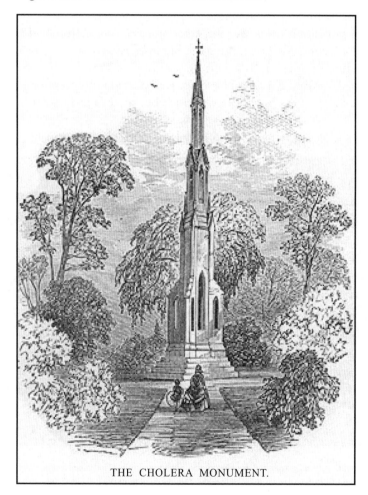

THE CHOLERA MONUMENT.

Source: http://public-art.shu.ac.uk/sheffield/unk126im.html

31

currently the surplus monies that are allowed to the best-off 1 per cent – over 15 per cent of all income in Britain, and over 20 per cent in the US – are largely wasted. The surplus could be used more efficiently if a larger part of it was redistributed. In unequal countries the very rich squander and waste far more monies than any government, other than a dictatorship, ever could.

In recent years not only have the 'worst inequalities of all', health inequalities, widened in many affluent countries including the UK and the US, but they have also become so entrenched that poverty is no longer a thing of the past but instead a ghost that has returned. For many postwar decades it was rapidly receding. Living standards are currently falling by both absolute and relative measures in the UK.

The concluding chapter of this section, Chapter 5, suggests that not only is it clear that improving living standards and hence the income share in the most disadvantaged areas is still necessary to alleviate health inequalities, but also that the living standards of those who remain stuck need to be raised – which did not happen in recent years because they were not enough of a priority for the New Labour government (Shaw et al, 2005).

Since New Labour lost power the situation has changed from bad to worse. But we should still conclude by counting our blessings. At least in 2010 a chalk artist can draw a picture of opened-up sewers on the floor of a train station in Manchester (see Figure 2.7; BBC, 2010) and his work be reported with no sense of irony – but perhaps that also shows how little we remember of our recent past?

Figure 2.7: Picture drawn in chalk by Joe Hill, Manchester Piccadilly

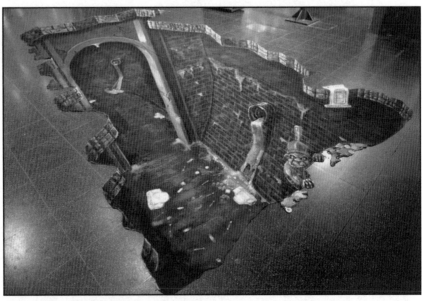

Source: BBC (2010): Temporary drawing made on the concourse floor. 'United Utilities say that Mancunians flush away thousands of incorrect items, such as make up wipes and ear buds, a year, causing sewers to block and toilets and drains to flood' (http://news.bbc.co.uk/local/manchester/hi/people_and_places/newsid_9135000/9135707.stm)

References

Acland, H.W. (1856) *Memoir on the cholera at Oxford, in the year 1854, with considerations suggested by the epidemic*, London: John Churchill (http://books.google.co.uk/ebooks/reader?id=aHEFAAAAQAAJ).

BBC (2010) 'In pics: artistic sewer opens at Manchester Piccadilly', 28 October (http://news.bbc.co.uk/local/manchester/hi/people_and_places/newsid_9135000/9135707.stm).

British Library (2012) Quotation and map made available of the 1832 cholera outbreak in Leeds (www.bl.uk/learning/histcitizen/21cc/publichealth/sources/source5/mapofleeds.html).

Brody, M., Russell Rip, M., Vinten-Johansen, P., Paneth, N. and Rachman, S. (2000) 'Map-making and myth-making in Broad Street: the London cholera epidemic, 1854', *The Lancet*, vol 356, pp 64–8 (www.casa.ucl.ac.uk/martin/msc_gis/map_making_myth_making.pdf).

Budd, W. (1931 [1874 originally]) *Typhoid fever, its nature, mode of spreading and prevention*, New York: American Public Health Association. [An excerpt can be found at www.ncbi.nlm.nih.gov/pmc/articles/PMC1556726/pdf/amjphnation00616-0128a.pdf]

Busteed, M. and Hindle, P. (2010) 'Angel Meadow: the Irish and cholera in Manchester, exploring Greater Manchester', Online pamphlet of the Manchester Geographical Society (www.mangeogsoc.org.uk/egm/3_2.pdf).

Census Bureau (2012) *The 2012 statistical abstract of the United States* (www.census.gov/compendia/statab/).

Davey Smith, G. (2002) 'Commentary: Behind the Broad Street pump: aetiology, epidemiology and prevention of cholera in mid-19th century Britain', *International Journal of Epidemiology*, vol 31, no 5, pp 920-32 (http://ije.oxfordjournals.org/content/31/5/920.full).

Davey Smith, G. (2012) Personal communication, referring in turn to articles published in the *Socialism and Health* journal dating from the 1970s.

Davey Smith, G. and Marmot, M. (1991) 'Trends in mortality in Britain 1920-1986', *Annals of Nutrition and Metabolism*, vol 25 (supplement 1), pp 53-63.

Davies, M. (2000) *Late Victorian holocausts: El Niño, famines and the making of the Third World*, London: Verso. [See famine timeline for India and review and summary at www.indicstudies.us/Demographics%20and%20Geopolitics/Famine.html]

Davies, N. (1998) *Dark heart: The shocking truth about hidden Britain*, London: Vintage.

Dorling, D. (2006) 'Infant mortality and social progress in Britain, 1905-2005', in E. Garrett, C. Galley, N. Shelton and R. Woods (eds) *Infant mortality: A continuing social problem*, Aldershot and Burlington: Ashgate Publishing, pp 213-28 (www.dannydorling.org/?page_id=2442) [reproduced as Chapter 4, this volume].

Dorling, D. and Thomas, B. (2009) 'Geographical inequalities in health over the last century', in H. Graham (ed) *Understanding health inequalities* (2nd edn), Buckingham: Open University Press, pp 66-83 (www.dannydorling.org/?page_id=2904) [reproduced as Chapter 5, this volume].

Dorling, D., Mitchell, R., Orford, S., Shaw, M. and Davey Smith, G. (2005) 'Inequalities and Christmas yet to come', *British Medical Journal*, vol 331, no 7529, p 1409 (www.dannydorling.org/?page_id=448) [reproduced as an annex to Chapter 3, this volume].

Dorling, D., Mitchell, R., Shaw, M., Orford, S. and Davey Smith. G. (2000) 'The ghost of Christmas past: health effects of poverty in London in 1896 and 1991', *British Medical Journal*, issue no 7276, vol 321, December, pp 1547-51 (www.bmj. com/content/321/7276/1547.full) [reproduced as Chapter 3, this volume].

Gaulter, H. (1833) *The origin and process of malignant cholera in Manchester, Considered chiefly in their bearing on the contagiousness and the secondary causes of the disease*, London: Longman (et al) (www.archive.org/details/originandprogre00gaulgoog).

Hamlin, C. (1998) *Public health and social justice in the age of Chadwick: Britain, 1800– 1854*, Cambridge: Cambridge University Press.

Hamlin, C. (2009) *Cholera: The biography*, Oxford: Oxford University Press.

Koch, T. (2011) *Disease maps: Epidemics on the ground*, Chicago, IL: University of Chicago Press.

Manchester City Council (2012) 'Manchester and the city centre: Cottonopolis', Information leaflet (www.spinningtheweb.org.uk/m_display.php?irn=5&sub=co ttonopolis&theme=places&crumb=City+Centre).

Moorhead, R. (2002) 'William Budd and typhoid fever', *Journal of the Royal Society of Medicine*, vol 95, no 11, pp 561-4 (www.ncbi.nlm.nih.gov/pmc/articles/ PMC1279260/).

Royal Commission (1854) *Health: Report from the Royal Commission on Cholera in Newcastle-upon-Tyne, Gateshead and Tynemouth, etc v.2* (British Parliamentary Papers), Dublin: Irish University Press (www.genuki.org.uk/big/eng/NBL/Cholera/index. html). [New issue of 1852-54 edition published in December 1970.]

Shaw, M., Davey Smith, G. and Dorling, D. (2005) 'Health inequalities and New Labour: how the promises compare with real progress', *British Medical Journal*, vol 330, no 7498, pp 1016-21 (www.dannydorling.org/?page_id=457).

Snow, J. (1855) *On the mode of communication of cholera*, London: John Churchill, New Burlington Street (www.ph.ucla.edu/epi/snow/snowbook_a2.html).

Subramanian, S.V., Ackerson, L.K. et al (2012) 'Association of maternal height with child mortality, anthropometric failure, and anaemia in India', *Journal of the American Medical Association*, vol 301, no 16, pp 1691-701.

Whitehead, H. (1855) *Special investigation of Broad Street* (Report note available at www.ph.ucla.edu/epi/snow/whitehead.html).

Young, B. (1977) 'Science is social relations', *Radical Science Journal*, pp 65-129.

Annex

Figure 2.8: Two pages from Gaulter's work on the 1832 Manchester cholera outbreak

118

because its sewers were in a worse condition. The truth is that in the greater part of Manchester there are no sewers at all, and that where they do exist they are so small and badly constructed that instead of contributing to the purification of the town, they become themselves nuisances of the worst description. Recently two or three have been formed or enlarged on a scale of dimensions somewhat more adequate to the functions which they have to fulfil, but to make the *subterranean* of this vast town what it ought to be, and to excavate under its whole surface a complete order of primary and secondary drains, would require an expenditure of not less than three hundred thousand pounds. The labours of the night-man and scavenger do something towards the abatement of this evil; but it is necessary that those of the latter should be placed under better regulations, while in the formation of new streets it ought to be imperatively required that the *subterranean* and pavement of the street be constructed and rendered complete before the houses are built.

Two more remarks are suggested by the consideration of the generating causes of cholera. First, it is to his complete protection from their influence that the rich man is indebted for his immunity from cholera quite as much if not far more, than to any remarkable freedom from the agency of the predisposing causes, which his wealth confers. The contrast between the localities which the rich and poor

119

inhabit, exhibits perhaps the most striking example of the substantial advantages, as far as health is concerned, which affluence can bestow, by enabling its possessor so to construct and fix his residence as to place himself and his family beyond the reach of every ordinary source of malaria. In ancient times the importance of such a choice was not understood, and in towns accordingly the better classes who inhabited dwellings almost as small, ill ventilated, and badly placed, as the poor of our own days, fell victims in far more equal numbers to the epidemics that then preyed upon the land. Even during the progress of cholera in some cities where the local partition between the two great classes of society has been less marked, the disease has attacked both rich and poor in their promiscuous habitations with almost indiscriminate severity, as in Moscow, where one hundred and twenty-four nobles died of the disease.

2.—It may be thought visionary perhaps, but I am disposed to ascribe a large share of the exemption from cholera, which the working classes of this town enjoyed during the epidemic, (an exemption which has been happily extended to the manufacturing districts generally) to the cotton factories in which they work. It was impossible, at least in this town, not to be struck with the fact, that of the whole number of the Manchester cases very few indeed were employed in factories at all, and that of these a pretty large proportion were at the

Source: www.archive.org/stream/originandprogre00gaulgoog#page/n128/mode/2up

3

The ghost of Christmas past: health effects of poverty in London in 1896 and 1991[1]

Dorling, D., Mitchell, R., Shaw, M., Orford, S. and Davey Smith. G. (2000) 'The ghost of Christmas past: health effects of poverty in London in 1896 and 1991', *British Medical Journal*, vol 321, no 7276, December, pp 1547-51.

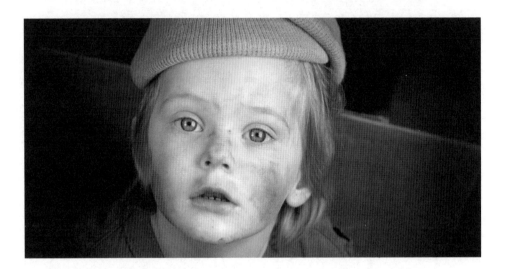

What is already known on this topic: People's health is strongly related to their material circumstances throughout their lives and particularly in childhood.

Places in which people had poor health in the past tend still to contain people with relatively poor health today.

What this study adds: At least in central London, a measure of the relative poverty and affluence of places made over 100 years ago is, for many causes of death, as useful a predictor of current inequalities in health as is the 1991 census.

Together, the last census and the Booth index of 1896 better predict inequalities in health seen across London in the 1990s.

The key message of *A Christmas Carol*—that redistribution of wealth reduces inequalities in mortality—is as relevant today as when it was written over 150 years ago; the fact that inequalities in health persist and match the 19th century pattern of inequalities in wealth so well suggests that that message has yet to be heeded.

---

[1] Editorial Note: This paper is reproduced as originally published other than the numbering of references, many of which are converted to footnotes here rather than left as originally listed in endnotes.

Abstract

Objectives: To compare the extent to which late 20th century patterns of mortality in London are predicted by contemporary patterns of poverty and by late 19th century patterns of poverty. To test the hypothesis that the pattern of mortality from causes known to be related to deprivation in early life can be better predicted by the distribution of poverty in the late 19th century than by that in the late 20th century.

Design: Data from Charles Booth's survey of inner London in 1896 were digitised and matched to contemporary local government wards. Ward level indices of relative poverty were derived from Booth's survey and the 1991 UK census of population. All deaths which took place within the surveyed area between 1991 and 1995 were identified and assigned to contemporary local government wards. Standardised mortality ratios for various causes of death were calculated for each ward for all ages, under age 65, and over age 65. Simple correlation and partial correlation analysis were used to estimate the contribution of the indices of poverty from 1896 and 1991 in predicting ward level mortality ratios in the early 1990s.

Setting: Inner London.

Results: For many causes of death in London, measures of deprivation made around 1896 and 1991 both contributed strongly to predicting the current spatial distribution. Contemporary mortality from diseases which are known to be related to deprivation in early life (stomach cancer, stroke, lung cancer) is predicted more strongly by the distribution of poverty in 1896 than that in 1991. In addition, all cause mortality among people aged over 65 was slightly more strongly related to the geography of poverty in the late 19th century than to its contemporary distribution.

Conclusions: Contemporary patterns of some diseases have their roots in the past. The fundamental relation between spatial patterns of social deprivation and spatial patterns of mortality is so robust that a century of change in inner London has failed to disrupt it.

Introduction

They [left the busy scene, and] went into an obscure part of the town, where Scrooge had never penetrated before, although he recognised its situation, and its bad repute. The ways were foul and narrow; the shops and houses wretched; the people halfnaked, drunken, slip shod, ugly. Alleys and archways, like so many cesspools, disgorged their offences of smell, and dirt, and life, upon the straggling streets; and the whole quarter reeked with crime, with filth, and misery.[2]

---

[2] Dickens, C. (1843) *A Christmas carol.* London: Chapman and Hall.

With these words Charles Dickens describes Scrooge's journey with the Spirit of Christmas Yet to Come into the poorest streets of London to view the body of Tiny Tim, the child his miserliness will kill if it continues unchecked. Dickens's *A Christmas Carol* also helped open the eyes of non-fictitious Londoners to the extent of poverty in their city at a time when social views were rapidly changing. Charles Booth was a contemporary chronicler of fact rather than fiction; together with his researchers he surveyed these same streets so that we can see today where the Tiny Tims of the past lived. Using Booth's map of poverty at the end of the 19th century we test the hypothesis of the Spirit of Christmas Yet to Come: that miserliness in the past and present leads to future inequalities in health.

Figure 3.1: Detail of *Charles Booth's descriptive map of London poverty 1889.*

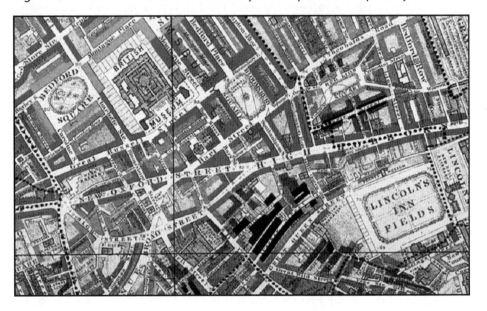

see colour version in plate section

Note: Light grey [yellow on colour plate] indicates the highest social class, black the lowest.

Source: *Charles Booth's descriptive map of London poverty 1889,* with introduction by D.A. Reeder, Publication No 130, London: London Topographical Society, 1984.

Today, poverty at all stages of life is implicated in determining the risk of mortality[3], and relationships between the spatial distribution of poverty and mortality are well known and robust.[4] It is also clear that there are specific relationships between adverse circumstances in childhood and the subsequent risk of particular causes of

[3] Davey Smith, G., Hart, C., Gillis, C., Hawthorne, V. (1997) Lifetime socioeconomic position and mortality: prospective observational study. *British Medical Journal,* 314: 547–52.
[4] Shaw, M., Gordon, D., Dorling, D. and Davey Smith, G. (1999) *The widening gap: health inequalities and policy in Britain.* Bristol: The Policy Press.

death in adulthood[5]. We seek to illustrate here one example of where the spirits of Christmases past—even those before childhood—have a strong influence on inequalities in health today.

Charles Booth's study of poverty in London was published between 1889 and 1903 in 17 volumes under the title of *Life and Labour of the People of London* (Aves, 1916; Bales, 1996, 1999; Booth, 1887, 1889, 1902a, 1902b; Cullen, 1979; Davies, 1978; Fried and Elman, 1969; O'Day and Englander, 1993; Pfautz, 1967; Simey and Simey, 1960; Spicker, 1990; Townsend, Corrigan and Kowarzik, 1987). Booth's survey covered over 120,000 households, an area bounded by Pentonville prison to the north, Millwall docks to the east, Stockwell smallpox hospital to the south, and Kensington Palace to the west. The information that Booth and his 20 researchers collected was projected on to a series of detailed and exact maps, the most important of which was the *Descriptive Map of London Poverty* (see Figure 3.1).[6] This map shows the streets of London, building by building, coloured to correspond to a classification of the resident population of the time. Booth's seven category classification scheme is described in Table 3.1.

This area of London was surveyed again in 1991 as part of the UK census of population. The registrar general's social classification scheme used in the census is similar to Booth's scheme[7]; indeed the former was in part derived from Booth's work (Stevenson, 1928; Szreter 1984, 1986). The similarity between the two schemes makes it possible to derive a hybrid which can be used as the basis for comparison between the two time periods. Table 3.1 shows how these two classification schemes fit together.

Method

To create an empirical measure of Dickens's fictitious description of 19th century London, Booth's map was digitised and its street-by-street data aggregated to contemporary ward boundaries using a Geographical Information System. Wards are administrative areal units used in UK local government. Booth's survey area included 104 complete modern wards and the major part of 28 additional wards. The distribution of household social class within each ward was calculated for both 1896 and 1991.

A ward index of poverty was calculated by computing the proportion of households in each social class, weighting that proportion by the relative position of the class in the social hierarchy of the time, and summing the weighted proportions. The index of poverty thus assumes (as Booth showed) that social class is a proxy for poverty and that the extent of poverty in a class is related to its position within the class hierarchy.

---

[5] Davey Smith, G., Hart, C., Blane, D. and Hole, D. (1998) Adverse socioeconomic conditions in childhood and cause specific adult mortality: prospective observational study, *British Medical Journal*, 316, 1631–5.

[6] (1984) *Charles Booth's descriptive map of London poverty 1889*, with introduction by D.A. Reeder, London: London Topographical Society (Publication No 130).

[7] Gillie, A. (1996) The origin of the poverty line. *Economic History Review*, 49, 715–30.

Table 3.1: Booth's classes and Registrar General's classes.

Colour on 1896 Map	Booth Description	% Households in 1896	Equivalent RG Class	% Households in 1991*	1896 SEP indicator×	1991 SEP indicator×
Black	Lowest class; vicious, semi-criminal	1.5 ⎫				
Blue	Very poor, casual, chronic wants	3.7 ⎬ 12.6	V+	6.9	0.937	0.965
Light Blue	Poor, 18s-21s a week for a moderate family	7.4 ⎭				
Purple	Mixed, some comfortable, others poor	16.2	IV	12.8	0.794	0.867
Pink	Fairly comfortable, good ordinary earnings	35.2	III	33.8	0.537	0.634
Red	Well to do. Middle Class	27.7	II	37.3	0.223	0.278
Yellow	Upper-middle and Upper classes. Wealthy.	8.4	I	9.2	0.042	0.046

* Excludes households with no social class allocation in the 1991 Census (those described as in the army, inadequately described and others without a social class).
× Socioeconomic position (SEP) indicators are cumulative proportions.

For Class I the wI is (I/2)/(I+II+III+IV+V)
For Class II the wII is (I+II/2)/(I+II+III+IV+V)
For Class III the wIII is (I+II+III/2)/(I+II+III+IV+V)
For Class IV the wIV is (I+II+III+IV/2)/(I+II+III+IV+V)
For Class V the wV is (I+II+III+IV+V/2)/(I+II+III+IV+V)

+ Includes people of working age who have not worked in the last 10 years.

The extent of poverty within a class has thus been estimated using the number of people in higher social classes. The index for a particular ward is:

Ward Poverty Index = (I★wI + II★wII + III★wIII + IV★wIV + V★wV)/(I+II+III+IV+V)

where I is the number of households in class I in the ward at that time and wI is the socioeconomic position indicator associated with that class shown in Table 3.1. This indicator relates to the proportion of the population that is at a higher socioeconomic level than the midpoint of the group. For 1991, 9.2% of households are in social class I, so 4.6% of them are above the mid point of this category and the indicator is 0.046; 37.3% of households are in social class II and it is assumed that all social class I households and half of social class II households are at a higher socioeconomic level than the midpoint of this group. Thus the indicator for social class II households is $0.092 + 0.186 = 0.278$. Similar logic is applied to calculation of the indicators for social classes III to V. The formulae to calculate indicators of socioeconomic position are given in the footnote to Table 3.1.

The index was low (approaching 0) in areas where large numbers of the resident households were in more affluent social classes and high in areas where they were in less affluent social classes. Similar formulae were applied to calculation of the 1896 indicators. The use of such indicators takes into account the fact that the distributions of socioeconomic groups in 1896 and 1991 were different (such indicators have been widely used in inequalities in health research (Pamuk, 1985; Kunst and Mackenbach, 1994; Davey Smith *et al.*, 1998). This index measures level of affluence for each ward in the study area and not inequality within them.

Figure 3.2: Providence Place (Islington), c. 1900 and 2000.

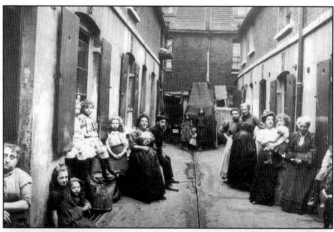

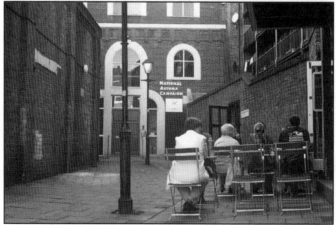

Source: More recent photograph by Mary Shaw, 2000, taken in similar position to archive photograph.

Figure 3.2 shows two images of Providence Place in Islington, north London, taken more than 100 years apart. Note how the number of people has fallen, as it has fallen in London as a whole over this period, and that the open drain has been covered. However, the social position of Providence Place in the geographical ranking of London streets remains much the same.

We compared the relative predictive power of the two poverty measures as they varied for specific causes of death and for different age groups. In particular, stroke and stomach cancer, as causes shown to be related to deprivation in early life, may be better predicted by a historical poverty measure.[8] Age and sex standardised mortality ratios for each ward were thus calculated for the causes of death shown in Table 3.2 and for all deaths which took place between 1991 and 1995. The analysis comprised simple weighted and partial correlations in which ward mortality ratios were predicted by the two measures of poverty. The population of each ward provided the weights. Partial correlation analysis was also used to ascertain the extent to which predictive power was duplicated between the indices. All analyses were carried out in SPSS.

Table 3.2: Strength of relationship (r values) between poverty in 1896 and 1991 and all-age SMR for deaths in 1991-95.

	Correlation of Booth-based index and mortality	Partial correlation of Booth-based index and mortality (controlling for Census-based index)	Correlation of 1991 Census-based index and mortality	Partial correlation of Census-based index and mortality (controlling for Booth-based index)
All Cause SMR	0.56 (p<0.001)	0.22 (p=0.012)	0.60 (p<0.001)	0.35 (p<0.001)
Coronary Heart Disease	0.58 (p<0.001)	0.211 (p=0.015)	0.65 (p<0.001)	0.41 (p<0.001)
Stroke	0.40 (p<0.001)	0.22 (p=0.013)	0.36 (p<0.001)	0.11 (p=0.20)
All Cardiovascular Disease	0.56 (p<0.001)	0.20 (p=0.023)	0.61 (p<0.001)	0.37 (p<0.001)
Chronic Obstructive Pulmonary Disease	0.58 (p<0.001)	0.24 (p=0.005)	0.61 (p<0.001)	0.35 (p<0.001)
Pneumonia	0.26 (p=0.002)	0.07 (p=0.450)	0.30 (p<0.001)	0.17 (p=0.055)
Lung Cancer	0.61 (p<0.001)	0.30 (p=0.001)	0.62 (p<0.001)	0.33 (p<0.001)
Stomach Cancer	0.49 (p<0.001)	0.24 (p=0.007)	0.47 (p<0.001)	0.20 (p=0.020)
Accidents and Suicides	0.05 (p=0.56)	-0.14 (p=0.100)	0.21 (p=0.012)	0.24 (p=0.005)

[8] Aves, E. (1916) Obituary: Charles Booth. *Economic Journal* 26: 537–42.

Results

Figure 3.3 shows three maps of the study area in inner London, allowing a comparison of the geography of poverty in the late 19th century (top) with that in the late 20th century (middle) and with mortality ratios for all causes for all ages (bottom). The correlation coefficient between the two measures is 0.73 (P < 0.001). The blank area in the middle of the maps marks the City of London, which was not surveyed by Charles Booth. Figure 3.3 shows that there has been little change in the distribution of poverty in inner London between the 19th and 20th centuries. Areas in which some groups of immigrants settled in the middle of the 20th century have moved down the social scale slightly, notably south of the River Thames, while others have gentrified. On the whole, though, affluent places have remained affluent and poor

Figure 3.3: London poverty (1896 and 1991) and mortality (1990s).

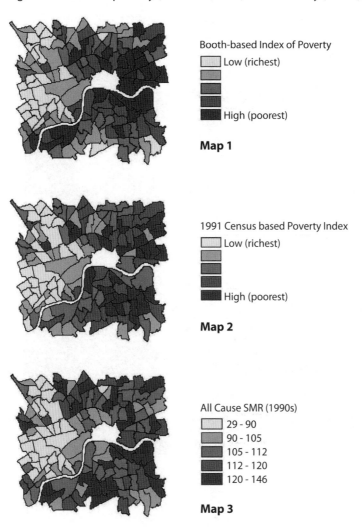

Booth-based Index of Poverty
- Low (richest)
- High (poorest)

Map 1

1991 Census based Poverty Index
- Low (richest)
- High (poorest)

Map 2

All Cause SMR (1990s)
- 29 - 90
- 90 - 105
- 105 - 112
- 112 - 120
- 120 - 146

Map 3

see colour version in plate section

places have remained relatively poor—two images of the Albert Bridge 100 years apart (Figure 3.4) show part of the reason for this continuity—the perseverance of transport infrastructure. The map of all age ratios, showing all cause mortality, demonstrates the close relation between poverty and mortality.

Table 3.2 shows the simple and partial correlations between the poverty measures and the standardised mortality ratios for 1991–95. Both indices of poverty were related to all cause ratios. The partial correlation coefficients in the table also show that the index of poverty derived from Booth's 19th-century observations (Booth

Figure 3.4: Albert Bridge, Chelsea, c.1900 and 2000.

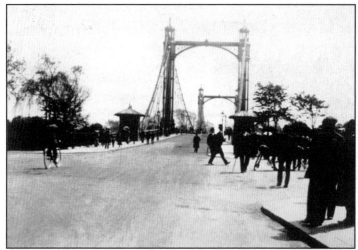

Note: These two images show that the main change is that trees have grown.

Souce: Recent photograph by Mary Shaw, 2000, taken from same position as archive photograph.

index) contributed more to predicting deaths from stroke and stomach cancer in the late 20th century than that derived from the 1991 census (modern index). For other causes of death, the modern index contributed more.

The results of further correlation analyses suggest that for deaths under the age of 65 the modern index makes a slightly greater contribution to predicting all cause mortality in 1991–95 ($r = 0.56, P < 0.001$) than does the Booth index ($r = 0.46, P < 0.001$). This is substantiated by the results of the partial correlation analyses, where $r = 0.39$ ($P = < 0.001$) when mortality is correlated with the Booth index, controlling for the modern index, but $r = 0.08$ ($P = 0.36$) when mortality is correlated with the latter, controlling for the former.

When only deaths at ages greater than 65 are considered, however, both indices make a similar contribution to the model; the correlation coefficients are $r = 0.56$ ($P < 0.001$) and $r = 0.57$ ($P < 0.001$) respectively. Here the results of the partial correlations also suggest a similar contribution from each index ($r = 0.28, P = 0.001$ for the Booth index, controlling for the modern distribution; $r = 0.26, P = 0.002$ when the indices are reversed).

Discussion

Almost everyone who was surveyed by Booth at the end of the 19th century will have died or left London before 1991. This means that the 19th-century poverty index is truly ecological—it describes 'area type' rather than the aggregate characteristics of the resident population. The fact that it performs so strongly as a predictor of mortality is perhaps partly because the median age of death of the people dying in the period 1991–95 is approximately 78. This means that, while very few would have been alive at the time Booth surveyed London, approximately half of these people would have been born before 1915. The Booth index is thus an indicator of the early life circumstances of those dying in the period 1991–95. The majority of those people, however, will have migrated in the intervening period. Thus the predictive power of the Booth index is also an illustration of how the nature (and hierarchy) of different parts of London has remained relatively stable despite constant changeover of the resident individuals (illustrated by the similarities between the top and middle maps in Figure 3.3). One might have expected to see considerable change in London's social and spatial structure given a century which included the Blitz in the Second World War and the development of London into an ever more dynamic major world city, but it is perhaps the continuity over this period which is most remarkable. Even the big wheel built to celebrate the millennium is not new—one just three quarters of its size was built a century ago in London (see Figure 3.5).

The social segregation of London is maintained through many processes. One that is particularly important is the maintenance of differential housing values across the capital, which help steer patterns of migration within London. However, we have no way of knowing the migration histories of the individuals who died between 1991 and 1995. Thus these results will not reveal whether the high rates of mortality found in areas which have been continuously poor throughout are due to the continuous

Figure 3.5: Big wheel at Earl's Court (1986) and the London Eye (2000).

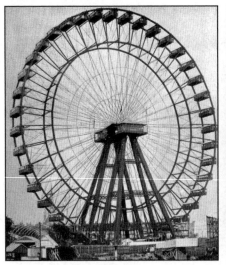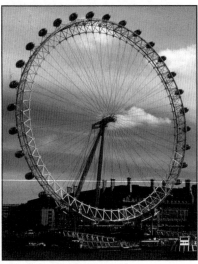

Souce: Recent ohotograph by Mary Shaw, 2000; photograph on left from archive.

inward migration of a population at relatively higher risk of mortality (perhaps forced into cheaper accommodation, for example) or to some accumulative mortality risk raising the effects of day-to-day life in the area. The fact that the index of poverty derived from Booth's survey is related more strongly to causes of death that have previously been shown to be sensitive to deprivation in early life—that is, stroke and stomach cancer[9]—suggests that to some degree the ecological associations with past and present deprivation levels of areas do reflect individual level associations of deprivation at different stages of the life course and health outcomes. In short, the longer people spend both in poverty and in poor places, the earlier they tend to die. The maps and models also show that 100 years of policy initiatives have had almost no impact on the patterns of inequality in inner London and on the relationship between people's socioeconomic position and their relative chances of dying.

We thus have a different ending to *A Christmas Carol* from that given by Dickens below. The hypothesis of the Spirit of Christmas Yet to Come seems to be true— inequalities in health have not declined, partly because miserliness in the past does lead to future inequalities in health. Dickens advocated redistribution of wealth at the end of his tale. Wilkinson has suggested that greater income equality is beneficial for the health of the whole population—including the relatively affluent—not just for those who are badly off.[10] In Dickens' story such redistribution not only aided the family of Tiny Tim, it also benefited Scrooge himself.

[9] Leon, D. and Davey Smith, G. (2000) Infant mortality, stomach cancer, stroke, and coronary heart disease: ecological analysis. *BMJ*, 320, 1705–6.

[10] Wilkinson, R.G. (1996) *Unhealthy societies: the afflictions of inequality*. London: Routledge.

A merrier Christmas, Bob, my good fellow, than I have given you for many a year! I'll raise your salary, and endeavour to assist your struggling family . . . Scrooge was better than his word. He did it all, and infinitely more; and to Tiny Tim, who did NOT die, he was a second father . . . His own heart laughed: and that was quite enough for him.[11]

References [excluding those in the footnotes above]

Aves, E. (1916) 'Obituary: Charles Booth', *Economic Journal*, 26, 537–42.

Bales, K. (1996) 'Lives and labours in the emergence of organised research, 1886–1907', *Journal of Historical Sociology*, 9, 113–38.

Bales, K. (1999) 'Popular reactions to sociological research: the case of Charles Booth', *Sociology*, 33, 153–68.

Booth, C. (1887) 'The inhabitants of Tower Hamlets (school board division) their condition and occupations', *Journal of the Royal Statistical Society*, 50, 326–401.

Booth, C. (1889, 1969) *Life and labour of the people. First series, poverty (i) east, central and south London*, London: Macmillan.

Booth, C. (1902a, 1969) *Life and labour of the people. First series, poverty (ii) streets and population classified*, London: Macmillan.

Booth, C. (1902b) *Life and labour of the people in London, Final Volume, Notes on social influences and conclusions*, London: Macmillan.

Cullen, M. (1979) 'Charles Booth's poverty survey: some new approaches', in Smout T.C. (ed) *The search for wealth and stability: essays in economic and social history presented to M.V. Flinn*, London: Macmillan, 115–74.

Davies, W.J.D. (1978) 'Charles Booth and the measurement of urban social character', *Area*, 10, 290–6.

Davey Smith, G., Hart, C., Hole, D., MacKinnon, P., Gillis, C., Watt, G., Blane, D. and Hawthorne, V. (1998) 'Education and occupational social class: which is the more important indicator of mortality risk?', *Journal of Epidemiology and Community Health*, 52, 153–60.

Fried, A. and Elman, R.M. (1969) *Charles Booth's London: a portrait of the poor at the turn of the century, drawn from his 'Life and labour of the people in London'*, London: Hutchinson.

Kunst, A.E. and Mackenbach, J.P. (1994) 'The size of mortality differences associated with educational level in 9 industrialised countries', *American Journal of Public Health*, 84, 932–7.

O'Day, R. and Englander, D. (1993) *Mr Charles Booth's inquiry: life and labour of the people in London reconsidered*, London: Hambledon.

Pamuk, E.R. (1985) 'Social class inequality in mortality from 1921 to 1972 in England and Wales', *Population Studies*, 39: 17–31.

Pfautz, H.W. (1967) *On the city: physical pattern and social structure: selected writing of Charles Booth*, Chicago: Chicago University Press.

---

[11] Dickens, C. (1843) *A Christmas carol*. London: Chapman and Hall.

Simey, T.S. and Simey, M.B. (1960) *Charles Booth: social scientist*. London: Oxford University Press.

Spicker, P. (1990) 'Charles Booth: the examination of poverty', *Social Policy and Administration*, 24, 21–38.

Stevenson, T.H.C. (1928) 'The vital statistics of wealth and poverty', *Journal of the Royal Statistical Society*, 91, 207–30.

Szreter, S.R.S. (1984) 'The genesis of the registrar general's social classification of occupations', *British Journal of Sociology*, 35: 522–46.

Szreter, S.R.S. (1986) 'The first scientific social structure of modern Britain 1875-1883', in L. Bonfield, R.M. Smith, K. Wrightson (eds.) *The world we have gained: histories of population and social structure*, Oxford: Blackwell, 337–54.

Townsend, P., Corrigan, P., and Kowarzik, U. (1987) *Poverty and labour in London: interim report of a centenary survey*, London: Low Pay Unit (Survey of Londoners' living standards No 1).

Annex:[12] Letter, 'Inequalities and Christmas yet to come'

Editor—On 10 November National Statistics released new life expectancy figures by area and announced that 'Inequalities in life expectancy persist across the UK'.[13]

'Persist' was an odd word to use. In Kensington and Chelsea, where it was already highest, it rose by exactly one year for both men and women (from 79.8 to 80.8 years and 84.8 to 85.8 years, respectively). In contrast, in Glasgow where it was lowest a year ago, life expectancy remained static at 76.4 years for women, and rose just slightly for men from 69.1 to 69.3 years. The range in life expectancy between the extreme highest and lowest areas thus increased from 8.4 to 9.4 years for women, and from 10.7 years to 11.5 years for men.

For men and women combined, the life expectancy gap between the worst- and best-off districts of the UK now exceeds 10 years for the first time since reliable measurements began. Of course more sophisticated measures are needed than this simple range, and the population denominators are problematic, especially in Kensington and Chelsea,[14] but the overall gap exceeding 10 years, and the first achievement of an average life expectancy over 85 years in women in one area whereas men's average expectancy remains below 70 years in another—should not pass without comment.

---

[12] *BMJ* (2005) 331:1409 (10 December), doi:10.1136/bmj.331.7529.1409-b; written by the same five authors as the article that forms the main text of this chapter.

[13] National Statistics (2005) Inequalities in life expectancy persist across the UK. Press release, 10 November. www.gnn.gov.uk/Content/Detail.asp?ReleaseID=177219&NewsAreaID=2 (accessed 1 Dec 2005).

[14] Shaw, M., Davey Smith, G., Dorling, D. (2005) Health inequalities and New Labour: how the promises compare with real progress. *BMJ*, 330, 1016-21 [reproduced as Chapter 7 in this volume].

Five years ago we wrote, in relation to historic trends in inequalities, and in reference to Dickens' *A Christmas Carol*, that 'The hypothesis of the spirit of Christmas yet to come seems to be true—inequalities in health have not declined, partly because miserliness in the past does lead to future inequalities in health'.[15] Christmas Yet to Come, it seems, is upon us.

---

[15] Dorling, D., Mitchell, R., Shaw, M., Orford, S. and Davey Smith, G. (2000) The ghost of Christmas Past: health effects of poverty in London in 1896 and 1991, *BMJ*, 321: 1547-51 [reproduced as the main text of Chapter 3 above].

4

Infant mortality and social progress in Britain, 1905–2005[1]

Dorling, D. (2006) 'Infant mortality and social progress in Britain, 1905–2005',
in E. Garrett, C. Galley, N. Shelton and R. Woods (eds) *Infant mortality*,
Aldershot: Ashgate, chapter 11

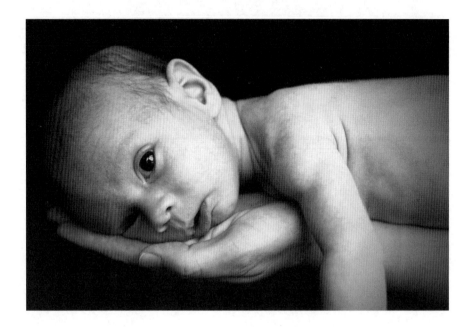

Introduction

In Britain by the end of the nineteenth century it became evident that birth rates
were falling and infant mortality was rising. This lead to a rapid decline in 'natality'
and consequently to a fall in the supply of 'infants for Empire'. By 1905, and in a
remarkably apposite observation, the medical officer for health in Battersea wrote
that within Britain:

> *"England is now regarded as the nucleus of a great Empire, with colonies which, though
> vast in extent are poor in population, and the fact must be faced that in view of our*

[1] I remain grateful to Tiffany Manting Tao who helped with drawing an earlier version of Figure 4.5,
to Graham Allsopp and John Pritchard who helped redrawing all figures and to Eilidh Garrett and
Nicola Shelton for their comments on two earlier drafts of this chapter.

declining natality, the stream of emigrants that formally left our shores cannot be expected to continue." (McCleary, 1905, quoted in Dwork, 1987: 6)

A century later, in 2005, there was great concern among some without imagination over a stream of immigrants coming to our shores. McCleary did not see that far ahead but in the century since he wrote it has become clear that fertility, mortality, natality and migration are all intimately linked over the course of lifetimes. However, society in Britain is still arranged very much in a hierarchy from those who 'think they know best' to those who are 'not to be trusted'. For instance, medical officers still treat much of the population with suspicion as became evident when the Department of Health, in 2005, said that, rather than increase benefit levels, mothers should be paid to eat, and give their infants to eat, 'healthy start food'; however, mothers could not be trusted to do this without vouchers requiring a statutory instrument laid before parliament. In the latest such instrument it was stated that within Britain:

A person … is entitled to benefit in accordance with these Regulations with a view to helping and encouraging her to have access to, and to incorporate in her diet, food of a prescribed description. The benefit to which a person described … is entitled is Healthy Start food to the value represented by a voucher… (Department of Health, 2005: 13)

For the ten possible categories of persons entitled to 'healthy start food' in 2005 see the draft regulations laid before Parliament under section 13(10) of the Social Security Act 1988 for approval by resolution of each House of Parliament (2005: Part II). However certain types of person were excluded, for example category 3(b) is:

a woman under the age of 18 who has been pregnant for more than ten weeks, provided that she is not a person to whom section 115 (exclusion from benefits) of the Immigration and Asylum Act 1999(b) applies.

Clearly pregnant teenagers who were claiming asylum were not to eat too healthily by 2005. Progress is a strange concept.

This chapter addresses the questions of how, in the space of just four generations, concerns of 'natality for Empire' moved on to 'healthy start foods'; why so many parents are still prevented from access to the resources needed to even properly feed their infants in Britain, and thus how much further still has to be gone. The main underlying cause of infant deaths in Britain was poverty at the beginning of the twentieth century and it remains poverty now. Infant health, and in particular, the unprecedented decline of infant mortality, is used here to begin to answer the questions of how far we have come and how far we have to go; starting with what was just beginning to be widely realised at the turn of the last century:

It is difficult to escape the conclusion that this loss of infant life is in some way related to the social life of the people. (Newman, 1906: vi).

The death of an infant, a child in the first year of its life, is extremely painful to imagine. It is even more painful when it is considered that in every year in the last century, and continuing into this, most of those youngest of deaths were caused by poverty. 'Healthy start food' is being introduced to replace the Welfare Food Scheme established in 1940 (Department of Health, 2005: 5) which itself was a response to the work of Newman, McCleary (whose concerns over Empire were quoted above) and others who pioneered better health for infants a century ago. McCleary (1905) argued that the propagation of clean milk for infants through depots was needed to reduce infant mortality. He recommended the establishment of the first milk depot in Battersea in 1902 (Dwork, 1987: 105). It then took forty years for a means tested right to clean milk to be established and sixty more years for that right to be extended to other forms of food so that poorer mothers who choose to breast feed are not discriminated against, as they do not need free milk; one rational for the 'healthy start foods' initiative. Perhaps in another century there will be no need for such targeted and inflexible 'benefits'. One day a substantial number of infants and children will not have to be fed by the state through various forms of benefit and free meals. However, in order to understand how this might be achieved, we need to first understand how the realisation, a century ago, that the social lives of people mattered, led to the poorest – excluding teenage asylum seekers – being allowed to choose a little cheap fruit in place of milk powder in 2005.

Background

For all of the period (1900–2005) considered here, poorer people have been much more likely than most to see their babies die, and the rich the least likely. A century ago the majority of people would have had first hand experience of infant mortality and of living in poverty. That is no longer the case, so a fictional account of a couple living at the turn of the last century likely to lose their baby is reproduced in Figure 4.1. It is worth reading this account before turning to the argument below as it is all too easy to forget what and who is involved when short lived lives are turned into digits. The account shows too why people such as McCleary were arguing for clean milk, not just for infants but to reduce the chances of mothers going hungry, and by 1905 for education on breast feeding (termed 'nursing' in the account). The contents of Figure 4.1 also, superficially, illustrate the problems of trying to imagine the change that has occurred over the course of the last century and how rapid that change has been.

One way to imagine change is to compare the fortunes of recent generations of one's own family. You are only reading this because your parents and their parents survived their first year of life. What were their chances of doing so?

My two oldest grandparents were both born in 1905, the year in which George Newman wrote the book [which inspired the writing of this chapter] and in which McCleary's 'Infantile mortality and infant milk depots' was published. My parents were both born during the Second World War. My partner and I were born around 1971 and our two children in the first three years of the present century.

There will hopefully never again be four generations in Britain who experience such different chances of surviving their first year of life. Rates are traditionally expressed as proportions of live births. The respective infant mortality rates (IMRs), per 1,000 live births, of the cohorts born in the same years as the pairs of my most

Figure 4.1: 1905: The meaning of poverty - extract from Tressell, 1914: 53-8.

They walked softly over and stood by the cradle side looking at the child; as they looked the baby kept moving uneasily in its sleep. Its face was very flushed and its eyes were moving under the half-closed lids. Every now and again its lips were drawn back slightly, showing part of the gums; presently it began to whimper, drawing up its knees as if in pain.

"He seems to have something wrong with him," said Easton.

"I think it's his teeth," replied the mother. "He's been very restless all day and he was awake nearly all last night".

"P'r'aps he's hungry."

"No, it can't be that. He had the best part of an egg this morning and I've nursed him several times today. And then at dinner-time he had a whole saucer full of fried potatoes with little bits of bacon it in."

Again the infant whimpered and twisted in its sleep, its lips drawn back showing the gums: its knees pressed closely to its body, the little fists clenched, and face flushed. Then after a few seconds it became placid: the mouth resumed its usual shape; the limbs relaxed and the child slumbered peacefully.

"Don't you think he's getting thin?" asked Easton. "It may be fancy, but he don't seem to me to be as big now as he was three months ago."

"No, he's not quite so fat," admitted Ruth. "It's his teeth what's wearing him out; he don't hardly get no rest at all with them."

They continued looking at him a little longer. Ruth thought he was a very beautiful child: he would be eight months old on Sunday. They were sorry they could do nothing to ease his pain, but consoled themselves with the reflection that he would be all right once those teeth were through.

"Well, let's have some tea," said Easton at last.

… [later] …

The woman did not reply at once. She was bending down over the cradle arranging the coverings which the restless movements of the child had disordered. She was crying silently, unnoticed by her husband.

For months past - in fact ever since the child was born - she had been existing without sufficient food. If Easton was unemployed they had to stint themselves so as to avoid getting further into debt than was absolutely necessary. When he was working they had to go short in order to pay what they owed; but of what there was Easton himself, without knowing it, always had the greater share.

extract from Tressell, 1914: 53-58

immediate relations were 151, 60, 18 and 5 per 1,000. These numbers translate to the following brief account of progress as applied to the cohorts corresponding to the four generations of my family and all other families born in Britain around the years 1901, 1941, 1971 and 2001.

In England and Wales in and around 1901, one in just over six babies died in their first year of life. The average chance of any pair surviving to age one was 72 per cent and most prospective pairs of grandparents did not survive, as a pair, from birth until they were old enough for it to be socially acceptable for them to have children of their own. Rates varied widely between poor and rich geographical areas and social classes; terms which were often synonymous with very small areas such as affluent streets or poor ones. In 1901 at the age of thirty, Benjamin Seebohm Rowntree reported that amongst the babies of the worse-off employees of his father's chocolate factory, 247 of their babies were dying for every 1,000 born. Thus a quarter of the children of the poorest working classes in York died before their first birthday in 1898; whereas, for Rowntree's servant keeping classes only 94 babies were dying for every 1,000 born (Newman, 1906: 189). The highest infant mortality rate Newman reports is 289 per 1,000 for illegitimate infants in London around the same time (Newman, 1906: 17). Thus depending on to whom and where a child was born, its chances of surviving to its first birthday ranged from around three quarters to better than nine tenths and infant mortality was the major influence on life expectancy at birth. Within towns, where health was often poorer than in parts of the countryside, life expectancy in total varied from 30 years in central Liverpool to 50 years in the Clifton district of Bristol by 1900 (figures from Szreter and Mooney, 1998: 90).

By 1941 one in just over sixteen babies died in their first year of life. The chances of an 'average' pair surviving to age one were 88 per cent. Great improvements in health during the childhoods of these children meant that the large majority were surviving to be old enough for it to be socially acceptable for them to have children of their own. Local statistics were hard to come by during the years of the Second World War. Much changed in the years during and immediately following the War for the 1941 cohort, weaned more equitably on rations and eligible for free milk if needed. By the early 1950s decennial reporting of mortality statistics by area had begun again. The Registrar General's decennial report for the period 1950-53 found that, by area, IMRs varied from being 68 per cent above the national average in Port Glasgow to being 68 per cent of the national average in Oxfordshire. Furthermore, and coincidentally, for 68 per cent of the population, local IMRs were no more than a quarter above or a fifth below the national average. Note that 5/4 and 4/5 are comparable reciprocals for comparing distributions around unity. Hence the ratio of the worse-off infants by area being 2.5 more likely to die in their infancy than the best-off did not vary markedly over this time period (247/94 = 2.62 in 1901 and 168/68 = 2.47 in 1951). In other words for every 5 infants who died in the worse-off areas in both 1901 and 1951, only 2 died in the best-off areas.

By 1971 fewer than one in fifty six babies died in their first year of life, the chances of a pair surviving to age one were 96 per cent. Thus there was only one chance in twenty five that both my partner and I would not live to see our first birthday (and hence later be able to meet if we ignore our much smaller chances of dying in childhood and younger adulthood). Whether children would survive long enough to have children of their own had largely stopped being an issue. What mattered now, for most that had a choice, was whether and, if so, when they choose to have children. At the extremes, geographically, 64 per cent more baby boys died in Coatbridge, Lanarkshire, than the national average and 57 per cent less in the rural districts of Buckinghamshire (Dorling, 1997). Although this variation may appear a little wider than before, some four fifths of the population lived in areas where rates did not exceed a quarter nor were a fifth below, the national average. Put another way, no matter where my partner or myself had been born, or to whom, we had a better chance of reaching age one than had almost anyone born in 1941 no matter how privileged their social or geographical circumstances. In contrast, those born into the worst situation in 1941 did 'only' as well as the most privileged babies born in 1901. By 1971 for every 2 babies dying in the best-off areas, 6 were dying in the poorest places (as compared to 5 above).

By 2001 less than one in 186 babies died in their first year of life, the chances of a pair of children surviving to age one were more than 99 per cent. IMRs had become so low that they were no longer routinely published at local authority level for individual years (ONS, 2005). For the year 2002 IMRs reported for very large areas were lowest at 3.8 per 1,000 live births in the Norfolk, Suffolk and Cambridgeshire Strategic Health Authority (SHA) and at 3.9 per 1,000 in Thames Valley SHA. Rates were highest at 7.0 per 1,000 in West Yorkshire SHA and 7.7 per 1,000 in Birmingham and the Black Country SHA. The extreme ratio is thus lower if these large areas are used but is wider when measured for cities (see below). However, three quarters of births, and a similar proportion of the population as in 1971 lived, in 2002, in areas with rates no more than a quarter above nor a fifth below the national average for England and Wales. A child born into the worst-off Strategic Health Authority in 2002 had a much better chance of reaching age one than did a child in the best-off district of the early 1970s. In many of the best-off districts as defined in the 1970s there are now years in which no infant dies in their first year of life. If progress were to continue at its present rate then this is what many of the currently poorest districts will experience, in just a generation's time. However note that as very low rates are achieved inequalities have risen over sixfold (10.3/1.5) between the largest of English cities by 2001 (see Figure 4.3 below). This translates to more than 6 infants dying in the worst-off cities in 2001 for every one dying in the best off cities, as compared to local authority areas in 1901 (2½:1), 1951 (2½:1), and 1971 (3:1). Ratios of probabilities are difficult entities to compare when the probabilities are reducing so quickly. However it is clear that as infant mortality has become more rare its association with poverty rather than chance (otherwise known as the more general environment) has widened. Probabilities are also difficult concepts to apply to individuals.

As any statistician will gleefully tell you, in hindsight your chances of being born are 100 per cent and thus also are those of all your past relations. However, far more of us are the product of more affluent parents and grandparents than would have been the case had these chances of death been more equal. The eugenicists of 1905 would be pleased by this outcome (see Dwork, 1987: Chapter 1, entitled 'Infant mortality and the future of the race'). Conversely, that most of us are largely the product of poor grandparents and great-grandparents is testament simply to how extensive poverty in the past was. There were very few, very affluent people living at the start of the twentieth century in Britain. They almost completely monopolised the telling of the past, certainly its quantitative recording, and only a tiny minority of them were interested in the poor or the idea of infant mortality as a social problem. The account given in the extract from Tressell above is a very rare example of a non-elite publication (Davey Smith *et al*, 2001: 135). To give an example of how enlightened health professionals approached these issues at the time, five years following Seebohm Rowntree's report on York, George Newman reported on the work of Dr Niven, the Medical Officer of Health of Manchester:

> *By means of a number of beer-traps Dr Niven contrived to count the flies in some dozen houses in Manchester during the summer months of 1904, and from these data he concluded that the advent of the house-fly in numbers precedes by a short time the increase in the number of deaths from diarrhoea. In the fortnight ending August 13th, for instance, the number of flies caught in these traps was 37,521, the maximum in any fortnight, and in the fortnight following the maximum number of deaths from diarrhoea occurred – namely, 192.* (Newman, 1906: 168-169; see also Dwork, 1987: 48-49).

Diarrhoea is now one of the major killers of infants worldwide but no infants die as a result of untreated diarrhoea in Britain now. One possible account of the geography and recent history of infant mortality in Britain would begin with the Battersea milk depot of 1902, the Manchester beer-traps of 1904, and other key events, such as the 1906 election, and work progressively forward through ever increased experimentation, autopsy, argument, realisation and intervention through to the situation in 2005 to produce a story of political, social, medical and technological achievement. Although such a story would be interesting, by concentrating on the nuts and bolts of what occurred to lower infant mortality so dramatically, it is possible that we would miss something quite remarkable in all the detail. That something we might miss concerns progress itself and what often has to be sacrificed in order to achieve it: the growth in the short term wealth of the richest. The remainder of this chapter thus concentrates on what happened that was coincident with the most and least rapid periods of the fall of infant mortality, to suggest why infant mortality fell when and where it did beyond the necessary but not sufficient improvements in public sanitation, private hygiene, state care, general finance and public medicine which occurred over this period.

Figure 4.2 contains 6 graphs. The first, Figure 4.2(a), of the decline of infant mortality 1841–1998 has been reproduced in many forms numerous times (this version is taken from Davey Smith *et al*, 2001: xxiii). The second, Figure 4.2(b), should be equally familiar but is now of exponential growth rather than decline, in this case of Gross Domestic Product per person (GDP per capita derived from

Maddison, 2005). The GDP per capita figures are produced such that they can be compared over time assuming equal purchasing power for a universal dollar at each point in time. When these two graphs are compared it would appear that as monies have risen mortality has fallen. The British population became wealthier as their incomes rose and they were able to afford and produce better medical, environmental and social care for their children, progressively more and more of whom survived to their first birthday. This improved care took numerous forms: cleaner milk, fewer flies, less exhausted mothers (and fathers), a decline also in parental mortality and family size, a rise in health visitors, maternity units, paediatric specialists, income support

Figure 4.2: Infant mortality and affluence in the UK: six views of 160 years (1841-2001).

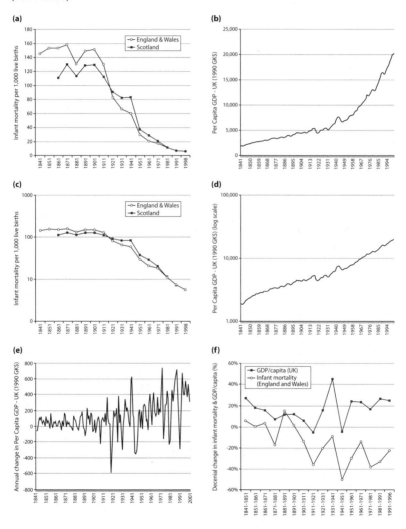

Sources: 1841-1971: Mitchell (1988); 1981, 1991 and 1998 Macfarlane *et al*. (2000) for data on infant mortality; Maddison (2005) for historical statistics on per capita GDP in 1990 international Geary-Khamis dollars (GK$).

payments and so on. These advances were some of the first expenditures made with the excesses of monies earnt from empire, and investment in child care continues, encompassing the wider care of families with children as a result. As standards of living rose exponentially, IMRs fell exponentially.

There is, however, a problem with this story and that problem is hinted at in Figures 4.2(c) and 4.2(d) which are simply the earlier two figures with the vertical axis drawn on a log scale. Log scales ensure that comparable rates of change are comparable lengths on the graphs. In Figure 4.2(c) it is easier to see that IMRs did not begin to fall continuously until after 1901 and fell fastest after 1941 with the most improvement being experienced in the two decades in which World Wars were fought (Dwork, 1987). In Figure 4.2(d) it is evident that, in real terms, GDP per capita rose steadily from 1841 to 2001 with no great break in slope around 1941. Most importantly it actually fell significantly during the final and immediately subsequent years of war – at the very times when the greatest progress was being made in reducing aggregate infant mortality. If improvements in the health of infants are so closely linked to rising living standards then why did infant health improve fastest when living standards, as measured by GDP per capita, fell?

Figure 4.2(e) shows the annual change in GDP per capita with local minima (measured using consistent international purchasing power dollars and in descending order of magnitude) in the years to 1919, 1945, 1931, 1991, 1980, 1908 and 1926, and 1973. The graph is simply the first derivative of Figure 4.2(b) and shows how economic fortunes oscillate in an ever more chaotic fractal pattern. What matters here is that it was these periods when GDP per capita actually fell the most that coincided in aggregate with the fastest proportionate decreases in infant mortality as shown in Figure 4.2(f). The two lines in Figure 4.2(f) show the decennial proportionate increase in GDP per capita and in infant mortality (which in most cases is a negative figure as the rate was decreasing). The most rapid decrease in infant mortality coincides with the decade 1941–1951 centred around the 1945 realisation (at least by those who held the purse strings) that Britain had emerged on the winning side of the war but had been 'bankrupted' by it. The next most progressive decade in terms of IMR decline, 1971–1981, included the start of the 1980s recession. Thus, in general, infant mortality fell fastest in Britain when GNP per capita rose most slowly. What then occurred? As a clue take one paragraph written at the start of the decade of most improvement – in infant mortality and much else – and ask: Were the reforms that were then introduced, introduced through altruism or supposed necessity?

> ... *facts ... should dominate planning for [the] future ... the low reproduction rate of the British community today: unless this rate is raised very materially in the near future, a rapid and continuous decline of the population cannot be prevented ... [which] makes it imperative to give first place in social expenditure to the care of childhood and to the safeguarding of maternity.* (Beveridge, 1942: point 15 of introduction)

The declines in infant mortality, through better infant health, through the 'safeguarding of maternity' and better 'care of childhood' were achieved as a result of a decision made to implement a plan. The plan itself was justified on the almost reverse Malthusian grounds that without such safeguarding and better care Britain would soon run out of people, or at least fit and able bodied people. Forty years earlier the concern was that the nation was running out of people to fill an Empire, now it was running out of people to fill a geographically tiny island! That, at least, was how the plan was sold to those with the traditional power over such plans, and to the population as a whole who had not had a vote for some ten years.

The landslide election of the 1945 Labour government allowed the plan's implementation, probably more completely than had been realised when the plan was proposed (Bevan, 1947). Four decades before, a landslide Liberal party victory followed an earlier national debate on poverty, infant mortality and the physical degeneration of the population that arose from the earlier war in South Africa (Dwork, 1987). When those in power in Britain thought they might begin to lose their Empire - they used the resources of that Empire, the national wealth arising from it, to improve domestic infant health. Wealth may be necessary but it is certainly not all that is sufficient to reduce infant mortality. This is most obviously seen in those poor countries where just a few individuals now hold almost all the wealth. It even appears to be the case, in England and Wales at least, that infant mortality falls fastest when national government are least effective or interested in maximising a more even overall wealth distribution.

Where most infants die

IMRs today remain relatively high in much the same places that they were high a century ago. Figure 4.3 shows the map of the cities with the largest populations in England at the beginning of the 21st century. Bar the slight effects of the locations of medical facilities that care for very sick infants – and therefore see elevated mortality rates – the map is mainly of a north-south divide. Figure 4.4 shows that divide again, but charts when rates of infant mortality by area in 1921 and 1931 are compared with age/sex standardized rates of mortality for all people under age 65 in the early 1980s and early 1990s respectively. A naïve, epigeneticist interpretation of these two graphs might be that high rates of infant mortality in the past are indicative of a poor inter-uterine environment in gestation which is reflected by relatively high rates of mortality amongst the population of those areas some sixty years later – and a consequent relatively higher mortality of their grandchildren's infancy. Of course, the majority of people living in Rutland county – the best-off area in health terms in the figure – were not born there, let alone will most of their children or grandchildren stay there. What the graphs instead show is that areas which are affluent tend to have remained relatively affluent over time whilst areas which were poor at the start of the last century remain so even today. In many cases the people currently living in the worse social conditions in some of our poorest northern mill towns bear almost no hereditary connection with those who lived there in the past. It is not just that they are not the same people, they are not even closely related to the same people but instead to people, say, in the Indian sub-continent. Some Northern mill towns

Figure 4.3: (a) and (b) Infant mortality in 2001 for the largest cities of England. (c) A key to their location in population space.

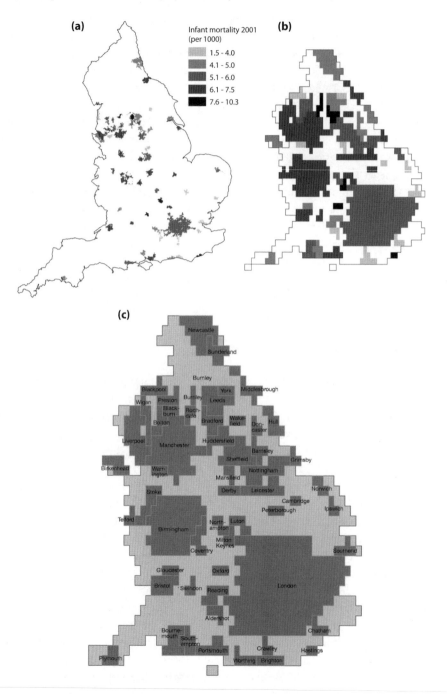

Source: State of the cities report 2005 for ODPM: Sheffield University Social and Spatial Inequalities Group. (www.shef.ac.uk/sasi/socr).

suffer relatively high infant mortality not because the current population is related to people who used to live there, nor because the large numbers of the current population are related to people living in what was India, but because of the social conditions of life in those towns today. Life in towns in Britain is mainly determined by where those towns are located, largely in relation to London, and the fact that British society is apparently organised mainly to maximize profit in London.

Figure 4.4: (a) shows the relationship between infant mortality rate around 1931 and SMR under age 65 by 1990–92. (b) shows the same but for 1921 and 1981–85 respectively.

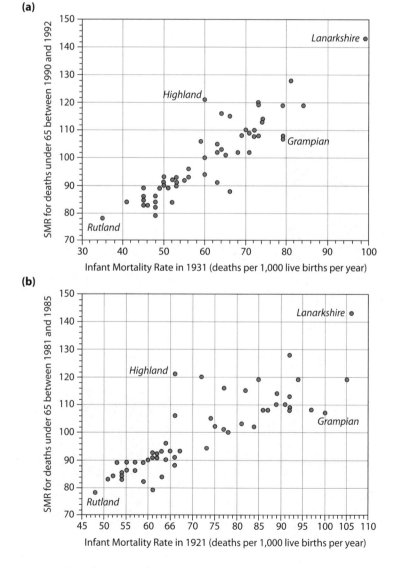

Source: Decennial Supplements and Dorling 1997.

The areas shown in Figure 4.3 are the built-up areas of the cities of England as defined in 2001. The geographic areas used in Figure 4.4 were 'historic' counties of Britain (as they are now termed) for which IMRs were published before the Second World War. Contemporary data can be re-aggregated to historic areas. In contrast the areas shown in Figure 4.5 are the contemporary local authority districts of England and Wales to which historic data has been approximated (see source of figure: www. visionofbritain.org.uk). Here rates are shown in 1881, 1911, 1931, 1951, 1981–85, 1990–91, 1996–97 and 2000–1. Care should be taken over interpreting these last three periods as by the end of the twentieth century, in some small districts, there were areas where no infant deaths occurred in some years. Figure 4.3 is a much better guide to the contemporary geography of IMR than Figure 4.5(h). However, even with this caveat in mind it could be argued that Figure 4.5 suggests that the north-south geography of mortality (which was always partly an urban-rural geography) is becoming more evidently urban-rural over time. High relative

Figure 4.5 **(a)** to **(d)**: Infant mortality in England and Wales 1881–1951.

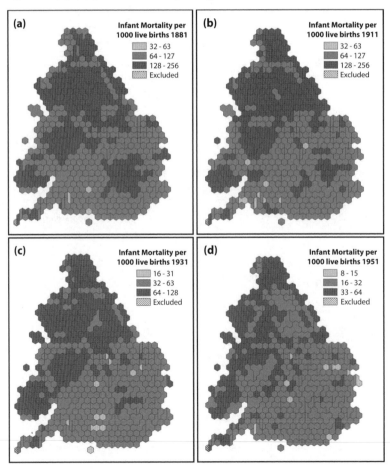

Source: Data was originally posted on the vision of britain website - www.visionofbritain.org.uk

rates of infant mortality have also returned to London after a century of better than usual improvement. However, in the main the relative picture is one of stability – as Newman had noted at the start of the twentieth century:

Figure 4.5 **(e)** to **(h)**: Infant mortality in England and Wales 1981–2001.

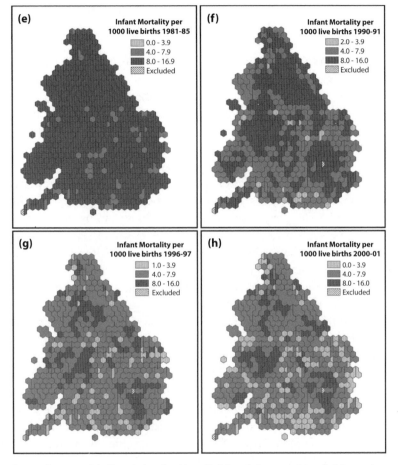

Source: Data was originally posted on the vision of britain website - www.visionofbritain.org.uk

The chief [infant] mortality occurs in the North and North-Midland districts, and the lowest mortality in the counties below a line drawn from the Wash to the mouth of the Severn. Each decennium shows some minor variation, but practically it may be said that during the whole last century this was in the main the general distribution. (Newman, 1906: 22)

Conclusions

*Last year (1905) there was a loss to the nation of 120,000 dead infants in England and Wales alone, a figure which is almost exactly one quarter of all the deaths in England and Wales in that year. That is to say, that **one quarter** of the total deaths every year is of children under the age of twelve months. And this enormous sacrifice of human life is being repeated year by year and is not growing less.* (Newman, 1906: 2, emphasis as in original).

In 2005 roughly 3,000 infants died in their first year of life in England and Wales, which is almost exactly one half of one per cent of all deaths in England and Wales in that year. Thus one in two hundred of the total deaths is of children under the age of twelve months. This sacrifice has been falling, with no exception, every year since 1951 and is expected to continue to fall. However, the toll is increasingly concentrated amongst the children of the poorest areas of Britain. For the sacrifice to continue to fall requires further social progress. We now have the means to reduce IMRs to near zero in affluent areas of Britain, but for the infants of poor areas the government consults on the costs of 'healthy start food' (Department of Health, 2005).

It was not until 1946, forty years after George Newman published his findings that sufficient measures were enacted to improve the health of new born infants and the number dying simultaneously – and thereafter without exception – fell year on year. Government officials often talk about time lags in health policy and how many years it might be before an improvement might be seen as a result of a particular measure being implemented but, in the case of mid-twentieth-century infant mortality, there clearly was no such lag. It is possible that improvements in health in their childhood of the women who gave birth in 1946 might have led to 3.1 fewer infants dying per 1,000 in that year as compared to 1945, but the timing just appears a little too fortuitous with the ending of the War and the small but immediate improvement in living standards which that engendered. Furthermore the largest drop ever recorded in infant mortality, of 7.5 fewer infants dying per 1,000 born in 1948 as compared to 1947 coincides far too conveniently with the introduction of the National Health Service and the rights and access to better care which that gave prospective and new mothers.

In the story of the fall in infant mortality the most important time-lag was not between policy change and result, but the forty years between the turn of the century escalation in calls for social justice, of which Newman's book was just a small part, and the winning of enough hearts and minds to prevent the continuation of the enormous sacrifice. That winning of hearts and minds was not just over the elite who had most power over resources but of people in general growing up in a much more infant health conscious society informed by the work conducted at the start of the last century and its propagation through books and magazines over the course of four decades. Of course, medical advances were made in the interim but, as seen above, by 1941 the poorest of children only had the chances of the best-off in 1901. What occurred after 1941 was possible with the medical knowledge of the previous century, but it required people to vote in 1945 and for them to know what they were voting for and why. Until it is made clear that infants die because of poverty rather than fecklessness, why vote against poverty, as happened in 1945, 1964 and 1997? No amount of medical knowledge, as is obvious from worldwide infant mortality figures today, is sufficient without the will and funds to implement it. The '*vast array of small human beings that lived but a handful of days*' that Newman found '*so difficult to make real to the mind*' (Newman, 1906: 3) has grown by millions worldwide in the century since he wrote. In 2005, the 'make poverty history' year, pop stars clicked their fingers on television screens every three seconds to signify the death of an infant through poverty. Infant mortality was first accurately measured globally in the 1970s. Worldwide since that date it has fallen fastest where it was lowest to begin with.

Back in Britain, the final piece of evidence presented here, Figure 4.6(a), shows the 1921–2001 national time series of infant deaths in England and Wales by age of the infant at their death in days, weeks, and months. Although there has been some change in the distribution of the ages at which infants are most likely to die, it has not been as dramatic as might have been the case were specific medical interventions key. Figure 4.6(b) shows that in 1921 13 per cent of infant deaths occurred in the first day of life, by 2002 that figure had reached 32 per cent. Of the far fewer babies who could not be saved by 2002, more as a proportion could not be saved in that first day and far fewer now die after living for six months. Congenital diseases, associated most with the earliest deaths, decline more slowly in the graphs than do the infectious diseases associated with deaths later in the first year of life. Figure 4.6(c) shows that the decline in the latter occurred fastest a generation before the decline in the former, but Figure 4.6(d) suggests that rates of decline of death at all ages are following much the same long term trajectory.

Each generation demands overall improvement. It occurs for each but different proximal mechanisms are at play. For the mothers of the 1940s it was diseases that their infants were freed from most quickly, perhaps partly due to increased availability of antibiotics. For the mothers of the 1970s, deaths in the first days and weeks of the lives of their infants fell fastest; perhaps greater access to incubators helped. For the mothers of the start of the present century deaths after a number of months became rarer again more quickly, perhaps associated with increased and better information on preventing Sudden Infant Death Syndrome and other once largely unknown causes. However, for most generations the best-off have enjoyed access to the kind of care that the worse-off only achieve a generation later.

Medical and almost all other innovations appear to take roughly a generation, some twenty-five years, to diffuse down social hierarchies in Britain. To achieve this for a fifth generation will require social progress equivalent to the ending of child poverty in Britain within the next two decades. Progress of a similar magnitude has been achieved before.

Figure 4.6: Infant mortality 1921–2002 in England and Wales by age of death: (a) rates per 1000 births per year (cumulative); **(b)** deaths by age as a proportion of all infant deaths per year (%); (c) deaths by age per 1000 births per year (not cumulative); (d) deaths by age per 1000 births per year (not cumulative, log scale).

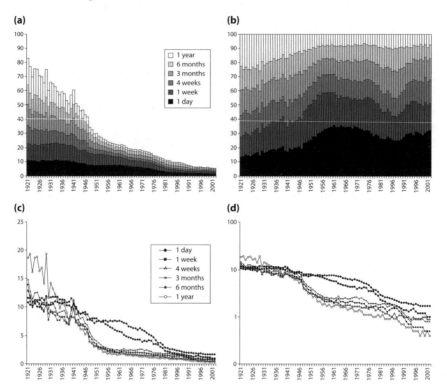

Source: ONS national statistics on stillbirth and infant death rates by age at death, 1921–2002. Taken from Table 33 published in Mortality Statistics: Childhood, infant and peri-natal (series DH3, number 35).

References

Bevan, A. (1947) *In place of fear*, London: William Heinemann.

Beveridge, W. (1942) *Social Insurance and Allied Services*, Cmnd 6404, London: HMSO (part 1).

Davey Smith, G., Dorling, D. and Shaw, M. (2001) *Poverty, inequality and health in Britain 1800–2000: A reader*, Bristol: The Policy Press.

Department of Health (2005) *Healthy Start: consultation on draft regulations* (Gateway Ref: 3936), London: HMSO.

Dorling, D. (1997) *Death in Britain: How local mortality rates have changed: 1950s–1990s*, York: Joseph Rowntree Foundation.

Dwork, D. (1987) *War is good for babies and other young children*, London: Tavistock.

Macfarlane, A., Mugford, M., Henderson, J., Furtado, A. and Dunn, A. (2000) *Birth Counts: Statistics of childbirth and pregnancy. Volume 2 – Tables*, London: The Stationery Office.

Maddison, A. (2005) The World Economy: Historical Statistics; website accessed: http://www.eco.rug.nl/~Maddison/ – 10 June 2005 (documented in The World Economy: Historical Statistics, OECD Development Centre, Paris 2003).

McCleary, G.F. (1905) *Infantile mortality and infant milk depots*, London: P.S. King (page 6).

Mitchell, B.R. (1988) *British Historical Statistics*, Cambridge: Cambridge University Press.

Newman, G. (1906) *Infant mortality: A social problem*, London: Methuen and Co.

ONS (2005) *Deaths 2002: Childhood, infant and perinatal mortality: Live births, stillbirths and infant deaths by area of residence (numbers and rates)*. Available via National Statistics Website (accessed 10 June 2005).

Szreter, S. and Mooney, G. (1998) 'Urbanization, mortality, and the standard of living debate: new estimates of the expectation of life at birth in nineteenth-century British cities', *Economic History Review*, 51, 1, 84–112.

Tressell, R. (1914, 1955) *The ragged trousered philanthropists*, London: Lawrence and Wishart.

5

Who cares in England and Wales? The Positive Care Law[1]

Shaw, M. and Dorling, D. (2004) 'Who cares in England and Wales? The Positive Care Law: cross-sectional study', *British Journal of General Practice*, vol 54, pp 899–903.

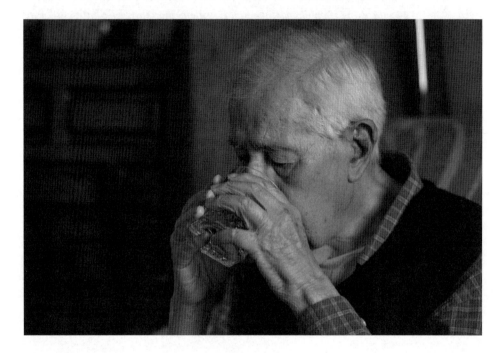

How this fits in

What do we know? An 'inverse care law', stating that medical services are distributed inversely to population health needs, has been repeatedly demonstrated since it was first suggested in 1971.

What does this paper add? Data from the 2001 census allow us for the first time to analyse the need for care in conjunction with the provision of both formal and informal care. This study demonstrates a 'positive care law', whereby formal

[1] We thanked Julian Tudor Hart, Helena Tunstall, and two anonymous referees for their constructive comments on earlier drafts of this chapter, and remain grateful for their help. At the time of writing Mary Shaw was funded by the South West Public Health Observatory, Bristol.

medical care is provided inversely to need, but informal care is provided in direct proportion to need.

Summary

Background: The inverse care law proposing that medical services are distributed inversely to population health needs, and that this law operates more completely where medical care is most exposed to market forces, was first suggested by Tudor Hart in 1971. This paper considers whether an inverse care law can be observed for the provision of informal care as well as for medical care.

Aim: Using data from the 2001 census we sought to investigate the contemporary relevance of the inverse care law.

Design of study: Cross-sectional study.

Setting: England and Wales.

Method: Data from the 2001 census for the population of England and Wales were analysed at the county, unitary, or former metropolitan authority level. The prevalence of the conjunction of general health status and limiting long-term illness was correlated with the percentage of the local population who were working as qualified healthcare workers (nurses, qualified medical practitioners, dentists, and other health professionals and therapists) and with the percentage of the population providing 50 or more hours of unpaid care per week.

Results: In 2001, 7.6% of people reported that their health was not good and that they had a limiting long-term illness (the need for care). Over one million people reported providing 50 or more hours of unpaid care per week. An inverse care law was found at the ecological level between the need for care and the proportion of the population who were working as qualified medical practitioners, dentists, and other health professionals. Informal care was almost perfectly positively correlated with the need for care ($r = 0.97$). These relationships were more marked for areas in the north of the country compared with the south. In the north more people provide unpaid care as more people need that care and because there are fewer working qualified medical professionals, other than nurses, providing such care per head.

Conclusions: Medical care is distributed inversely to need, whereas the provision of informal care is positively related to need — where care is most needed, informal care is most likely to be provided. The greater the market forces that are allowed to intervene in the relationships between the need for care and its provision, the more likely the inverse care law is to be found to apply. Where no market forces apply, where people give up their time for free to provide care, an almost perfectly positive care law is found to apply.

Keywords: censuses; delivery of health care; dentists; nurses; physicians.

Introduction

The 'inverse care law' was first suggested by Julian Tudor Hart in 1971, stating that medical services were distributed inversely to population health needs and, moreover, that this law operates more completely where medical care is most exposed to market forces:

> *In areas with most sickness and death, general practitioners [GPs] have more work, larger lists, less hospital support, and inherit more clinically ineffective traditions of consultation, than in the healthiest areas; and hospital doctors shoulder heavier caseloads with less staff and equipment, more obsolete buildings, and suffer recurrent crises in the availability of beds and replacement staff. These trends can be summed up as the inverse care law: that the availability of good medical care tends to vary inversely with the need of the population served.*[2]

This inverse care law has subsequently been found to apply to a range of health service provision; for example, the uptake of childhood immunisations, the use of child health services, the provision of coronary artery revascularisation and waiting times for cardiac surgery, transport accessibility in rural areas, the management of depression in primary care, the provision of health promotion clinics, GP consultation times in relation to the presence of psychological symptoms, advice giving in community pharmacies, and the take-up of annual health checks for the elderly (Lynch, 1995; Webb *et al.*, 1996; Payne and Saul, 1997; Black *et al.*, 1995; Pell *et al.*, 2000; Lovett *et al.*, 2002; Chew-Graham *et al.*, 1994 and 2002; Gillam, 1992; Stirling *et al.*, 2001; and Rogers *et al.*, 1998). As Julian Tudor Hart himself commented in 2000: '*You name it, there's now some inverse law for it, or soon will be. The world never runs out of injustice*'.[3]

Three decades on from the original paper, as the debate over the role of market forces in the National Health Service (NHS) intensifies, this observation continues to ring true. Here we consider the inverse care law in a new context: a) with data covering the whole of England and Wales, and b) considering not only medical care but also informal care. We ask the question 'does empirical evidence support the notion that those most in need receive the least care?'.

Method

Our analysis is based on data for England and Wales from the 2001 census, aggregated to county, unitary, or former metropolitan authority level. These areas were used in this analysis to minimise the influence of cross-border commuting. For the first time, the census in 2001 asked questions on general health status as well as

---

[2] Hart, J.T. (1971) Inverse care law, *Lancet*, 1: 405-412.
[3] Hart, J.T. (2000) Commentary: three decades of the inverse care law. *British Medical Journal*; 320: 18-19.

limiting long-term illness, on the qualifications and current employment status of healthcare workers (nurses, qualified medical practitioners, dentists, and other health professionals and therapists), and on the care provided by the population as a whole (those providing 50 or more hours of unpaid care per week, see Table 5.1). We calculated unweighted and weighted (for population size) correlation coefficients for these variables, to investigate the relationship between health and care.

Results

In England and Wales in 2001, 3,894,870 people (7.6% of the population) stated that their health was not good and that they also lived with a limiting long-term illness (defined by the census as an 'illness, health problem, or disability which limits your daily activities or the work you can do'[4]). Although these are self-reported and hence subjective assessments of health, and some of these answers will have been imputed from forms that were not completed, the 2001 census is the most accurate and comprehensive source of information on this topic to date.[5] For the purposes of this article we consider this group (7.6% of the population) as being those most in need of health care. Of this group of almost 4 million people, 54% are

Table 5.1: Number and rates of people providing 50+ hours of care per week, by age, in England and Wales, 2001.

Age (years)	n	%	Total population
0-4	-	-	3 091 047
5-7	792	0.04	1 945 633
8-9	863	0.06	1 358 612
10-11	1360	0.10	1 380 278
12-14	2982	0.15	2 014 759
15	1272	0.20	650 764
16-17	3684	0.29	1 273 506
18-19	4999	0.44	1 127 392
20-24	18 262	0.61	2 969 687
25-34	102 707	1.40	7 328 760
35-44	178 359	2.32	7 701 510
45-49	91 081	2.78	3 278 446
50-54	116 178	3.25	3 572 315
55-59	113 027	3.84	2 945 765
60-64	108 608	4.29	2 530 113
65-74	199 266	4.61	4 321 768
75-84	121 371	4.33	2 806 237
85-89	16 785	2.90	578 595
90 and over	3728	1.60	232 452
Total	1 085 324	2.12	51 107 639

Source: Data from the 2001 census.

women (women make up 51% of the population as a whole), 54% live in the north (where only 44% of all people live) (Table 5.2; notes to Figure 5.1 and the discussion below give the definition of the north), one-third are aged over 70 years, a sixth are over 85 years, but 10% are aged under 40 years. Other than mothers giving birth, children in the first few months of life, and adults suffering an accident or injury, this group clearly includes the bulk of healthcare need in England and Wales.

---

[4] Office for National Statistics (2003) *Census 2001: National report for England and Wales*, London: HMSO.
[5] Dorling, D. and Rees, P. (2003) A nation still dividing: the British census and social polarisation 1971-2001. *Environment and Planning A* 35(7): 1287-1313.

Table 5.2: Proportion of the population reporting limiting long-term illness and poor health ('ill-heath'), percentage of population providing 50+ hours care per week, percentage working in various healthcare professions and unweighted and weighted correlations of those variables with ill health, England and Wales, 2001.

	Percentage of total population	Percentage females	Percentage in north	Correlation with ill health	P-value	Weighted correlations*	P-value
Total population (n = 51 107 639)		51.3	44.4				
Limiting long-term illness and poor health	7.6	54.2	53.8	1.0		1.0	
Carers 50+ hours unpaid per week	2.1	60.0	52.9	0.968	<0.001	0.961	<0.001
Working nurses	0.8	90.6	46.5	0.310	0.001	0.275	<0.001
Working medical practitioners	0.2	35.3	39.2	-0.219	0.022	0.171	<0.001
Working dentists	0.04	32.2	41.5	-0.415	<0.001	-0.414	<0.001
Other working health professionals and therapists	0.2	76.0	39.8	-0.480	<0.001	-0.598	<0.001

* Weighted for population size in 2001. Units of analysis are county, unitary or former metropolitan authorities.

Source: Data from the 2001 census.

Over 1 million people in England and Wales stated on their census form that they provided at least 50 hours a week of unpaid care. This care was principally for people's health needs and included looking after and giving help or support to family members, friends, neighbours or others because of long-term physical or mental ill-health or disability or health problems relating to old age. Of these million carers, 7269 were aged 5–15 years; 8683 aged 16–19 years; 120 969 aged 20–34 years; 269 440 aged 35–49 years; 337 813 aged 50–64 years; 199 266 aged 65–74 years; 121 371 aged 75–84 years (for a complete age breakdown see Table 5.1); 20 513 were aged over 85 years; 60% were women; 21% were not in good health themselves but provided care to someone else in spite of that.

Figure 5.1 shows the remarkably close relationship, at the ecological level, between the provision of unpaid care and the need for that care. On average, one person provided 50 or more hours of unpaid care a week for every 3.58 people with the health needs described above. This ratio hardly varies at all across England and Wales. Clearly, some individuals in need of care will find that friends and family are more generous with their time than others, and this care is more likely to be provided by women. On a population level, however, there is no evidence that people are more or less altruistic in their care, when given for free, within any particular area of the country — it is provided (geographically) on the basis of need. We term this the 'positive care law', whereby informal care is provided in direct proportion to the degree that care is needed; the correlation coefficient for these two variables is 0.97 (P<0.001) (see Table 5.2 for all correlations calculated).

Figures 5.2 to 5.5 are similar to Figure 5.1 except that the y-axis of each graph is the proportion of qualified health professionals, from various specialisations,

Figure 5.1: The relationship between the population with health needs and those providing care, areas in England and Wales, 2001.

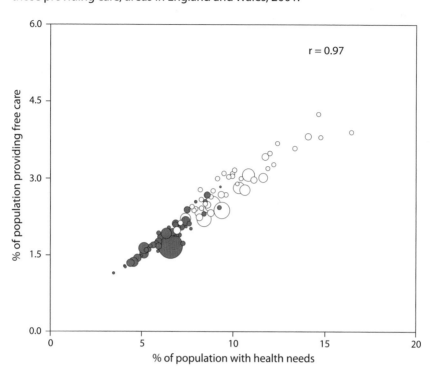

Note: Each circle is a county, unitary, or former metropolitan authority drawn in proportion to its population in 2001. Circles are shaded white if they lie west or north of the counties of Gloucestershire, Warwickshire, Leicestershire, and Lincolnshire (the Severn–Wash divide). Circles are drawn with area in proportion to total population (with the largest circle representing London). Each circle is positioned on the x-axis according to the proportion of the population who live there who have both poor health and limiting long-term illness, and on the y-axis according to the proportion of the population who live there who provide 50 hours' or more per week unpaid care, which includes: looking after, giving help or support to family members, friends, neighbours or others, because of long-term physical or mental ill-health or disability or problems relating to old age. On each of the graphs that follow only the y-axis alters. The x-axis position and the size of each circle remains constant.

Source: Data from the 2001 census.

in employment in that occupation and living in each area. Obviously, many people commute, and so any disparity between need and care might be caused by commuting patterns. However, the vast majority of the disparities shown occur over the north–south divide. Doctors and nurses do not live in Oxford and Bristol and commute to Easington or Salford to work. The health professionals shown are, respectively: nurses, medical practitioners, dentists, and other health professionals with a professional qualification. Of these four groups only nurses (the largest in number and predominantly female) are geographically distributed roughly in proportion to need (r = 0.31, P = 0.001). Weighting the correlations for population size does not alter their rank order. An inverse care law applies (correlation coefficients are negative) to the distribution of people working in all of the more highly paid forms

Figure 5.2: The relationship between the population with health needs and working qualified nurses, midwifes and health visitors, England and Wales, 2001.

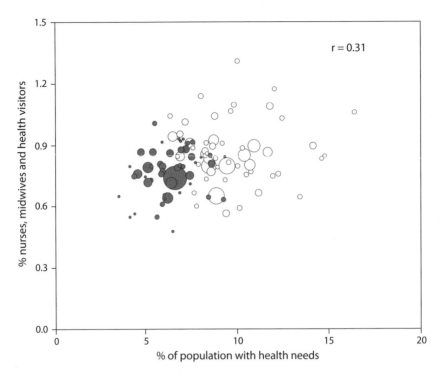

Note: Each circle is a county, unitary, or former metropolitan authority drawn in proportion to its population in 2001. Circles are shaded white if they lie west or north of the counties of Gloucestershire, Warwickshire, Leicestershire, and Lincolnshire (the Severn–Wash divide). Circles are drawn with area in proportion to total population (with the largest circle representing London). Each circle is positioned on the x-axis according to the proportion of the population who live there who have both poor health and limiting long-term illness, and on the y-axis according to the proportion of the population who live there who work as nurses, midwives and health visitors.

Source: Data from the 2001 census.

of healthcare, with that distribution being strongest for the fourth group — the group most likely to be providing private services (such as chiropractors and osteopaths).

If formal care were distributed according to need, as with informal care, each circle in each figure would lie on the diagonal line running from the bottom left to the top right of the graph. Instead, below, there is a large amount of deviation from that line. It is notable that those in the southern part of England (dark grey circles) tend to be positioned above the line and those elsewhere below the line.

Discussion

The census reveals that a considerable amount of care is provided by the friends and families of those in need. This care is provided at no cost to the state save the benefit payments and allowances that are paid to some carers. This care is provided

Figure 5.3: The relationship between the population with health needs and working qualified medical practitioners, England and Wales, 2001.

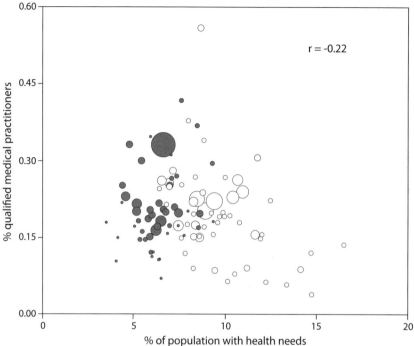

Note: Each circle is a county, unitary, or former metropolitan authority drawn in proportion to its population in 2001. Circles are shaded white if they lie west or north of the counties of Gloucestershire, Warwickshire, Leicestershire, and Lincolnshire (the Severn–Wash divide). Circles are drawn with area in proportion to total population (with the largest circle representing London). Each circle is positioned on the x-axis according to the proportion of the population who live there who have both poor health and limiting long-term illness, and on the y-axis according to the proportion of the population who live there who are qualified medical practitioners and employed a such.

Source: Data from the 2001 census.

in almost direct and exact proportion to need — defined here as the geographical distribution of people both suffering poor health and living with a limiting long-term illness. The observation of the 'inverse care law', as originally stated, can thus now be supplemented with additional data referring to the provision of informal care. We propose that an additional regularity, observed from analysis of the 2001 census data, can be stated as a 'positive care law', a law that takes into account not only medical care in the formal sector of paid work, but health care in its broadest sense. We suggest that the 'positive care law' can be stated thus:

> *In contemporary society, both informal and professional care are provided to those in need. When we consider these very different types of care, informal and formal, we observe that in those areas with most people in need, people disproportionately receive even more care from the informal, unpaid sector — the least skilled form of care. This is also the*

75

Figure 5.4: The relationship between the population with health needs and working qualified dental practitioners, England and Wales, 2001.

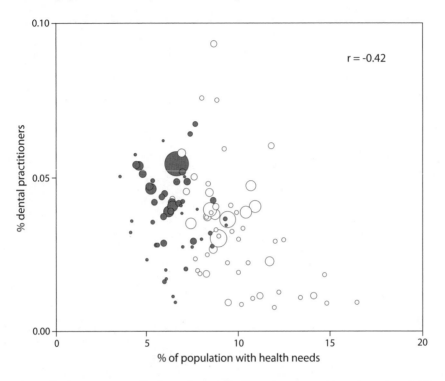

Note: Each circle is a county, unitary, or former metropolitan authority drawn in proportion to its population in 2001. Circles are shaded white if they lie west or north of the counties of Gloucestershire, Warwickshire, Leicestershire, and Lincolnshire (the Severn–Wash divide). Circles are drawn with area in proportion to total population (with the largest circle representing London). Each circle is positioned on the x-axis according to the proportion of the population who live there who have both poor health and limiting long-term illness, and on the y-axis according to the proportion of the population who live there who are working and qualified as dentists.

Source: Data from the 2001 census.

cheapest form of care (for the state) and constitutes a group of carers without power or representation. Conversely, those people living in areas least in need of care (as defined here) receive the most specialised and skilled medical care through the formal paid sector. Between these two extremes there is a continuum. Formal medical care is thus distributed inversely to need whereas informal care is positively related to need — where care is most needed it is informal care that is most likely to be provided. Where market forces are allowed to intervene in the relationships between the need for care and its provision, the more likely the inverse care law is found to apply.

These findings concern the motivations that underpin human actions, and the value that we ascribe to the services that we provide for each other. A key motivation for the provision of personal or medical care is traditionally considered to be altruism.

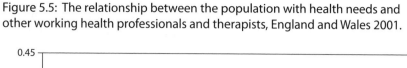

Figure 5.5: The relationship between the population with health needs and other working health professionals and therapists, England and Wales 2001.

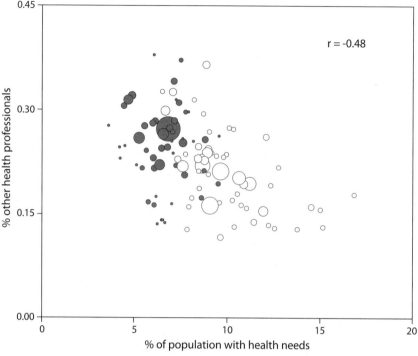

Note: Each circle is a county, unitary, or former metropolitan authority drawn in proportion to its population in 2001. Circles are shaded white if they lie west or north of the counties of Gloucestershire, Warwickshire, Leicestershire, and Lincolnshire (the Severn–Wash divide). Circles are drawn with area in proportion to total population (with the largest circle representing London). Each circle is positioned on the x-axis according to the proportion of the population who live there who have both poor health and limiting long-term illness, and on the y-axis according to the proportion of the population who live there who work as 'other' qualified health professionals (not including doctors, dentists, nurses, midwives or health visitors).

Source: Data from the 2001 census.

The issue of whether the fundamental basis of human relationships operates through altruism or exchange, and the consequences of that, was central to the analysis in *The Gift Relationship*.[6] Titmuss' analysis of the donation of human blood in the United Kingdom and the selling of human blood in the United States, has relevance for understanding 'gift relationships' — or how and why people help one another — more generally. When someone gives their blood to another person the act is altruistic, unselfish and unconditional. When a donor sells their blood, however, then the relationship is mechanical, impersonal and responsive to pressures of demand and supply.

---

[6] Titmuss, R.M. (1970) *The gift relationship: From human blood to social policy*. Harmondsworth: Penguin Books.

However, the truly altruistic act, such as the gift relationship of giving blood, appears to be rare and is not easily measured, as Murray points out[7]. Altruism implies a lack of connection and lack of reciprocation between the carer and the cared for, which characterises the giving of blood, and to some extent the provision of medical services, but is unlikely to be the case with informal care. In fact, it may be because people are connected, because they experience reciprocation, that they care for each other. Conversely, there are many collective actions that suggest that the population may be more altruistic than this simple reciprocal model would suggest, and that altruism is partly learnt behaviour. In the north of England more middle-class people tend to vote for left-wing politicians advocating redistributive policies, despite the implementation of these policies being to their direct immediate disadvantage. Perhaps the more you can see the benefits of altruistic behaviour, the more likely you are to act altruistically. On the other hand, the greater the role of the market, the more likely people are to be driven by motives other than altruism; the contrast between nurses and doctors, in terms of their choice of occupation, their salaries and in our results presented here, are an example of this.

It is important to note that this paper is only concerned with ecological data: the number of medical practitioners per head of the population as they vary between areas, the number of informal carers as a proportion of the population and the number in need of medical care. Within any area it is almost certainly the case that those most in need of care will be cared for by medical practitioners more than those who are in less need of care. It is important not to invoke the ecology fallacy and suggest that the sickest people in England and Wales are not cared for by paid carers. Nevertheless, this analysis does reveal that where there are more ill people there are fewer people, per head, being paid to provide medical care. There are also very large geographical distances between the areas where more doctors and dentists live and where the population is most in need of their services. Thus it is certainly the case that, by area, there is less paid care available overall where it is most needed, and most paid care available where it is least needed. Conversely, and everywhere in England and Wales, almost exactly the same proportions of people give up 50 or more hours per week of their time to care for those in need, unpaid. Altruism is found everywhere, but in greatest quantities where it is most needed.

This geographical division of England and Wales revealed through the data used in this paper is a division familiar to those who have studied the human geography of these countries over the last century. As the land rises to the north and west of Gloucestershire, Warwickshire, Leicestershire, and Lincolnshire, more people are ill and fewer medical professionals (other than nurses) are in work. People of all professions are more likely to live in the southeast of England; they are more likely to have achieved access to university from there, to return there if they trained in the north, or to move there later in their working lives. What is unusual about medical professionals is that, as a group, they manage to achieve this same south-eastern bias

---

[7] Murray, T.H. (2003) Are we better than we can say? Altruism in general practice. *British Journal of General Practice*; 53: 355-357.

despite the majority of their most needy client group living in the north and despite the large majority of them working for the NHS, which partly allocates resources in relation to the needs of area populations. The 2001 census figures would suggest that a greater proportion of those resources are used to employ nurses in the north and doctors in the south of England.

References

Black, N., Langham, S. and Petticrew, M. (1995) 'Coronary revascularisation: why do rates vary geographically in the UK?', *Journal of Epidemiology and Community Health*, 49: 408-412.

Chew-Graham, C.A., Mullin, S., May, C.R., *et al.* (2002) 'Managing depression in primary care: another example of the inverse care law?', *Family Practice*, 19(6): 632-637.

Chew, C., Wilkin, D. and Glendinning, C. (1994) 'Annual assessments of patients aged 75 years and over: views and experiences of elderly people', *British Journal of General Practice*, 44: 567-570.

Gillam, S. (1992) 'Provision of health promotion clinics in relation to population need: another example of the inverse care law?', *British Journal of General Practice*, 42: 54-56.

Lovett, A., Haynes, R., Sunnenberg, G. and Gale, S. (2002) 'Car travel time and accessibility by bus to general practitioner services: a study using patient registers and GIS', *Social Science and Medicine*, 55(1): 97-111.

Lynch, M. (1995) 'Effect of practice and patient population characteristics on the uptake of childhood immunisations', *British Journal of General Practice*, 45: 205-208.

Payne, N. and Saul, C. (1997) 'Variations in use of cardiology services in a health authority: comparison of coronary artery revascularisation rates with prevalence of angina and coronary mortality', *British Medical Journal*, 314: 257-261.

Pell, J.P., Pell, A.C., Norrie, J., *et al.* (2000) 'Effect of socioeconomic deprivation on waiting time for cardiac surgery: retrospective cohort study', *British Medical Journal*, 320: 15-18.

Rogers, A., Hassell, K., Noyce, P. and Harris, J. (1998) 'Advice-giving in community pharmacy: variations between pharmacies in different locations', *Health and Place*, 4(4): 365-373.

Stirling, A.M., Wilson, P. and McConnachie, A. (2001) 'Deprivation, psychological distress, and consultation length in general practice', *British Journal of General Practice*, 51: 456-460.

Webb, E., Naish, J. and Macfarlane, A.. (1996) 'Planning and commissioning of health services for children and young people', *Journal of Public Health Medicine*, 18(2): 217-220.

SECTION II
The liberal record

6

Paving the way for 'any willing provider' to privatise the NHS

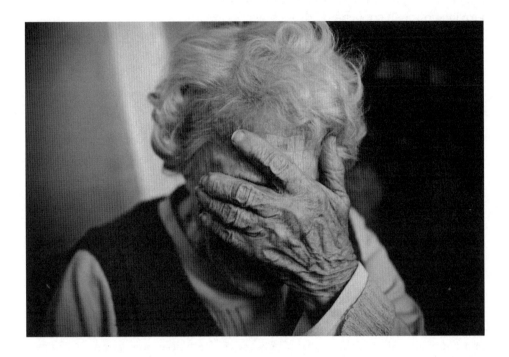

Privatisation of the NHS began under the 1979–90 Thatcher government, with fiddling at what were thought to be the edges. First came contracting out the cleaning. This initial round of privatisation was a means of saving money as firms employed cleaners with poorer contracts than those that they had when working for the NHS. During the mid-1980s older children attending my secondary school regularly worked at weekends as cleaners on both hospital wards and in operating theatres as a result of these first privatisations. Those who employed them gave them more and more to clean in a shorter and shorter amount of time. Infections within hospitals became more common.

The second Blair and Brown period of privatisation was dressed up as a series of short-term plans aimed at achieving laudable goals such as reducing hospital waiting list times. Specialist providers were brought in but, like the private finance initiative (PFI), these measures proved uneconomic in the medium term (let alone in the long term). The not-so-prudent Gordon Brown may have thought he was increasing efficiency by increasing apparent competition, but private companies will only take on work for the NHS if it profits them; they are not charities. Their 'efficiency savings' profit the shareholder, not the NHS, and healthcare is not like other goods and services. Much of the training of doctors and nurses occurs within the NHS, and by avoiding these training costs, private companies can easily undercut the NHS. Another way in which healthcare differs is that in many other forms of consumption you can pick up most goods at bargain prices, expecting that a mistake in your 'choice' would just affect your pocket. With health, if the quality is low, you might die. I argue that health, education and some aspects of housing are far better provided through cooperation than competition.

We are now in a third round of privatisation. Is it different again? Some think it is a plan to use NHS monies to profit private companies and their shareholders. This would provide value for money to a particular group of people with whom the current government (often accused of being out of touch with most people) are very much and very closely in touch. Of course they have not said this, but it is an interesting coincidence, one that is worth thinking about. Just how in touch so many British Conservative politicians are with 'private providers' is demonstrated by listing at the end of this chapter some of the private health connections of many Conservative members of the House of Lords.

The Coalition government says it needs to save a lot of money in the short term. Cutting services does that, but major restructuring of an organisation is most unlikely to save money in the short term. So why do it, especially if it is not in your manifesto, and when you end up in coalition with a party, the Liberal Democrats, who say they do not want to do it (but a party that backed the privatisation nevertheless)?

The Health and Social Care Bill was said by the Coalition government, using New Labour-style rhetoric, '… *to restructure the health service in the hope of reducing costs, improving quality and cutting bureaucracy'*. Among these plans the founding principle of the NHS had been forgotten, that principle being to provide free healthcare of a national quality at the point of delivery to the whole population. As the Bill became an Act, passed into law on 20 March 2012, the way healthcare services were to be commissioned became set to undergo major restructuring. The clinical commissioning groups (CCGs) created by the Act were not simply metamorphosed primary care trusts (PCTs). Instead, they now hold the powers once held by the Secretary of State for Health.[1]

From 2012 onwards CCGs act in place of the Secretary of State rather than on behalf of him or her. This means the government's current legal duty to secure comprehensive healthcare is passed to the local commissioners and providers of care. It is a step back in time to an era before the NHS was established, to a time when what you received depended far more on the vagaries of what local charity boards and hospitals might provide. Those vagaries in turn depended on how affluent an area you lived in and on how miserly or how kind was the local disposition. Furthermore, unlike PCTs, CCGs are not responsible for all children and adults in contiguous

---

[1] Strangely the opposite appeared to be occurring in education where the Secretary of State, Michael Gove, was taking on more and more powers for himself. Possibly as an incentive for the future further privatisation of schools, the only way to avoid being directly answerable to Gove or his successors would be to privatise a school completely. There appeared to be no single, coherent, well-thought-out but devious plan across all of government.

geographical areas. Instead, patient populations are selected from general practitioners' (GPs') lists, and CCGs will have to provide care for this selected population rather than a pre-determined geographical area. In other words, not everyone need be included any more.

To an extent it was possible not to be on a patient list before the 2012 Act was passed, and refugees not recognised as asylum-seekers were often officially excluded. However, in practice many clinicians chose to follow the Hippocratic oath and provided treatment. Officially, all patients needed to be on a GP's list to receive treatment. In practice, however, if you turned up at A&E (Accident and Emergency) or a drop-in centre you were treated, and there was an obligation on local GPs to take patients allocated by an over-arching PCT whose job it was to ensure that every person living in their area could be assigned to a GP. Using a map on which PCT boundaries are shown and where population density has been made even, Figure 6.1 shows how evenly spread PCTs were over the population of the country. Some PCTs served larger populations; some smaller ones, depending on local circumstances. Some worked in cooperation with other parts of government and their boundaries. Figure 6.1 shows what the geography of a planned healthcare system looks like.

The new system changes the ethos. It leaves the CCGs to decide what services are provided and how. The loss of clearly defined area responsibilities means that those most in need may well not have services allocated for them. Furthermore, some current NHS services will cease to be free and much of the delivery will become privatised. Under the new Act, up to 49 per cent of an NHS hospital's beds can become full private beds. It was a great concern of many of the commentators on the Bill's passing that this reorganisation would increase the inequality of service access and provision. And, as they stated as an additional objection, all this would do nothing to tackle the ongoing health inequalities faced by Britain's population (Pollock *et al*, 2012).

Origins of the Coalition government's Health and Social Care Bill

The 2012 Bill to further privatise the NHS had its roots firmly planted by the previous (New Labour) government that in turn had built on Margaret Thatcher's privatising legacy. On 13 May 2009 the New Labour government announced that the then new Care Quality Commission (CQC, not to be confused with CCGs) would '*do a bit of a number*' on the '*worst performing providers*' (*Health Service Journal*, 2009). Other sources suggested that NHS Chief Executive David Nicholson had held a meeting for all chief executives in the NHS on 12 May 2009 to announce the need for cost savings and that, from that point until the 2010 General Election, all trusts were required to produce QIPP (quality, innovation, productivity and prevention) plans. This has continued to be a requirement under the Coalition government. Furthermore, under the new government it was claimed that NHS 'productivity' had been falling (Grice, 2012), although the validity of such claims has been hotly disputed by independent academic research (Black, 2012).

Figure 6.1: Primary care trusts as they existed in 2011 drawn on an equal population projection (these areas were abolished in 2012).

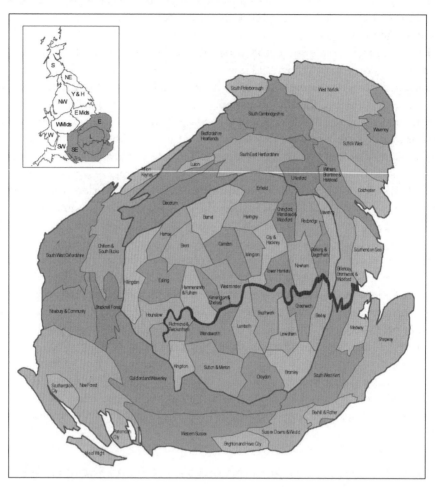

Note: Each area is a primary care trust. The size of the area is drawn in proportion to the number of patients served. Here only the south eastern group is shown.

Before the May 2010 General Election, one of the then Opposition leader David Cameron's key election promises was '*I'll cut the deficit, not the NHS*'. Some believed him then and also later when, as Prime Minister, he said that the NHS budget was to be ring-fenced ... it turned out it was in a way – the costs of direct patient care were ring-fenced, but that ring-fencing did not take account of the increasing cost of drugs and other treatments. The Coalition's first NHS White Paper was published in July 2010.

At a superficial level privatisation can appear positive. It should mean that GPs are able to buy the services they want from whoever they want, provided that the provider meets the quality criteria set down by the government. Why would you want to wait for an operation at an NHS hospital when you can have it at the local private one next week? One answer might be that many other people would have to each wait longer if you were to jump the queue.

It is also often claimed that NHS hospitals waste lots of money and are inefficient, and that better care may be available outside the NHS. However, other than the known huge proportion of US GDP spent on private medicine both by the state and by millions of individuals in the US, estimates are rarely published of the true cost of private care. Specialist private services tend to only be used by very rich people because of their very high costs. These high costs are despite competition in the private sector and the claim that competition reduces costs.

In Britain the high cost of private health care also continues despite the NHS having previously trained many of their staff, and the NHS continuing to provide the necessary back-up, such as intensive care beds, when private health care has insufficient resources. The private sector gets both the training and the medical back-up for free. The privatisation theory suggests that if part of the NHS sees its business going elsewhere it will drive up efficiency and drive down costs in order to win back business, and that, in theory, patients have more choice of where they can be treated. However, without private health care providers having to pay for the benefits they get for free from the NHS, it is not a level playing-field.

Private care providers were allowed to enter the NHS 'family' under the 1997–2010 New Labour administration – just as New Labour introduced student fees, which the Coalition then tripled to £9,000. Private health 'competition' introduced by New Labour has, later, been more than tripled in future costs to patients by the new Bill. But there was a point at which this could have been avoided. As Chapter 7 on income inequalities concludes: '... *if there were the political will, the reduction in income inequalities seen for 2002–03 could signal a turning point in this vitally important trend'*. The political will was not there; in its place was the will to privatise.

Reasons not to privatise

There are numerous reasons put forward not to privatise. They include the fact that most GPs do not have the time or the skills needed for clinical commissioning. It is also widely recognised that patients do not always want choice; most just want to be told what is wrong and how to get better, and to have any necessary treatment, locally, if possibly. The arguments against privatisation made at the time of the 2012 Bill also included:

- We should be looking at all hospitals being great, not pushing competition.
- It means *yet another* major restructure for the NHS, which is costing billions already (NHS, 2012).
- None of the major professional groups think it is a good idea, including nurses and the General Medical Council and even the Royal College of General Practitioners who would get much of the power and profit!
- NHS staff are fed up with being reorganised and do not see this as an improvement in any way, even the 'Conservative Home' website argued against the idea in

February 2012 – not on principle (which it agreed on), but over how many votes might be lost.

But the Bill got passed. And part of the reason it got passed was that the previous New Labour government had not shown that another route was possible. Health inequalities had continued to increase under its authority and throughout its period in office (they had fallen under all previous Labour governments). As Chapter 8 argues later, many of the Labour Members of Parliament (MPs) whose constituents had suffered most due to the failure to narrow inequalities had the power to change policy back in 2005, 2006 and 2007 when it became clear that policy was failing

Perhaps because Labour MPs knew it was partly their fault that privatisation was spreading there was far more concerted opposition from the media than from Her Majesty's Official Opposition in Parliament (*Guardian*, 2012).

Journalist Polly Toynbee's response to Secretary of State Andrew Lansley's determination to force the Bill through was: *'he's running into such deep trouble … every single part of the NHS is up for sale'*. And, she continued, *'The market ideology of the Health and Social Care Bill shows that the pragmatic prime minister is on another planet.'*

Figure 6.2: David Cameron and his Health Secretary, Andrew Lansley, meet nurses during a visit to the Royal Salford Hospital in Manchester on 6 January 2012

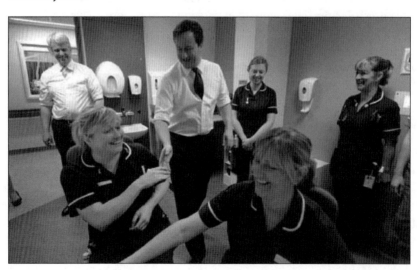

see colour version in plate section

Source: Photograph: John Giles/Press Association (2012)

She went on, her story illustrated by the photograph in Figure 6.2, to explain that:

Andrew Lansley's last refuge is his most disreputable argument so far: his Health and Social Care Bill must pass as so much has already been implemented without waiting for Royal Assent. None can recall such flagrant flouting of Parliament. All but abolished are 151 primary care trusts – replaced by 279 clinical commissioning groups – while strategic health authorities are to become four hubs. The new national commissioning board already has a chief executive and finance director with seven board members recruited on salaries of up to £170,000 before the bill is passed. Brass plate shifting has squandered £2bn, while the NHS suffers cuts of £20bn. McKinsey and KPMG already have fat contracts to take over much commissioning supposed to be done by GPs. Which sector will they instinctively favour for contracts? Yet none of it has yet passed into law. The health economist Professor Kieran Walshe says £1bn could still be saved by stopping it now. "Too late," the health secretary says with grim glee, and Lansley's alarmed party believes it's so. (Toynbee, 2012b)

A week earlier Toynbee had explained that:

… this should make your hair stand on end: only 6% of public service cuts have happened yet. Another 94% are still to come, with cascades more public servants sacked. In benefits, 88% of cuts are still to come. But Tory and Lib Dem MPs voted through an £18bn benefit cut for the 'squeezed' bottom half with few qualms, taking £1,400 from disabled children and £94 a week from the sick who don't die or recover within a year. The IFS [Institute for Fiscal Studies] says these cuts are 'almost without historical or international precedent'. 'How deliverable these will prove remains to be seen,' it adds. The answer is blindingly obvious. Cuts of these dimensions are impossible. Austerity will not be politically tolerable in a rich country in peacetime where boardrooms pay themselves 49% rises. The Attlee government was toppled by peacetime austerity that voters no longer trusted. The government reassures itself that the country is muddling along, coping with cuts, getting by. But the frightening truth is that it's hardly begun … The aim of cuts is to 'incentivise' people out of 'dependence'. Presumably the way kicking away crutches incentivises the lame to walk. (Toynbee, 2012a)

A day later the *Daily Mail* wrote up another version of the story – appearing to be moving even further to the left than *The Guardian*. It concerned McKinsey & Company, a global management consulting firm, *'the trusted advisor to the world's leading businesses, governments, and institutions'*. Here is what *Mail* journalists described:

A Mail on Sunday investigation, based on hundreds of official documents disclosed under the Freedom of Information Act, has revealed the full extent of McKinsey's myriad links to the controversial reforms.

Many of the Bill's proposals were drawn up by McKinsey and included in the legislation wholesale. One document says the firm has used its privileged access to 'share information' with its corporate clients – which include the world's biggest private hospital firms – who are now set to bid for health service work.

McKinsey's involvement in the Bill is so great that its executives attend the meetings of the 'Extraordinary NHS Management Board' convened to implement it. Sometimes

McKinsey even hosts these meetings at its UK headquarters in Jermyn Street, Central London.

The company is already benefiting from contracts worth undisclosed millions with GPs arising from the Bill. It has earned at least £13.8million from Government health policy since the Coalition took office – and the Bill opens up most of the current £106 billion NHS budget to the private sector, with much of it likely to go to McKinsey clients. (Rose, 2012)

Or, as the medical correspondent of the magazine, *Private Eye*, put it,

If Lansley had wanted evolution, rather than revolution, he would simply have slimmed down the existing Primary Care Trusts, put clinical staff on the board alongside the best of the NHS managers and let them figure out how best to spend the money and focus on the quality and safety of care. By throwing all the cards up in the air, he's created chaos, uncertainty and the perfect storm for another Mid Staffordshire scandal. The fact that even the more moderate health unions – the Royal College of Nurses and the Royal College of Midwives – now oppose the Bill outright and are calling for its withdrawal should make the Government reconsider. But it won't. (Hammond, 2012)

Two months later, Health Secretary Andrew Lansley, speaking at a meeting of 150 (clinical commissioning) leaders in London on 24 April 2012, explained how the funding formula for CCGs would change with a greater emphasis on the population's age rather than deprivation (Durham, 2012). The deprivation indexes used in health care traditionally include a factor for the proportion of elderly in the population. It is probably the only deprivation factor that is likely to disproportionately benefit Conservative voters, who, on average, will have greater life expectancy than the rest of the population

Conclusion and collusion

It is hardly surprising that the NHS 'reforms' have met such hostility given that their aims were to increase choice and competition. I can remember when the NHS was a 24/7 healthcare system, when GPs would visit you in your bed if you were ill, any day or night of the week. By May 2012, on one night, two thirds of the county of Cornwall was covered by only a single GP *'in a car west of Bodmin'* working for a private profit-making company undertaking work now contracted out of the NHS (Lawrence, 2012a). A UK citizen is currently most likely to die under the care of the NHS at the weekend, purely as a direct lack of resources. Ironically, given Lansley's apparent concerns, this particularly impacts on older people who need a more comprehensive social care system, which the 2012 Health and Social Care Bill seemed largely to neglect. More must be done to create greater cohesion between the healthcare service and the social care sector. It has already been shown how the privatisation of sheltered accommodation and care homes for older people has left individuals in unaffordable, substandard conditions. This should not be allowed to happen to the NHS.

The privatisation of health services is likely to further stoke the increase in health inequalities that exist in UK society. Much political endeavour has been employed to implement various policies over the last century to reduce health inequalities but, although overall health has generally improved, inequality in health both remains and grows, and this Bill is not the least interested in such inequalities. A GP who had been *'... one of the most prominent supporters of Andrew Lansley...'* turned out to have been de-registering elderly and disabled patents from his list because they were more time-consuming to treat; this is a taste of privatisation to come (Ramesh, 2012).

Many revelations came out after the Bill was passed, not just revealing the acts of the selfish, but also the failures of New Labour. Inequalities in health between areas had not been falling before 2010. Given this and 13 years of New Labour rule it was possible to suggest that a change in direction would be beneficial. A similar duplicity was seen earlier in the 2006 Mental Health Bill, described later in Chapter 9, introduced to the House of Lords by the then Minster of Health, Lord Warner. But when duplicity becomes normal, how can one political party effectively complain about the other? The New Labour government's targets were symbolic, rather than addressing the issue of rising health inequalities which were increasing alongside income and wealth inequalities.[2] And monetary inequalities matter greatly because they have an effect on health. Chapter 10 charts how geographical health inequalities rose during the later New Labour years. That government's failure to reduce inequalities in health set the scene for the events that followed.

On Monday, 20 February 2012, the columnist Jackie Ashley wrote: *'In the real world of individual NHS hospitals, if they are able to gain up to 49% of their income from private health, we will see a growing health apartheid with those who have cash or insurance policies walking up the corridors past those who haven't.'* (Ashley, 2012). Following this, and exactly a week after the Bill was passed, the 'risk register' concerning it was leaked. It stated that there was a risk of *'Greater costs if new GP-led consortiums make greater use of the private sector. One example of an area where the system could be more costly is if GP consortia makes use of private sector organisations/staff which adds costs to the overall system'* (Watt and Ramesh, 2012). At the same time it was revealed that *'... in 22 of the new clinical commissioning groups (CCGs), at least half and sometimes all of the GPs that dominate their boards have a personal financial interest in a private or other non-NHS provider'*

---

[2] Inequality in health between areas is best measured by the Slope Index of Inequality, which tends to be about half as wide as the range between the worst-off and best-off district. It takes into account all areas and not just the extremes. For England by local authority district, this index of inequality rose from 3.65 years of life expectancy between the hypothetical poorest and richest place in 1992–94, to 3.77 in 1995–97, to 3.83 in 1998–2000, and then reached 3.98 by 2001–03, when the measure was last updated (Shaw et al, 2005). There was improvement in the trend following the 1997 General Election. See Chapter 10, this volume, for recent figures. During 2012 there have been reports of mortality rates falling more quickly in some of the poorer areas of England than elsewhere. These falls appear to date from around 2008 and may be due to lower rates of out-migration from these areas. Most affected are Blackburn with Darwen, Liverpool, Trafford, the Wirral, Hatton and St Helens, Blackpool and Wigan – all thought to have seen increasing life expectancy (personal communication, Tom Hennell, 2012).

(Campbell, 2012a). Partly because of the time commitments involved, most of these GPs will actually only be part-time healthcare providers, and part-time financiers.

Just a fortnight earlier, details of 62 Conservative peers in the House of Lords who had officially declared interests in companies involved in the private healthcare industry had been listed on the web, alongside details of how loyally they had voted the Bill through (Social Investigation, 2012). Here are a few details.

BUPA, possibly Britain's largest health insurance, private hospital and care group, was closely connected to many members of the House of Lords, including Baroness Bottomley of Nettlestone, better known when she was the former Conservative Health Secretary Virginia Bottomley, a director of BUPA since May 2007. She voted on key amendments of the Health and Social Care Bill, despite normally having a below average vote turnout in the Lords, turning up for less than a quarter of most other votes. On the Bill she said: *'I give this Bill an unequivocal and extraordinarily warm welcome.'* There are many other Lords, Baronesses and Barons with an interest in BUPA, and many probably use BUPA in preference to the NHS, but they do not have to list that in their financial interest statements.

The other Conservative Lords' declared interests in private healthcare ranged from having shares in companies set to benefit from the Bill to being chair of (or adviser to) healthcare companies. Some worked as advisers for investment companies that invested heavily in companies that would benefit from the Bill. Others were directors of companies in direct competition to the NHS. The list includes the former Conservative Party Treasurer Lord Ashcroft, and Lords Ashton, Bell, Blackwell, Brittan, Chadlington, Coe, Feldman, Fink, Forsyth, Freeman, Garel-Jones, Griffiths, Hamilton, Howard, Lang, Lawson, Lloyd-Webber, Macfarlane, McColl, Magan, Maple, Marland, Naseby, Newton, Patten, Popat, Ribeiro, Saatchi, Selborne, Sheikh and Tugendhat, Baroness Cumberlege, Baron Higgins and Viscount Goschen. Many who voted for the Bill had previously shown little enthusiasm for voting in the House of Lords, but without their support, it would have been very difficult for the government to get the Bill through Parliament. By contrast, if you are an elected councillor in local government, you are expected to not take part in a debate, or to vote on matters in which you, or your partners, have a financial interest.

None of those who at the last hurdle helped secure the privatisation of the NHS were even voted into power, and no rules prevented them from voting in their own self-interest. Internationally, for selecting members to the upper house, only 15 countries predominantly use appointments instead of being democratically elected, countries such as Jordan, Belize and Burkina Faso. The very detailed list referred to above only covers Conservative peers; no doubt there were also some Labour, Liberal Democrats and so-called cross-benchers with similar personal financial interests, interests that could be construed as likely to improve were the Bill to be passed. So how did they vote?

If you are worried about the NHS in the future, remember that the Secretary of State for Health is no longer directly responsible for its provision. It is no longer national. It is often more a business than a service. And all this has very little to do with improving health. To conclude I repeat the story of the one GP working west of Bodmin in Cornwall, for a private service that had tendered for a dramatic cut in funding to win the bid, and whose '... *profit-making ethos has left the service beset by serious problems and have made it unsafe. Staff say they have been pressurised to downgrade their assessment of the urgency of calls.*' (Lawrence, 2012b). An ill woman had to wait six hours in great pain for the GP to arrive. She died later within a few weeks of that delayed visit. The thousands of stories of the other patients who no longer get seen, the people who have stopped trying to use the service and of the mistakes made when people hurry so that their bosses are able to profit, all remain to be told.

Shortly after the infamous privatisation Bill was passed into law, a study reported that it was so badly drafted that 'It would seem that the recently enacted Health and Social Services Bill has some very serious 'real world' flaws in that it is not possible to do in the real world what the bill purports to achieve' (Jones, 2012). However, the accuracy of such a view depends on what the Bill's real purpose was. In September 2012 it was revealed that private firms were already bidding for £20 billion of NHS 'business' (Campbell, 2012b).

References

Ashley, J. (2012) 'Only fear of losing face keeps this mad NHS gamble going', *The Guardian*, 19 February (www.guardian.co.uk/commentisfree/2012/feb/19/nhs-gamble).

Black, N. (2012) Letter to *The Guardian*, 19 February (www.guardian.co.uk/theguardian/2012/feb/19/jb-priestley-was-a-northerner).

Campbell, D. (2012a) 'GPs' shares in private healthcare firms prompt conflict of interest fears', *The Guardian*, 27 March (www.guardian.co.uk/society/2012/mar/27/gps-private-health-firm-shares).

Campbell, D. (2012b) 'Health firms told to get set for £20bn bonanza', *The Guardian*, 17 September (www.guardian.co.uk/business/2012/Sept/16/health-firms-nhs).

Durham, N. (2012) 'Lansley promises CCGs autonomy in return for results and financial responsibility', *GP News*, 25 April (www.gponline.com/News/article/1128559/lansley-promises-ccgs-autonomy-return-results-financial-responsibility/).

Grice, J. (2012) Letter to *The Guardian*, 17 February (www.guardian.co.uk/theguardian/2012/feb/17/military-camp-healthcare-work-schemes).

Guardian, The (2012) 'Politics Weekly podcast: the future of the NHS', 9 February (www.guardian.co.uk/politics/audio/2012/feb/09/politics-weekly-podcast-nhs).

Hammond, P. (2012) 'Medicine balls', *Private Eye*, issue 1306, 26 January (http://drphilhammond.com/blog/2012/01/26/private-eye/medicine-balls-private-eye-issue-1306/).

Health Service Journal (2009) 'NHS and Health Management News Blog', 13 May (www.hsj.co.uk/comment/blogs/hsj-news/nhs-and-health-management-news-blog/5001072.bloglead).

Jones, R. (2012) 'End of life and financial risk in GP commissioning', *British Journal of Healthcare Management*, vol 18, no 7, pp 374-81.

Lawrence, F. (2012a) 'Cornwall out-of-hours case study: Eve Tonkin', *The Guardian*, 25 May (www.guardian.co.uk/society/2012/may/25/cornwall-case-study-eve-tonkin).

Lawrence, F. (2012b) 'Cornish complaints raise questions over national drive to outsource NHS care', *The Guardian*, 25 May (www.guardian.co.uk/society/2012/may/25/questions-outsource-nhs-care).

NHS (2012) Calderdale NHS (www.calderdale.nhs.uk/get-involved/board-meetings/).

Pollock, A.M., Price, D. *et al* (2012) 'How the Health and Social Care Bill 2011 would end entitlement to comprehensive health care in England', *The Lancet*, vol 379, no 9814, pp 387-9.

Ramesh, R. (2012) 'GP practice "offloaded vulnerable patients to save money", practice run by supporter of Andrew Lansley's health reforms let go of 48 patients who needed high levels of care', *The Guardian*, 31 May (www.guardian.co.uk/society/2012/may/31/gp-health-reform-cost-cut).

Rose, D. (2012) 'The firm that hijacked the NHS: MoS investigation reveals extraordinary extent of international management consultant's role in Lansley's health reforms', *The Daily Mail*, 13 February (www.dailymail.co.uk/news/article-2099940/NHS-health-reforms-Extent-McKinsey--Companys-role-Andrew-Lansleys-proposals.html).

Shaw, M., Davey Smith, G. and Dorling, D. (2005) 'Health inequalities under New Labour: author's reply', *British Medical Journal*, vol 330, pp 1507-8.

Social Investigation (2012) 'Conservative Lords and their financial links to companies involved in private healthcare' (http://socialinvestigations.blogspot.co.uk/2012/03/conservative-lords-and-their-financial.html).

Toynbee, P. (2012a) 'The welfare reform bill will incentivise people to turn on David Cameron', *The Guardian*, 2 February (www.guardian.co.uk/commentisfree/2012/feb/02/welfare-reform-bill-cameron-frightening).

Toynbee, P. (2012b) 'The NHS bill could finish the health service – and David Cameron', *The Guardian*, 6 February (www.guardian.co.uk/commentisfree/2012/feb/06/nhs-bill-finish-cameron-ideology).

Watt, N. and Ramesh, R. (2012) 'Reforms could damage NHS, warns draft risk register', *The Guardian*, 27 March (www.guardian.co.uk/politics/2012/mar/27/health-reforms-damage-nhs-risk-register?newsfeed=true).

7

Health inequalities and New Labour: how the promises compare with real progress[1]

Shaw, M., Davey Smith, G. and Dorling, D. (2005) 'Health inequalities and New Labour: how the promises compare with real progress', *British Medical Journal*, vol 330, pp 1016-21.

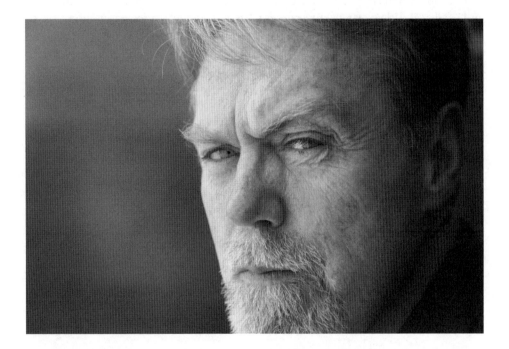

Summary points

Inequalities in health widened in the 1980s and 1990s, and the current government has repeatedly expressed its intention to reduce these inequalities.

The health inequalities targets that have been set are symbolically important, but may be little more than that.

New analysis shows that inequalities in life expectancy between rich and poor areas of the UK continued to widen in the first years of the 21st century, alongside widening inequalities in wealth, suggesting that more potent and redistributive policies are needed.

---

[1] In the original article, we thanked Francis Jones at the Office for National Statistics for providing detailed income inequality data. The article appeared in the 'Education and Debate' section of the *BMJ*.

It is not adequate simply to compare the worst off with the average, nor to pull some of the worst off out of poverty and assume inequalities in health will reduce.

Raising the living standards of some of the poorest people in Britain has not reduced overall inequalities in health, while inequalities in wealth have continued to grow and are likely to be transmitted to the next generation.

Introduction

Despite government rhetoric to the contrary, inequalities in health and wealth have continued to increase in Britain.

Inequalities in health between rich and poor areas of Britain widened in the 1980s and 1990s, and the current government has repeatedly expressed its intention to reduce these inequalities. In this chapter, however, the authors report that inequalities in life expectancy have continued to widen, alongside widening inequalities in income and wealth, and argue that more potent and redistributive policies are needed.

This year marks the 20th anniversary of the World Health Organization's Global Strategy for Health for All by the Year 2000, which proposed 38 targets to reduce inequalities in health.[2] These targets were taken up by the governments of many countries, including Margaret Thatcher's Conservative government in the United Kingdom, which, just like Tony Blair's current administration, wished that inequalities in health would fall (see box).

The four cornerstones of the Health for All policy[3]

- Ensuring equity in health by reducing gaps in health status between countries and between population groups within countries
- Adding life to years by helping people achieve, and use, their full physical, mental, and social potential
- Adding health to life by reducing disease and disability
- Adding years to life by increasing life expectancy

In Britain the observation of and preoccupation with health inequalities has a much longer history than the last two administrations (Davey Smith *et al.*, 2001) and many recent studies have documented a social and spatial polarisation of life chances continuing into the 1980s and late 1990s from a possible lull in the 1970s. (Shaw *et al.*, 1999; Acheson, 1998; Davey Smith *et al.*, 2002; Donkin *et al.*, 2002), Clearly then, the Health for All aim of reducing inequalities between groups of the population had not been reached by the end of the 1990s—in fact, the opposite had occurred even though the fourth goal of increasing life expectancy has been attained.

---

[2] World Health Organization (1985) *Targets for health for all*, Copenhagen: WHO.
[3] World Health Organization (1998) *Health in Europe 1997*, Copenhagen: WHO (www.euro.who. int/document/e60594.pdf).

Increasing health inequalities have been shown to reflect trends in income inequality, which also increased substantially over the last decades of the 20th century (Shaw *et al.*, 1999; Lakin, 2004). While in opposition, the Labour party had made political capital out of the non-implementation of the recommendations of the Black report (Shaw *et al.*, 1999; DHSS, 1980; Davey Smith *et al.*, 1998). The New Labour government that came to power in 1997 did not initially shy away from acknowledging the wider (social and even structural) determinants of health (although the recent public health white paper 'Choosing Health' very much places the responsibility for health with the individual[4]). In 1997 Tessa Jowell, then minister for public health, criticised the previous administration for its 'excessive emphasis on lifestyle issues' that 'cast the responsibility back onto the individual' (Shaw *et al.*, 1999).

Labour has repeatedly expressed rhetoric directed at tackling health inequalities: 'Tackling health inequalities is a top priority for this government', according to Hazel Blears, parliamentary under secretary of state for public health (DH, 2002). Indeed, the government has launched repeated and unprecedented initiatives signalling its intent to tackle health inequalities through an independent inquiry, (Acheson, 1998) a 'cross-cutting review'(DH, 2002) and a 'programme for action' (DH, 2003). In February 2001 it announced two headline national targets for 2010—to reduce the gap in infant mortality across social groups and to raise life expectancy in the most disadvantaged areas faster than elsewhere[5].

The original wording of the latter target, as announced by the Secretary of State in February 2001, was: '*Starting with **health authorities**, by 2010 to reduce by at least 10 per cent the gap between the quintile of areas with the lowest life expectancy at birth and the population as a whole*' [emphasis added].[6] This is not simply a health target but, arguably (given that Frank Dobson, then secretary for health, stated in 1997: 'Inequality in health is the worst inequality of all. There is no more serious inequality than knowing that you'll die sooner because you're badly off'), is the most basic of all government targets for 'bringing Britain together'.[7]

Technically, however, this is only a partial target for health inequalities because it concerns people with the worst life expectancy in comparison with the average rather than the worst compared with the best. Although comparing worst and best can be used to good effect to convey the extent of inequalities (Figure 7.1; Shaw *et al.*, 1999), better still is the slope index of inequality, which takes into account the position of all groups across the gradient simultaneously (see below).

The progress towards the life expectancy target can be monitored by means of the statistics that the government now makes available (www.statistics.gov.uk), but it should be noted that the target now states: '*Starting with **local authorities**, by 2010 to*

[4] Department of Health (2004) *Choosing health: making healthier choices easier.* London: Stationery Office.
[5] Exworthy, M., Stuart, M., Blane, D. and Marmot, M. (2003) *Tackling health inequalities since the Acheson inquiry.* Bristol: The Policy Press.
[6] Department of Health (revised 2002) Health inequalities—national targets on infant mortality and life expectancy—technical briefing. www.dh.gov.uk/assetRoot/04/07/78/96/04077896.pdf (accessed 11 Apr 2005).
[7] Social Exclusion Unit (1998) *Bringing Britain together: a national strategy for neighbourhood renewal.* London: Stationery Office (Cm 4045).

reduce by at least 10 per cent the gap between the fifth of areas with the lowest life expectancy at birth and the population as a whole' [emphasis added] (because health authorities as defined at the time of the original target no longer exist). The baseline for the target has been set at 2001, and the most recent life expectancy data available are for 2001–3, so we cannot yet, even eight years after the election of New Labour, assess progress completely— but we can look at the trend up to the end of 2003.

Figure 7.1: Mapping the best and worst health in Britain.

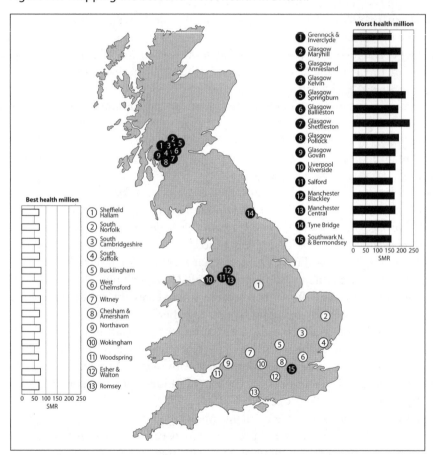

Note: The areas (parliamentary constituencies) containing the million people with the highest and lowest premature mortality (standardised mortality ratios (SMR) for deaths under 65 years of age) in Britain, 1991-5. (Average standardised mortality ratio for England and Wales = 100).

Source: Original research by authors.

Tracking progress towards (sensible) targets

[In this chapter progress is assessed] by using a modified version of the government's target that can be calculated for different times and which is less sensitive to changes in geographical boundaries and population deciles. We use the published life expectancy data for local authority districts that are aggregated to three year periods (revised figures published in October 2004)[8] and mid-year estimates of population for the same areas and times (revised figures published in September 2004).[9]

Note the importance of using the revised population data. Until late 2004, population figures (and thus life expectancy figures) from the early 1990s onwards were still being revised to account for the finding from the 2001 census that almost a million men thought to be living in the UK were not actually here (and that they tended not to be living in poorer areas, as was previously thought). Any study that does not use the final revised population estimates by area for the late 1990s will (erroneously) tend to produce results suggesting that health inequalities were declining in this period.[10] *[See appendix to the original article on bmj.com for the rationale behind the revisions to the census data.]*

The government target does not refer specifically to male or female life expectancies, but these can be combined as a weighted average, as well as analysed separately. Many of the health inequalities initiatives relate only to England, and it is not entirely clear whether the targets refer to England, England and Wales, or the UK. As some of the areas in the UK with the highest premature mortality and worst health are found outside England, we have here included the data for England, Wales, and Scotland. It is also possible to include Northern Ireland here, which previous analyses of inequalities had not been able to include (Shaw *et al.*, 1999; Davey Smith *et al.*, 2002; though its relatively small population size means that it has only a small influence on the findings). Any investigators wishing to replicate this work will find that they have to exclude the City of London and the Isles of Scilly because the Office for National Statistics does not publish life expectancy data for these small areas.

Taking poverty into account

Having obtained life expectancy and population data by area over time, we then need to order areas in some way. The official method is to rank areas, at each time

---

[8] Office for National Statistics. (2005) *Life expectancy at birth by health and local authorities in the United Kingdom 1991-1993 to 2001-2003, including revised results for England and Wales 1991-1993 to 2000-2002, 2004.* www.statistics.gov.uk/statbase/Product.asp?vlnk = 8841 (accessed 11 Apr 2005).

[9] Office for National Statistics (2005) *Population estimates for England and Wales.* www.statistics.gov. uk/statbase/Product.asp?vlnk = 601&More = N (accessed 11 Apr 2005). (Included link to data for Scotland and Northern Ireland.)

[10] Bajekal, M. (2005) Healthy life expectancy by area deprivation: magnitude and trends in England, 1994–1999. *Health Statistics Quarterly*, 25:18-27.

point, by life expectancy. An alternative, and arguably better practice[11], is to rank the areas by a measure that reflects the residents' socioeconomic circumstances at the start of the period studied; we use a measure of poverty.

Poverty in 1991 can be best indexed by a modified version of the 1991 Breadline Britain index, based on lack of basic amenities and access to a car, unskilled and semiskilled manual occupations, unemployment, households that are not owner-occupiers, and lone parent households. This index has the advantage of being based on what a sample of the population consider to be the conditions and extent of poverty and is a validated indicator of poverty.[12]

We therefore ranked local authority districts according to this poverty measure and grouped them into 10ths of equal population size on the basis of this ranking. We used the same 10ths, based on the 1991 census data, for each of the time periods so that, all else being equal, inequalities should attenuate over time as the poverty rate is for areas ranked at the start of the study period. In practice the choice of census date is immaterial as the geography of poverty has changed little since 1991 (the correlation coefficient of the 1991 Breadline Britain index and a preliminary version of the 2001 index for local authorities in Britain being r = 0.97[13]); indeed there is some evidence that the broad geography of poverty in Britain has changed little over the past century.[14]

Note that a poverty ranking of areas tends to be robust—in contrast with the official measure of health inequalities, which sorts areas into 10ths on the basis of the contemporary life expectancies. The official measure is highly volatile because individual authorities can enter or leave the worst-off fifth of areas as the result of a tiny number of events.[15]

The most inclusive measure of inequality in life expectancy is the slope index of inequality, which we calculated for each three year period from the slope of the regression line from the hypothetically poorest individual to the hypothetically richest individual derived from the relative poverty ranks of life expectancy for each local authority district, weighted for population size.[16] The slope index of inequality takes into account all measures for all areas and not, say, simply the worst-off and best-off 10th or fifth of areas. The index is most effective as a summary measure when the two measures are linearly related, as is the case with the data we analysed.

---

[11] Low, A. and Low, A. (2004) Measuring the gap: quantifying and comparing local health inequalities, *Journal of Public Health*, 26:388-95.

[12] Gordon, D. (1995) Census based deprivation indices: their weighting and validation. *Journal of Epidemiology and Community Health* 49 (supplement 2):S39-44.

[13] Dorling, D. and Thomas, B. (2004) Appendix. In: *People and places: a 2001 census atlas of the UK.* Bristol: The Policy Press.

[14] Dorling, D., Mitchell, R., Shaw, M., Orford, S., and Davey Smith, G. (2000) The Ghost of Christmas Past: the health effects of poverty in London in 1896 and 1991. *BMJ* 321:1547-51 [reproduced as Chapter 3 in this volume].

[15] Department of Health (revised 2002) Health inequalities—national targets on infant mortality and life expectancy—technical briefing, www.dh.gov.uk/assetRoot/04/07/78/96/04077896.pdf (accessed 11 Apr 2005).

[16] Wagstaff, A., Paci, P., and van Doorslaer, E. (1991) On the measurement of inequalities in health, *Social Science and Medicine*, 33:545-57.

The index has a further advantage that it is, by definition, unaffected by general increases or decreases in life expectancy over time (in this case the constant changes but not the slope).

Table 7.1 shows the life expectancy for males, females, and both sexes combined by poverty. Over the 10 years studied life expectancy has risen for all poverty groups. However, the slope index of inequality for both sexes has also edged upwards, from 3.71 in 1992–4 to 3.87 in 2001–3. The absolute difference in life expectancy between the top and bottom poverty groups has increased to more than four years. Similarly the difference between the individual local authority areas with the highest and lowest life expectancies (Kensington and Chelsea and Glasgow City) has risen to 9.4 years by 2001–3. [*See appendix to original article on bmj.com for a list of the local authorities with the highest and lowest life expectancies.*]

Table 7.1: Life expectancy in Britain by poverty, slope index of inequality, and difference between poorest and richest areas, 1992–2003 (values are life expectancy in years unless stated otherwise).

	Both sexes combined				Males				Females			
	1992-4	1995-97	1998-2000	2001-3	1992-4	1995-97	1998-2000	2001-3	1992-4	1995-97	1998-2000	2001-3
Poverty group*												
1	74.4	74.8	75.5	76.2	71.2	71.7	72.5	73.3	77.4	77.8	78.3	79.0
2	75.4	75.9	76.4	77.1	72.3	73.0	73.6	74.5	78.2	78.6	79.0	79.5
3	75.7	76.1	76.7	77.4	72.8	73.4	74.0	74.8	78.4	78.7	79.3	79.8
4	75.7	76.1	76.6	77.3	72.8	73.3	74.0	74.9	78.4	78.7	79.2	79.7
5	76.2	76.6	77.2	77.7	73.4	73.9	74.5	75.3	78.9	79.2	79.6	80.0
6	76.9	77.3	77.8	78.4	74.1	74.6	75.4	76.1	79.5	79.8	80.2	80.6
7	77.2	77.6	78.3	79.0	74.6	75.2	75.9	76.8	79.7	79.9	80.6	81.1
8	77.5	78.0	78.6	79.3	74.9	75.6	76.3	77.1	80.0	80.4	80.8	81.4
9	78.0	78.4	79.0	79.7	75.4	76.0	76.8	77.7	80.3	80.6	81.1	81.7
10	78.3	78.8	79.5	80.3	75.9	76.5	77.3	78.3	80.6	81.0	81.5	82.2
Slope index of inequality	3.71	3.69	3.80	3.87	4.47	4.50	4.57	4.64	3.00	2.94	3.08	3.12
Difference between highest and lowest												
Poverty group	3.91	3.95	4.02	4.06	4.73	4.84	4.89	4.97	3.16	3.15	3.20	3.17
Local authority†	8.9	8.6	8.7	9.4	9.8	10.0	10.7	11.0	8.1	7.8	7.5	8.4

* Groups formed by ranking local authority districts according to poverty and grouping them into 10ths of equal population size on the basis of this ranking.
† Individual local authority areas with the highest and lowest life expectancies.

For males the slope index of inequality increased from 4.47 to 4.64 over the period studied, and the difference in life expectancy between the top and bottom poverty groups rose from 4.73 to 4.97 years (table). When individual local authority districts are compared, the difference between the one with the lowest life expectancy (Glasgow City) and the one with the highest (East Dorset) has risen to 11 years. Since Victorian times, such inequalities have never been as high.[17]

---

[17] Dorling, D. (1998) *Death in Britain: how local mortality rates have changed: 1950s–1990s*. York: Joseph Rowntree Foundation, 1997. And: Szreter, S. and Mooney G. (1998) Urbanization, mortality, and the standard of living debate: new estimates of the expectation of life at birth in nineteenth century British cities. *Economic History Review*, 51:84-112.

For females the slope index of inequality increased from 3.00 to 3.12, but the difference in life expectancy between the top and bottom poverty groups remained stable (table). Comparison of individual local authorities, however, showed that the difference between the one with the lowest life expectancy (Glasgow City) and the one with the highest (Kensington and Chelsea) has risen to 8.4 years from 8.1 years in 1992–4.

Figure 7.2: Slope index of inequality (SII) for life expectancy (by area level poverty) 1992–94 to 2001–03, and income ineqalities (gini coefficient) 1981 to 2002–03.

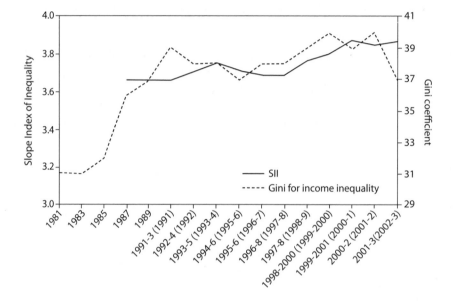

Note: The first years shown relate to income inequality trend, the years in brackets relate to life expectancy data, which are three year aggregates. The gini coefficient (the ratio of the area under the Lorenz curve to the area under the diagonal on the graph of the Lorenz curve) is a measure of inequality where 0 represents complete equality (all people have the same income) and 100 represents the most extreme inequality (one person receives all the income).

Source: Life expectancy data from analysis by authors, income inequality from Lakin (2004).

Figure 7.2 shows the trend in the slope index of inequality in life expectancy alongside trend data for income inequalities from the early 1980s to the early 2000s. We derived time series data on income inequality from work by Lakin (2004). Trends in both series of data fell slightly in the early 1990s—when John Major's Conservative government was in power. The current New Labour government thus inherited a slightly improving situation in terms of both mortality and income inequalities. Since the mid-1990s, however, and (as can be seen from these new results) continuing into the first years of the 21st century, both mortality inequality (by poverty by area) and income inequality increased. The notable exception to this is that in the most recent period for which data are available income inequalities decreased. Closer investigation of the factors contributing to this suggests that direct taxation may have become slightly more redistributive, alongside increases in benefits for those at the lower end of the income distribution, since the 2001 budget announcements were implemented in April 2002.

What does all this show?

The new data and the use of conventional measures such as slope index of inequality show increases in health inequalities in the early years of the 21st century in the UK: life expectancy continues to rise in the most advantaged areas of the country at a greater pace than in the poorest areas. This is despite much government rhetoric during the two terms of its administration [New Labour's first two terms, 1995–2005] proclaiming its intention to tackle health inequalities.

Moreover, for almost 20 years now, income inequality has remained at a historically high level. Income inequalities rose markedly in the 1980s and have been sustained throughout the 1990s and into the 2000s (Lakin, 2004). These inequalities are such that the poorest 10% in society now receive 3% of the nation's total income, whereas the richest 10% receive more than a quarter (Goodman and Shephard, 2002). Income inequality is only part of the picture, however.

Wealth (which can be financial, such as savings, or in terms of other assets, such as house ownership) is more unequally distributed than is income. From a life course perspective wealth—which reflects lifelong circumstances—is a more salient measure than income. The distribution of wealth became more equal through much of the 20th century, but since the 1970s wealth inequality has increased, particularly so since 1995–6.[18] Between 1990 and 2000 the percentage of wealth held by the wealthiest 10% of the population increased from 47% to 54%, and the share of the top 1% rose from 18% in 1990 to 23% in 2000 (Goodman and Shephard, 2002). In Britain by area between 1993 and 2003, the housing wealth of the best-off 10th of children increased by 20 times more than that of the worst-off 10th of children.[19]

Clearly for some health outcomes there will be a delay in terms of the effect of material circumstances; the full impact of present income inequalities on population health may not be immediately apparent. Wealth inequalities, on the other hand, better reflect the accumulation of lifetime (dis)advantage, and the growing inequalities in wealth seen in recent years do not bode well for future trends in health inequalities.

---

[18] Cabinet Office (2005) *Strategic audit: progress and challenges for the UK*. London: Prime Minister's Strategy Unit.

[19] Dorling, D. and Thomas, B. (2004) Know your place: housing wealth and inequality in Great Britain 1980–2003 and beyond. The Shelter policy library, 26 November. http://england.shelter.org.uk/files/docs/7970/Knowyourplace.pdf (accessed 11 Apr 2005).

Are these inequalities inevitable?

Inequalities vary between countries, and some have reduced their internal inequalities in recent years (Hills, 2004). Inequalities in income and wealth are determined by policies on tax and benefits. Our levels of social security benefit for those out of work are relatively low compared with EU poverty standards (Hills, 2004) and too low to sustain good health.(Morris *et al.*, 2000, 2004).

Are these inequalities acceptable?

The British Social Attitudes Survey series has tracked the population's opinion on the key issue that underlies health inequality since 1983 (Bromley, 2003) asking: 'Thinking of income levels generally in Britain today, would you say that the gap between those with high incomes and those with low incomes is too large, about right or too small?'

In 1983, 72% of the population said that this gap was too large, and since 1989 this has been the view of 80% or more; in 2002, 82% of people thought this gap too large. Moreover, most people in each socioeconomic group, income group, and self-rated hardship group thought that the gap between people on high and low salaries was too large (77% of those 'living comfortably', 84% of those 'coping', and 90% of those 'having difficulty'). There is also consensus with this view across the broad political spectrum, by party identification (71% of Conservative voters, 88% of Labour voters, 84% of Liberal Democrats voters, and 81% of those with no affiliation; Bromley, 2003).

Yet 'redistribution' is a dirty word in British politics, and we are a far cry from Denis Healey's threat to 'tax the rich until the pips squeak'. In the run up to the general election [of 2005] Labour and the Conservatives will not even hint at any tax rises; only the Liberal Democrats have a manifesto policy to increase the income tax of those earning more than £100 000 a year (1% of the total population). Despite their commitment to tackling health inequalities, when it comes to underlying income inequalities, New Labour have been prepared only to try lifting some sections of the population out of poverty; they have yet to effectively tackle the wider issue of inequality. The small changes towards redistribution of income that (may) have recently occurred need to be seen in the context of increasing inequalities in wealth (which may partly be a lag effect of increased income inequalities over the preceding decade; Lakin, 2004), although only large reductions in inequalities in income can lead to a long term reduction in inequalities in wealth.

Have policy changes been sufficient to redress these inequalities?

In the light of the evidence from 100 years of poverty research in Britain it was recently claimed of the government's strategy on poverty that: 'Though the treatment is good and getting better, the dose needs strengthening.... If the government is going to be able to deliver on poverty it is going to need to raise more from our tax system and make it more redistributive.'[20]

Despite favourable economic circumstances, and inroads made by initiatives such as the national minimum wage, new deal, and tax credits, more substantial redistributive policies are needed that address both poverty and income inequality.

What do recent changes suggest for inequalities in the future?

The current trend of growing inequalities in wealth suggests that we are likely to see growing inequalities, transmitted to and magnified among future generations. However, if there were the political will, the reduction in income inequalities seen for 2002-3 could signal a turning point in this vitally important trend.

References

Acheson, D. (1998) *Independent inquiry into inequalities in health*. London: Stationery Office.

Bromley, C. (2003) Has Britain become immune to inequality? In: Park A., Curtice J., Thomson K., Jarvis L. and Bromley C., eds. *British social attitudes: continuity and change over two decades*. London: Sage.

Davey Smith, G., Dorling, D., Mitchell, R. and Shaw, M. (2002) 'Health inequalities in Britain: continuing increases up to the end of the 20th century', *Journal of Epidemiology and Community Health*, 56:434-5.

Davey Smith, G., Dorling, D. and Shaw, M. (2001) *Poverty, inequality and health in Britain: 1800–2000: A reader*. Bristol: The Policy Press.

Davey Smith, G., Morris, J.N. and Shaw, M. (1998) 'The independent inquiry into inequalities in health', *British Medical Journal*, 17: 1465-6.

DH, Department of Health (2002) *Tackling health inequalities: 2002 cross-cutting review*. www.dh.gov.uk/assetRoot/04/06/80/03/04068003.pdf (accessed 11 Apr 2005).

DH, Department of Health (2003) *Tackling health inequalities: a programme for action*. London: DoH, 2003. (www.dh.gov.uk/assetRoot/04/01/93/62/04019362.pdf)

DHSS, Department of Health and Social Security (1980) *Inequalities in health: report of a working group*. London: DHSS (Black Report).

Donkin, A., Goldblatt, P. and Lynch, K. (2002) Inequalities in life expectancy by social class, 1972-1999. *Health Statistics Quarterly*, 15 (autumn): 5-15.

Goodman, A. and Shephard, A. (2002) *Inequality and living standards in Great Britain: some facts*. London: Institute for Fiscal Studies.

Hills, J. (2004) Policy challenges and dilemmas for the next 20 years, in: Glennerster, H., Hills, J., Piachaud, D. and Webb, J., eds. *One hundred years of poverty and policy*. York: Joseph Rowntree Foundation.

Lakin, C. (2004) 'The effects of taxes and benefits on household income, 2002-2003', *Economic Trends*, 607:39-84.

---

[20] Bradshaw, J. (2004) Understanding and overcoming poverty, Keynote address given at Joseph Rowntree Foundation Centenary Conference, University of York, 13 December.

Morris, J. and Deeming, C. (2004) 'Minimum incomes for health living (MIHL): next thrust in UK social policy?', *Policy & Politics*, 32: 441-54.

Morris, J., Donkin, A., Wonderling, D., Wilkinson, P. and Dowler, E. (2000) 'A minimum income for healthy living', *Journal of Epidemiology Community Health*, 54: 885-9.

Shaw, M., Dorling, D., Gordon, D. and Davey Smith, G. (1999) *The widening gap: health inequalities and policy in Britain*. Bristol: The Policy Press.

8

Closer to equality? Assessing New Labour's record on health after 10 years in government[1]

Dorling, D. (2007) 'Health', in J. Crudas *et al* (eds) *Closer to equality? Assessing New Labour's record on equality after 10 years in government*, London: Compass.

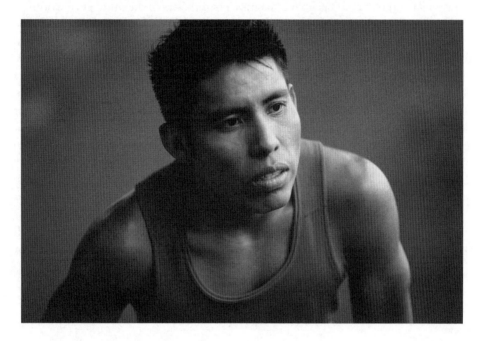

"I say to the doubters, judge us after ten years in office. For one of the fruits of that success will be that Britain has become a more equal society. However, we will have achieved that result by many different routes, not just the redistribution of cash from rich to poor, which others choose as their own limited version of egalitarianism ..." (Peter Mandelson, Labour's Next Steps: Tackling Social Exclusion, Speech to the Fabian Society, 1997)

---

[1] Editorial Note: The chapter title here has been reworded to include the title of the report it was drawn from.

When New Labour came to office of all the inequalities they had to tackle they knew what mattered most.[2] The new health secretary, Frank Dobson, spelt it out to the House of Commons. He said:

> *"There are huge inequalities in our society. Poor people are ill more often and die sooner. And that's the greatest inequality of them all – the inequality between the living and the dead."*[3]

The Government identified two 'body counts' as targets to measure the success of their policies in reducing health inequalities. The first was of the number of working-class infants dying in their first year of life as compared to the number that would be expected to die were the infants born to middle-class parents. The second concerned the differences in life expectancy found between different areas across the country.

The definitions of both targets were altered over time. But, almost no matter how you measure the two targets, in general their progress has been in one direction only – toward the greatest inequality. Health inequalities have increased year on year under New Labour. Health inequalities reflect inequalities in society in general but are the most obvious and important outcome of the government's failure to tackle inequality locally[4].

Target 1: Infant mortality rates

Figure 8.1 shows for babies born to working-class parents the percentage by which their infant mortality rates have been above average levels in England and Wales for

---

[2] Editorial Note: In his introduction to the report this chapter is reproduced from, Jon Cruddas MP quoted the words of Peter Mandelson, who managed to so damage egalitarianism by his supposedly 'less limited' vision. By 2007 Peter had become a European Commissioner for Trade. Within Europe trade suffered shortly afterwards. In 2008 Peter became UK Secretary of State for Business, Enterprise and Regulatory Reform, just about the time of Lehman Brothers' crash and when a lack of regulatory reform in Britain became evident. By 2009 he become Lord President of the Council and took on a great many other titles of pomp. Peter was one of the principal architects of New Labour. It is not that everything Peter touched turned bad, but it is worth learning to beware people who not only think they have an especially unlimited vision, but who also think it is a good idea to tell others of their great ability. Peter, born in the same year as Tony Blair, 'read' PPE at St Catherine's College Oxford (1973-1976). Tony was 'reading' Jurisprudence at St Johns around the same time.
[3] Jack Warden, *BMJ*, 1998, 316: 493 (14 Feb) http://www.bmj.com/cgi/content/full/316/7130/493/d
[4] There is, of course, a far greater body count that will dominate the history of New Labour until the last of its architects are themselves dead, and which puts our local body counting into context: See Kim McPherson, 2005, 'Counting the dead in Iraq' *BMJ*, 330, 550-551, 'Counting the dead is intrinsic to civilised society. Understanding the causes of death is a core public health responsibility'. doi:10.1136/bmj.330.7491.550

each year between 1996 and 2004 inclusive[5]. If there were no differences between the chances of working-class and middle-class babies dying during the first year of life (most in their first few weeks) the bars would have zero height. That is the direction, towards equality, the direction that the statistics were taking from 1996 to 1998. However, from 1998 on, apart from two 'blips', the gap has relentlessly grown.

Figure 8.1: Infant mortality rates in England and Wales 1996–2005.

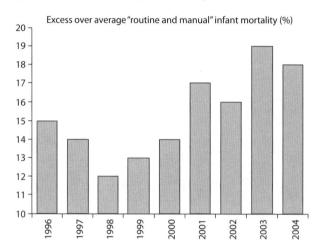

Source: Official target to reduce inequalities in health, excess mortality amongst the infants to parents labelled as being of 'routine and manual' social classes.

The growth of the gap in the survival chances of infants born to working class parents and infants born to middle class parents reflects well the growth of the gap between the material living standards of their parents and prospective parents. It is important to note that the government's decision to differentiate non-working individuals without children from those with children in the welfare and benefit system has led to many infants being born to parents without the means to care for themselves during pregnancy, or properly for their child after birth. Tax credits, child and other benefits associated with having children kick in too slowly for most of these children who die so soon after birth. There is a correlation between that

---

[5] The source of data used to draw Figure 8.1 is: Tackling health inequalities: Status report on the Programme for Action, London: Department of Health, 11 August 2005, p 27 (note infant mortality figures are for England and Wales only; figures for three year period ending December of the date shown, last period being 2001-2003 in that data). Note also that by very large area, reported infant mortality rates, 2002, were lowest at 3.8 per thousand live births in the Norfolk, Suffolk and Cambridgeshire Strategic Health Authority (SHA) and at 3.9 per thousand in Thames Valley SHA. Rates were highest at 7.0 per thousand in West Yorkshire SHA and 7.7 per thousand in Birmingham and the Black Country SHA. The latest 2003–2005 national figures are derived from: Tackling health inequalities: 2003-05 data update for the national 2010 PSA target, London: Department of Health, 21 December 2006. The change was slight, a 1% drop, and within the bounds of error (which the rise is not). Being published in August and just before Christmas neither report has received much attention.

financial punishment and the rising relative numbers of dead bodies of poor infants under New Labour[6].

Figure 8.2: A measure of social integration between geographical areas: Life expectancy estimates diverging in the United Kingdom 1995–2005.

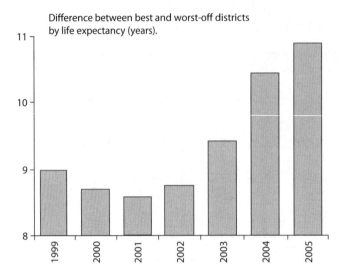

Source: Office for National Statistics, General Registrar's Office (Scotland) and the Northern Ireland Statistics & Research Agency.

Target 2: Life expectancy comparisons by area

Figure 8.2 shows the difference of life expectancy between the best-off and worst-off districts in the UK in the years between 1999 and 2005 (inclusive)[7]. The government uses complex measures to calculate inequalities in life expectancy by area, and their preferred measures have changed in definition. But the government's own figures highlight the same trends of rising inequalities as are seen in infant mortality rates. Figure 8.2 illustrates the trend more simply by comparing life expectancies of the

[6] Editorial Note: To see Figure 8.1 updated with the next six years of data, turn to Figure 44.1 on p 432 of Chapter 44. The high rates of inequality reached by 2002 were matched or exceeded through to 2008. After that there were two years of rapid improvement in the statistics and finally, by 2010, the ratio was better than it had been in 1998. As noted in footnote 4 of Chapter 2 (on p 30), the recent falls may not be the final effect of progressive social policy but emergency action taken as social disintegration increased. The falls are also coincident with the increased number of children being taken into care following the death of 'Baby P' on 3 August 2007 and the subsequent investigation into his death but geographically there is no correlation between fallin infant mortality and increases in numbers of children being taken into care (see footnote 2 in Chapter 44, this volume).

[7] Source: ONS details in Dorling, D., Mitchell, R., Orford, S., Shaw, M. and Davey Smith, G. (2005). Inequalities and Christmas Yet to Come. *BMJ*, 331 (7529): 1409 [reproduced as Chapter 3, this volume]. Also see http://sasi.group.shef.ac.uk/ publications/2005/BMJ_letter_dec05.pdf. Figure 2 in Dorling, D. (2006) Class Alignment Renewal, *The Journal of Labour Politics* 14(1), 8-19. Open access version available here: http://sasi.group.shef.ac.uk/publications/2006/dorling_class_alignment.pdf

populations of the most extreme districts year on year. Again the largest increases have been in the most recent years. Figure 8.2 is hardly good evidence that the continuing widening of the gap is merely a legacy of a past era of Conservative policies[8].

In 2006, a Department of Health report stated:

> *Nationally, life expectancy is increasing for both men and women, including in the Spearhead areas. But it is increasing more slowly there, so the gap continues to widen, and it is widening more for women than men. For males the relative gap is 2% wider than at the baseline (compared to 1% wider in 2002-2004), for females 8% wider (the same as in 2002–2004). The 2003–2005 relative gaps show little change over the 2002–2004 figures, and data are subject to year-on-year fluctuation.[9]*

When these figures were first released, my colleagues and I wrote this [stated above on page 48 but worth stating again]:

> *On 10 November National Statistics released new life expectancy figures by area and announced that 'Inequalities in life expectancy persist across the UK'.*
>
> *'Persist' was an odd word to use. In Kensington and Chelsea, where it was already highest, it rose by exactly one year for both men and women (from 79.8 to 80.8 years and 84.8 to 85.8 years, respectively). In contrast, in Glasgow where it was lowest a year ago, life expectancy remained static at 76.4 years for women, and rose just slightly for men from 69.1 to 69.3 years. The range in life expectancy between the extreme highest and lowest areas thus increased from 8.4 to 9.4 years for women, and from 10.7 years to 11.5 years for men. For men and women combined, the life expectancy gap between the worst and best off districts of the UK now exceeds 10 years for the first time since reliable measurements began.'*

A year's data later and the range in life expectancy has increased again to 9.5 years for women and 12.3 years for men – and the combined gap is now almost 11 years (10.9) – just twelve months after it passed the 10 year point[10]. The overall life expectancy of a population is a health indicator that responds more slowly to policy

---

[8] It was of course the Conservative governments of 1979–1997 that saw and helped the gap widen from historically low levels of inequality experienced in the 1950s, 1960 and early 1970s.

[9] Tackling health inequalities: 2003–05 data update for the national 2010 PSA target, London: Department of Health, 21 December 2006, p 6 (on which it also shows the gap in life expectancy between the Spearhead group and the rest widening from 2.60% to 2.61% for men in the most recent period, and from 1.90% to 1.91% for women). See http://www.dh.gov.uk/en/Publicationsandstatistics/Publications/Public ationsStatistics/DH_06368

[10] 21 November 2006 press release, ONS: http://www.statistics.gov.uk/ pdfdir/liex1106.pdf. 'Of the ten local authorities with the highest male life expectancy at birth all are in England: five in the South East, three in the East of England, and one each in the South West and London. Eight of the ten local authorities with the lowest male life expectancy are in Scotland. Glasgow City (69.9 years) is the only area in the UK where life expectancy at birth is less than 70 years. The local authority with the highest male life expectancy is Kensington and Chelsea (82.2 years), 12.3 years more than Glasgow City. Kensington and Chelsea also has the highest life expectancy for females (86.2 years), 9.5 years more than Glasgow City, the lowest at 76.7 years.'

interventions than does infant mortality[11]. Part of this widening gap will include the legacy of the different rates at which smoking for instance declined by social class in the past. However, the exacerbated sorting of people by class and ability to pay for housing between areas under New Labour has greatly magnified any such legacy effects.

Just as the rising inequalities in the chances of working-class babies dying as compared to the middle class reflect the rising material inequalities between poor parents (and most importantly prospective parents) and the rest, so rising inequalities in life expectancy between areas are a mirror of the rising economic inequalities that have emerged so clearly between different parts of Britain under New Labour. Regional geographical inequalities have risen faster under New Labour than they did under Margaret Thatcher. This may not have been the plan, but the effect in terms of the relative inequality body count has been devastating.

Conclusion

Current rates of growth in area health inequalities are unsustainable. They are unsustainable because immortality is not possible and so life expectancy cannot carry on rising so quickly where it is highest to begin with. Similarly there are limits beneath which infant mortality cannot fall (probably of around 1 infant dying per 1000 born). Because of this we should expect inequalities in infant health to improve in the future. The fact that human beings and infant babies are not immortal should not be a comfort to those in New Labour who hope to eventually welcome the turning of the trend in these graphs as proof that their policies have finally worked. What has been allowed to occur over the last ten years has been an abject failure, a dereliction of hope, when compared to the stated aims of New Labour when it came to power in 1997.

If New Labour has achieved anything positive in terms of health inequalities, they can claim to have presided over an era when health inequalities in Britain have not been transformed into the terrible absolute gaps that can be seen to have emerged in recent years in the United States of America – but that is hardly an achievement.

At some point soon the calculation will be made of the actual absolute number of babies that would have lived to see their first birthday, of men who would have made it to at least a year of retirement, and of women who would not have seen their children die before them – had New Labour achieved its ambitions to reduce

---

[11] Editorial Note: This is now evident from the recent changes discussed in footnote 6, where it is suggested that policy intervention did have an effect, but not the interventions planned when this chapter was written. There has been no similar move towards target 2. Figure 41.3, on p 381 in Chapter 41, updates Figure 8.2 in this chapter with the latest data, showing the overall life expectancy gap to have grown to more than 12.5 years of life by 2010. Very recently there have been unpublished suggestions that the gap between areas might finally be falling because the absolute number of deaths in the poorest areas has been falling, but this could be due to increased out migration and emigration as the long economic recession continues. Until detailed 2011 census data are released during 2013 we cannot be sure. Even then we may not know how many people who are now recorded as living in the UK only live there for part of the year.

inequalities in health in the period May 1997 to May 2007. All these infants and children and adults are now dead. In by far the greatest proportion will be those that voted Labour in 1997, or whose parents and grandparents had voted Labour in both that year and were the basis of that party's success in the past. Perhaps each Labour MP and Minister needs this list[12] to help them understand who amongst those they represented from 1997 is no longer here as a result of this policy failure?

Many of those Labour MPs whose constituents have suffered most due to the failure to narrow inequalities have had the power to change policy. Notable in the [1997 or 2007] government are Hazel Blears, who loses over 100 potential voters a year due to the continuation of such inequalities: one thousand excess young deaths in her constituency since she first contended her Salford seat. There are 750 fewer folk to vote for John Reid now where he has been MP since 1997; 640 fewer for Jack Straw; 590 less for Harriet Harman; and 360 less in the Dunfermline East constituency of Gordon Brown. These deaths are all due to the continued extent of inequalities in life chances in the United Kingdom. These figures all represent people who have died before they reached age 65 because rates in their area remain so much in excess of the national average. When these figures were first calculated they were the hypothetical body counts that would result from policy failure. Now they are gravestones in cemeteries and plaques in crematoria and, of course, thousands upon thousands of fairly fresh memories of lives that need not have ended so soon.

For a few MPs, enough of their constituents have died both prematurely and unnecessarily since 1997 to have been able to fill the House of Commons from their constituency's toll alone. It may well have been worse had another party won power in 1997, but for so many it could have been so much better. If we do not learn that what has been achieved since 1997 was not enough for so many people then there is little point in counting the dead.

---

[12] The list of potential victims of policy failure was drawn up shortly after the 1997 election victory: see Dorling, D. (1998) Whose voters suffer if inequalities in health remain?, *Journal of Contemporary Health*, 7, 50-54. The full paper is available here: http://www.sasi.group.shef.ac.uk/publications/1998/dorling_voting_and_inequalities.pdf. Table 5 in the paper listed the number of voters who would continue to die young 1997 onwards, by their MPs, in the worst-off areas, were inequalities to remain so high.

9

Social harm and social policy in Britain[1]

Dorling, D. (2007) 'Social harm and social policy in Britain', in Roberts, R. and McMahon, W. (eds) *Social justice and criminal justice*, London: Centre for Crime and Justice Studies, chapter 10

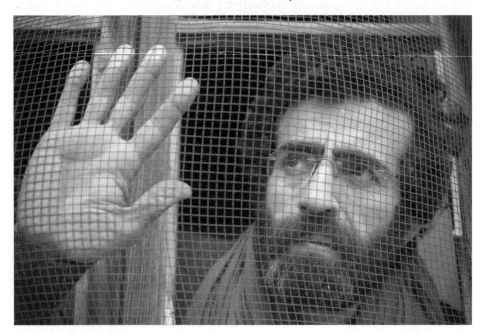

Introduction

'The distinction', Dupuy says, 'between a killing by an intentional individual act' and killing as a result of 'the egoistic citizens of rich countries focussing their concerns on their own well-being while others die of hunger' is becoming less and less tenable. (Bauman's 2006, page 100, translation of Jean-Pierre Dupuy's statement)

In Britain, France, and no doubt almost everywhere, part of the understanding and study of crime is slowly refocusing on studying social harms more widely defined and often more damaging than those acts we currently choose to criminalise. The most devastating acts of social harm concern the preventable deaths of one hundred

---

[1] A longer version of this argument appears as an editorial in the *Journal of Public Health Medicine*, autumn 2007 (Dorling, 2007a). A copy is available here: http://www.dannydorling.org/?page_id=514 and an extract from that paper is included in Chapter 15 of this volume.

million children under the age of five globally that occur every decade. Locally, premature deaths that could be prevented if we cared can be counted each decade in Britain in only hundreds and thousands by area – but still the vast majority who die even in this country due to the callousness of others do not die directly at their hands. It is not murder that accounts for the ten fold 'variations' in infant mortality between areas at the extremes.

In practise much of the harm is institutionalised. Welfare spending in Britain is set so that those reliant on it live in poverty. The government aims to abolish poverty by getting folk 'who can' into work and one way they do this is by making life outside of work very hard to live for those the government thinks should work. One effect of this is to damage the bodies of, (and subsequent survival chances of the babies of) those who become pregnant while living in poverty. Eating, resting and living well while pregnant is not possible when living in poverty. However, what possibly matters even more than physically damaging their bodies though such treatment is damaging young adult minds.

If the government tells you through your own welfare payments how little you are worth a week why have much respect for yourself? And what pleasures can you expect in life? You may as well have a smoke, or worse. If you think I'm making this case too strongly walk past the line of new teddy bear shaped grave stones in any large municipal cemetery of a poor town and then look at the odd one or two such stones in the cemetery near where you live. You can't blame the infants for dying, so do you think the harm was caused by apparently feckless parents?

Current inequalities in infant mortality in Britain are the most obvious manifestation of the social harm poor social policy can bring. The statistics of the last century show that previous Labour (and Liberal) governments had a better record of narrowing the gap than the current [2007] one has (Dorling, 2006a); and in more than just our mortality (Dorling, 2006b).

In this short commentary I want to try to show how the banal process of public policy creation is currently often skewed to result in outcomes that in turn result in greater social harm for little meaningful benefit. There is also much that is good and well meaning in current policy creation, but a streak of particularly nasty inhuman market idolisation runs though much of what is today being proposed on this richest of islands to deal with its poorest of people.

Many know this to be the case. Some of the civil servants insert clues to their discontent by giving fatuous examples of the implications of proposed policy in even the pages of published Green Papers! I give a few references below. I suspect that at the heart of some of our current stupidity is the naivety of a few who do not realise that we are all human and those who are poor are not some other species that can be treated differently. In contrast there are also plenty of signs of good intent and of those involved in the process who still see people as people and the error of the relentless pursuit of ever more wealth and work.

The new welfare reform bill

The *Mental Health Bill 2006* was introduced to the House of Lords by the then Minister of Health, Lord Warner. Part of the extremely long debate over its clauses concerned changes to the ways in which individuals could be deprived of their liberty. It was a mess and denounced by 77 charities and other members of the most concerned 'policy-alliance' as '*a missed opportunity for legislation fit for the twenty-first century*' (Mental Health Alliance, 2007). Depriving individuals of their liberties of course requires serious debate and members of parliament (and their civil servant advisors) should have done better than they did, but what was introduced by Lord Warner in November 2006 was not, I argue, the real mental health bill. That came later with *The Welfare Reform Bill 2006* designed to alter the lives of hundreds of thousands of people who have not worked for at least the last two years, mostly because of mental illness.

There are currently over two million people surviving due to receiving Incapacity Benefit (Freud[2], 2007, page 4, Figure 2 and PFMHTWG, 2006, page 8). The majority are too mentally ill and demoralised to work (while others are working with such illness, and many others are ill and not working nor claiming). I have documented some of the bizarre process of public consultation over the Bill elsewhere (Dorling, 2007a), it is now law and effects far more people with mental illness than the Bill but received far less attention.

Despite the Welfare Reform Bill (2006) having become law, much of its potential effects are still to be determined. As with the Mental Health Bill, the actual law does not determine the codes of practice and other mechanisms that will now be put in place[3]. It simply enables them to be. In this way members of parliament do not get to scrutinise what will actually happen at the point when they could have most effect.

The key policy turning point was obscure: the Minister's (then Jim Murphy's) acceptance of the Physical Function and Mental Health Technical Working Group's (PFMHTWG, 2006) Report on the Transformation of the Personal Capability Assessment of the Department of Work and Pensions (DWP). The remit of the Minister's department's working groups included, especially for the mentally ill, to '*accurately identify those who in spite of their condition are fit to continue to work*' (*ibid* page 2). They did this by attempting to assess the level of functional limitation at which it is unreasonable to require a person to engage in work.

What level of cognitive and intellectual function is too low; what degree of learning disability too high; of autistic spectrum disorder too severe; or of acquired

---

[2] Editorial Note: These figures were written when 'currently' was 2007 and David Freud was the New Labour appointed advisor on 'Welfare to Work'. By 2012 he had become Baron Freud, the Conservative Party's unelected Parliamentary Under Secretary of State for Work and Pensions. He did not appear to need to change any of his views or recommendations as he changed political allegiance from New Labour to Tory.

[3] Editorial Note: See Figure 15.1, on p 168 in Chapter 15 for an example of the new points systems introduced where 'being too frightened to go out alone' is only worth half of 'my mental problems impair my ability to communication with other people'. Agoraphobia is no excuse for not going out to work in twenty-first century Britain.

brain injury too poor scoring on their new system, to excuse a working age adult from the compulsion to labour in the New Britain to come? As I say, despite the Welfare Reform Bill having now passed into law we don't know the precise answers because their main recommendation involves testing and further developing, and full piloting of various claimant questionnaires and forms of medical evidence certification throughout 2007 (*ibid* page 4) and I am writing this in August of that year, but already there are enough clues to guess at the outcomes (Dorling, 2007a).

The current Personal Capability Assessment (PCA) is too physically based for the liking of the technical groups. Currently an assessment is made as to the extent that your limbs work; you can see, talk, and hear enough for whatever it is you might do; you can remain conscious; and can control your bowel and urine voluntarily. Points are given for how well (or badly depending on your point of view) you score on these and hit the magic number of 15 such that you are entitled to benefit. At that number, or above, they currently consider it would be unreasonable to expect you to work. Below that number and they have ways of making you work. It's not called 'New Labour' for nothing.

Not all work is good for you

The impetus for changing the rules in Britain over who has to undertake paid work has been the rise in benefit claimants suffering from mental health problems, depression and anxiety; and the falls in the number suffering back pain (PFMHTWG, 2006, page 8, paragraph 13). As our industrial employment continues to collapse at a rate as fast as it ever did in the 1980s it is hardly surprising that fewer folk have been developing serious musculoskeletal conditions (Dorling, 2006b)[4].

Changing industries and technology is not the reason more people are unable to work due to mental illness. Instead it is the rise in mental illness itself along (possibly) with a fall in our tolerance of difference. The huge rise there has been at work has been in employment with very low skilled service jobs (Elliott and Atkinson, 2007). So what could be contributing to the rise in mental illness? Illness rates have risen among children and the elderly in Britain, not just for those of working age, and they are highest where most people also spend most time providing unpaid care, so if the rise is partly deceit it is a very well organised deceit involving children, carers and pensioners too!

One possibility is that it is the substantive nature of the recent change in the nature work and society that literally made people ill. It is not a superficial difficulty with saying the words '*would you like to go large with that, sir?*' that presents the mental challenge. It's the mind-numbing drudgery of serving folk with crap, having to say

---

[4] Editorial Note: Industrial employment continued to fall through to 2012, which continued to increase sickness amongst the marginally employed. For the trend to 2009, see Minton, J., Pickett, K. and Dorling, D. (2012) "Health, Employment and Economic Change, 1973–2009: a repeated cross-sectional study", *BMJ*, 340:e2316 doi: 10.1136/bmj.e2316 (published 9 May).

crap, having to wear crap[5], and be demeaned through doing all that which would make any individual depressed if they were to work as an automaton on show for too long. One of the government's responses to the problem of *worklessness* is to work closely with the fast-food chain McDonalds (DWP, 2007, page 6) to help them fill jobs nobody wants to do possibly through forced (and not necessarily paid) employment. This is one example of those clues to disenchantment left by civil servants in the recent *welfare* Green Paper. Another is their example of getting black women to work (again possibly by compulsion and not necessarily paid) as care assistants for those taking out private health insurance (*ibid* page 34).

When I read about DWP forcing black people to labour for either very little or no money I thought 'what a nice way to celebrate one of the centenary anniversaries of the abolition of directly sponsored British slavery'[6]. These are a few examples, but I would have found it hard to make them up or some of the many other ridiculous ideas clearly inserted to show how even many of those putting policy together within the heart of government dissent so much from the 'everyone must labour' mantra.

Think about it. It is not an enjoyable (or easy) or particularly rewarding process claiming Incapacity Benefit due to mental illness. It is not something you would boast about in the pub, after all, success does not fund many pints for anyone. How often do you hear people celebrating the fact that they managed to convince a DWP contracted private doctor to believe that they really do feel 'tired all the time', look forward to almost nothing in the future and think they personally have no significant contribution to make?

This rise in mental illness is no great scam to claim higher benefits. This is not the feckless masses conspiring to live it up on an enhanced dole. It is also not occurring in many places because there is a lack of jobs of any kind, just a lack of reasonable jobs. It has been many years since we have had so many jobs available and so many in work in Britain that people are free to chose their labour. But exactly what kind of jobs are these, those that we want the mentally ill in particular to take? What are the jobs left unsold at the bottom of the labour market? I'll give some examples below, but many more are given in the Green Paper through the websites of the firms that are the DWP's partners – those firms that obviously offer work that is so bad, they cannot easily find labourers (DWP, 2007, page 36).

One of the firms listed provides 'manned guarding services' – a boom industry, and much of the work is of that nature, shelf stacking or till serving. However, the same firm needing those currently on benefits due to mental illness to work as security guards is also contracted to decommission some of the 'ponds' at Sellafield, the future's

---

[5] A colleague who kindly commented on an earlier draft of this piece told me they once worked for a multinational firm where the uniform included trousers with no pockets below management level. Only the managers were trusted not to steal. When you are next in a cinema, fast-food restaurant, or similar establishment, have a look for the pockets (but please try not to be obvious in your glances).

[6] Editorial Note: Five years later the next government was introducing what came to be recognised by numerous commentators, trade unionists and activists as slavery, through the 'Skills Conditionality Next Step placement' schemes and similar; see Chapter 36, this volume.

bright in nuclear waste. But the majority of unfillable jobs are not quite so exciting, take former 'mining' and industrial areas and the new leisure industry for example.

The mining industry had been in decline for sixty years before its obliteration in the 1980s. In 1991 the area with the largest number of people working in the mining industry was the potteries, and these 'miners' were mostly women[7], presumably hand-painting ceramics of one kind or another (Dorling and Thomas, 2004). Monotonous work, and far better done by robot spray brush than human hand, but work nonetheless that did not involve a constant feeling of being devalued while having to appear something you are not: happy.

By 2001, around the potteries, as much as anywhere – services of one kind or another now employ almost all who are employed. The best known perhaps is the theme park of Alton Towers. And the person most likely to greet you as you take your seat for a meal there grew up in Warsaw rather than Stoke. For those with hope and a future, university students, well-educated Polish immigrants, gap year migrant working-tourists, asking minute after minute exactly the same questions of groups of people taking their plastic seats to eat plastic food – people who quickly blur into exactly the same customers – becomes not only a monotonous, but a very demeaning occupation.

Being a servant in the new economy is demeaning because the interaction is directly and repeatedly with people and their money, not with putting colours on white clay. Factory work is brain-numbing, but other than in Cadbury's Bourneville Chocolate factory (where tourists can pay to see those who help run the conveyor belts) it is not a spectacle. Today's acts of service are. And you are no longer the servant of a rich family, who might at least get to see you as slightly human out of familiarity. Today's service worker is the 'annoying' voice of the call centre, never the same twice; the 'surly' receptionist; 'slow' bar tender; or 'immigrant' restaurant

---

[7] People's jobs can be classified by the industry they work in. Thus in the mining industry, although for decades only adult men were allowed underground, it was (mainly) women who cooked the food that miners ate after their shift, clerks who worked on the surface, managers, and cleaners among many other occupations employed. The industry was repeatedly decimated to such an extent before, and especially after the miners' strike of 1984, that by 1991 the largest single group of people classified as working in the industry of mining by the Office for National Statistics (ONS) in any one local authority then were women working in districts in the potteries region. Ceramics were included in the extractive mining industries as clay has to be extracted from the ground, just as coal is. When this decision was made it is almost certain that no one in the bodies that preceded ONS ever thought that the greatest concentration of 'miners' would be women in Staffordshire. Incidentally the industry continued to collapse to 2001 employing only a seventh of the workforce of 1991. The potteries (and the Stoke area) suffered most, and the greatest concentrations remaining by 2001 were of people associated with the North Sea oil industry working in Scotland, and a rise of people working in 'mining' in the centre of London and out in Guildford – these being consultants associated with multinational mining companies working with bankers there (all recorded in the 2001 population census as 'miners'). Britain makes more money from mining than it ever did – it's just that most of the miners are now in copper, coal, iron and diamond mines in very far flung parts of the globe. The future for mining in Britain was far worse than anyone envisaged in 1984: there was no fall in the numbers of people working in dangerous conditions down holes in the ground – they were just working in holes in the ground in other countries – and many of the new miners are, of course, children.

worker in a theme park. You don't really like them – and they have to be nice to you and what you blow your money on: valueless stuff that they could not afford.

Every time they return your change for that drink in the chain-pub they are reminded by their hourly wage, they are worth less than a minute's profit that passes through their fingers. Every time they listen to you on the phone transferring money between your bank accounts, ordering consumer goods, holidays, hotel rooms, they are aware of how little they have. Look how old the next person serving you is or ask them on the phone. They are almost always under or around age thirty. I don't think that is because of an ageist recruitment practice. Almost no one could take the drudgery for long who could see there were better things to be had, all around them.

If it was you, and you did not know it would only be temporary, how would you begin to feel? For an extra 10 pounds an hour wouldn't you rather work around the nuclear waste ponds in Sellafield? If it were me, I would. If I had to face the idea that demeaning service work was my only option, for year after year, I'd begin to feel tired all the time. Think about doing it yourself, the hours, the pay, the conditions. Doing this kind of work makes people ill, as will the thought of doing it. Of course pre-industrial agricultural toil will have been almost as boring and more backbreaking, and seemed as interminable, but it might have been more consistent with dignity and self-respect. It is the servile, inferior, low-status of the jobs, in a society where we are very conscious of other possibilities which is new, not just the jobs, but the kind of society their existence and growth represents (Wilkinson, 2007).

Direct visual contact is not all that is required to feel demeaned. Those working in call centres only hear the (not 'their') customers. Those changing the sheets in hotels only get to smell the customer. But the constant realisation that so many people can afford the luxuries they order through your ear, or don't have to make their own beds, begins to grate. It was only a few years ago that people applied for a mortgage, rather than shopped around for one. Then the building society clerk looked down on, or more often across to, you as customer. In most cases a local customer. It was not much further back in time that only the very rich stayed in hotels. Far fewer beds needed changing by others' hands each morning (leaving aside who made beds in the home – and who was most depressed back then?).

Providing badly paid service labour is less and less a respectable profession, career, or something that makes you part of the old working class majority – cohesive at least in the collective experience of living at the whim of a small minority of the affluent. If you knew that most other people were reading scripts in answer to customer queries, changing bed sheets, serving at tables, or repeatedly asking whether folk wanted to 'go large' or not, you might convince yourself that this is as good as it gets. But you'd have to be quite unaware of how much many others get, let alone how much today's most affluent get, to be happy with your lot.

And then the magazines and daytime TV shows are filled with detail on the lifestyles of the rich and famous. Popular culture is obsessed with what kind of home or second home you can purchase for that odd extra couple of hundred thousand in your 'budget'; or with locations for exotic holidays; with quick fixes whereby nobodies can become famous; with a message that says that if you are not beautiful, thin, non-smoking, rich, attractive, interesting and enjoying a great job – it is your fault for not trying hard enough. We are surrounded by advertising for what we cannot afford. State schools charge for school trips to embarrass the poorest of children and their parents. And we have a regressive taxation system whereby those who get more pay are taxed less once indirect taxes such as VAT are taken into account. Only a fool would not feel hard done by.

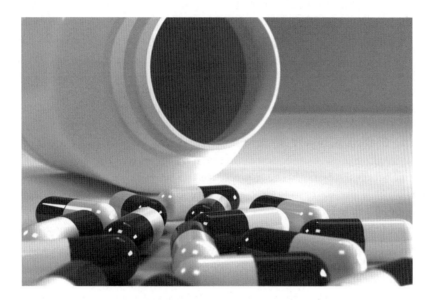

The solutions – mass medication?

In contract to my musings, the government's PFMHTWG report does not concern itself too much with the cause of the main component of the huge rise in mental illness; instead it just says that such depression is 'very amenable to therapeutic interventions' (PFMHTWG, 2006, page 8). It used to be psychoanalysis, but today there is medication, and if the drugs don't work, evidence can be created to show that they do (Dumit, 2005). There is a huge danger in implying that mass medication may be needed to get hundreds of thousands of depressed working age people to work.

What is needed, but lacking in almost all of this debate, is an understanding of how we came to organise our working lives to exclude so many who would like to work and to compel so many more to do jobs that might well make them ill. In the remainder of this commentary I concentrate on what is being suggested for the non-working mentally ill of working age in Britain to illustrate why that need for better understanding has become so vital now.

There are some sensible suggestions in the PFMHTWG report that imply less draconian ways in which more of the mentally ill can be coerced to work. It says that a new assessment regime should not be so biased against the mentally ill, scoring their afflictions so lightly; it could concentrate on the positive rather than the negative; it could involve practical help for people to find work rather than just simply assess their benefit entitlement status; it could be better linked to the pathways to work initiatives lauded as so successful in another more recent and much public DWP Report (Freud, 2007).

Incidentally don't be fooled by the figures in the (DWP-commissioned) Freud report suggesting spectacular falls in the number of Incapacity Benefit claimants in pathways pilot areas (a 9.5% fall on page 44 of his report). David Freud got his numbers wrong (to verify this simply read the sources he cites – they do not apply to all claimants as he implies, most of whom have been claiming for years, but apply only to a small minority of recent claimants), but then he is not a social scientist but a banker.[8]

David's report is titled *Independent*, but was both commissioned and published by the DWP. Independent no longer means independent. The point of independent reports to government and ministers is that they are not written by people who are independent of government but by folk whose lives and connections are intimately wound up in the machinery of government and elite civil society. For those who enjoy unravelling these connections, and given the origins of the Centre for Crime and Justice Studies[9] (formerly the Institute for the Scientific Study and Treatment of Delinquency), it is relevant to point out that David is the great grandson of Sigmund, and Sigmund was briefly associated with the Institute (CCJS, 2007). Delinquency was thought then and still by many now, to be a mental illness, possibly inherited. Although such thinking is today discredited the use of some of Sigmund's thinking to sell ideas to the public is continuous and underpins a huge consultancy industry: it is the basis of public relations (PR).

The DWP Working Group's report on the PCA (Personal Capability Assessment) was not written as an exercise in public relations. It is not all advertisers' bluff to try to get the public to purchase ideas that they should not really want to buy (if an idea is good it does not need PR which is needed the most the worse an idea or product is for you). Also parts of the report are not all carrot and stick. For instance, it suggests that as the PCA currently stands, it writes off too quickly people deemed to have learning disabilities and other conditions affecting their ability to think as not being able to work without considering their rights to work and support

---

[8] This is not an isolated example of innumeracy in the Freud report. That report will have been checked by civil servants so again I think their leaving of obvious gaffs in the text is an indicator of dissent in the policy maker ranks. Earlier in his report, on page 37, he suggested that: 'By 2009, over half the new entrants to the labour market are anticipated to be people in ethnic minorities.' Again Freud has misread the source he quotes (which is referring to half the increase, not half the total for new entrants). These errors do need pointing out as we should record how poor the 'evidence base' became in the dog days of the Blair government, when – presumably, as I suggest above, because so few civil servants had managed to maintain enthusiasm for the spin and were bothering to fact-check even simple things any more – such errors could emerge. For this error to be true would require (say) all new jobs to only be in London. And even then for their distribution to be skewed towards ethnic minorities dramatically, to redress old inequalities in employment in that city. Put another way, the only way David Freud could be correct is if Ken Livingstone became prime minister. I may be missing something here – but I really don't believe Ken's ascendancy is the establishment plot.

[9] Editorial Note: This chapter was originally given as the Eve Saville lecture at that Centre, hence the reference given here to the Centre's origins.

to work. Having a series of the most minor levels of physical ailment that can be recorded by the current system can entitle an individual to benefits whereas the same is not true of mental illnesses. The report also identifies the current self-assessment questionnaire as being 'hardly user-friendly', but then advocates a widening of the approach currently being piloted in 'Pathways to work' areas where a doctor is tasked with carrying out the PCA reports on each 'claimant's residual functional ability' PFMHTWG (2006, page 19). 'Residual functional ability' is not a phrase someone working in PR would applaud.

Conclusion: residual functioning ability

I suspect that the phase 'residual functional ability' will not make it to the final wording of the codes the proposed law is to enable: there is much work yet to be done on the language. But although the wording will change, it is unlikely that the underlying thinking and prejudices behind much of this current policy making will alter a great deal. These are not policies being made for the people making them – but with others in mind. When reading the report it became clear to me, that most of those who wrote it never expected to be assessed by these criteria, nor did they expect that for their children, lovers or friends. But they should, because the current numbers and trends make it very likely that all of us, or someone very close to us, will one day soon be assessed for whether our mental health means we are up to labouring.

So how can new social harms be averted such as those about to be inflicted through the *Welfare Reform Bill 2006* and far worse if the Green Paper is unopposed? During the final debate on the bill in the House of Commons on 17 May 2007 there was no dissent from the cross-party committee considering DWP's aims, including their aim of getting four out of five folk into paid work, almost regardless of what that work might do to these workers. One member of the government said:

> *The whole Committee agrees that the 80% target is wonderful; …* (Engel, 2007)

Perhaps all other MPs and folk in cyberspace (even the then DWP minister's blog went quiet) were keeping their heads down? Better not to be identified as a dissenter in this brave new world where more people will get better, more will work harder, more will be responsible, even if Natascha Engel ended her sentence above with a tiny note of caution. Here is what she said in full:

> *…The whole Committee agrees that the 80% target is wonderful; it was just the way to reach it that we had slight concerns about.*[10]

---

[10] Natascha was appointed parliamentary private secretary to Peter Hain MP a few weeks later. Hopefully she will still raise a few concerns as she climbs the ladder, but it is usually at this point of initial promotion that younger MPs become acquiescent.

Figure 9.1: **(a)** Number of dispensed items - Scotland, 2000/01 to 2009/10; **(b)** Number of DDDs per 1000 population (aged 15+) per day, 2000/01 to 2009/10; **(c)** Gross ingredient cost (£) of antidepressant drugs, 2000/01 to 2009/10.

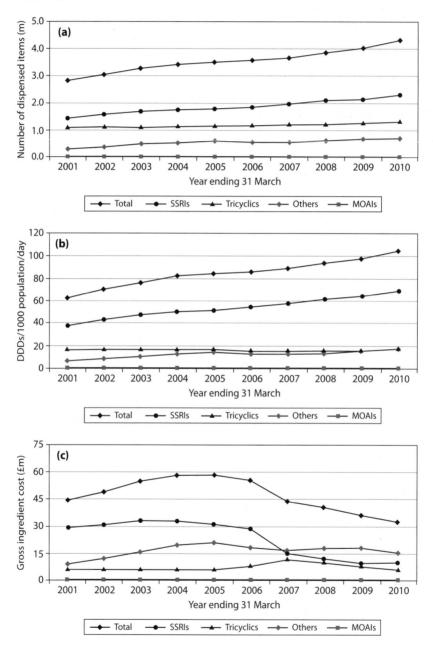

Note: DDD = Defined Daily Dose of antidepressant drugs.
      SSRI = Selective Serotonin Reuptake Inhibition.
      MOAI = Monoamine Oxidase Inhibitor

Source: Prescribing Information System, ISD Scotland. www.isdscotland.org.

One day soon such slight concerns need to be expressed a little more clearly. The more policy documents on health, work and well-being I read the more I come to believe more than ever that we need to be thinking more carefully about why so many of us have become so ill in recent years (Wilkinson, 2005). The alternative to more careful consideration is that '*in the not too distant future we will have mass medication, 80% in work, and wake up one morning and wonder what we are all working for*' (Anon, 2006)[11].

References

Anon (2006) Comments, http://www.dwp.gov.uk/welfarereform/blog/index. php/2006/10/19/ mental-health-action/#comments

Bauman, Z., (2006) *Liquid Fear*, Cambridge: Polity Press.

Beatty, C., Fothergill, S., Gore, T., and Powell, R. (2007) *The Real Level of Unemployment*, Sheffield: CRESR, http://www.shu.ac.uk/cresr/downloads/publications/The%20 Real%20Level%20of%20Un employment%202007-.pdf

Centre for Crime and Justice Studies (2007) *History of the CCJS*, http://www.kcl. ac.uk/depsta/rel/ccjs/history.html

Dorling, D. and Thomas, B. (2004) *People and Places: a Census Atlas of the UK*, Bristol: The Policy Press.

Dorling, D. (2006a) 'Infant mortality and social progress in Britain, 1905–2005', E. Garrett, C. Galley, N. Shelton, and R. Woods (eds) *Infant mortality*, Aldershot: Ashgate, Chapter 11 [reproduced as Chapter 4 of this volume].

Dorling, D. (2006b) Inequalities in Britain 1997-2006: The Dream that Turned Pear-Shaped. *Local Economy*, 21(4), 353–361, http://sasi.group.shef.ac.uk/ publications/2006/dorling_inequalityinBritain1997_corrected.pdf

Dorling, D. (2007a) Guest Editorial: The real mental health bill, *Journal of Public Mental Health*, 6(3), 6-13 [reproduced as Chapter 15 in this volume].

Dorling, D. (2007b) Health, in Compass (eds) *Closer to equality? Assessing New Labour's record on equality after 10 years in government*, London: Compass, http://clients. squareeye.com/uploads/ compass/documents/closertoequality.pdf [reproduced as Chapter 8 in this volume].

Dorling, D., Rigby, J., Wheeler, B., Ballas, D., Thomas, B., Fahmy, E., Gordon, D., and Lupton, R. (2007) *Poverty, Wealth and Place in Britain, 1968 to 2005*, Bristol: The Policy Press.

Dumit, J. (2005) The de-psychiatrisation of mental illness, *Journal of Public Mental Health*, 4(3) 8-13.

---

[11] Editorial Note: Figure 9.1 illustrates the rise in mass medication prescriptions of just one set of drugs for just one country within the United Kingdom, Scotland. It shows that by 2010 well over four million antidepressants were being dispensed a year, more than one recommended daily dose for every one in ten Scots, and this is just the NHS prescriptions, ignoring the many other drugs that are taken legally and illegally, led by self-medication through alcohol and the harm that causes. This figure was not included in the original paper but illustrates just how rapid the rise in use has been over and beyond the period being described here. Part (c) of the figure shows that the costs of mass medicating the population are falling.

DWP (2007) 'In work, better off: next steps to full employment', in Green Paper, Cm 7130, London: HMSO:.

Elliott, L. and Atkinson, D. (2007) *Fantasy Island*, London: Constable and Robinson. http://books. guardian.co.uk/extracts/story/0,,2082838,00.html

Engel, N., MP for North East Derbyshire (2007) Contribution to Westminster Hall debate on the Government Employment Strategy, 17 May, London, *Hansard*, col 341WH, http://www.publications.parliament.uk/pa/cm200607/cmhansrd/cm070517/halltext/70517h0003.htm

Freud, D. (2007) *Reducing dependency, increasing opportunity: options for the future for Work and Pensions*, 'Independent' report for DWP, London: HMSO.

Mental Health Alliance (2007) *Mental Health Alliance gives final verdict on 2007 Mental Health Act* (7 August), http://www.mentalhealthalliance.org.uk/news/prfinalreport.html

PFMHTWG (2006) Physical Function and Mental Health Technical Working Groups, Transformation of the Personal Capability Assessment, Department of Work and Pensions, September, http://www.dwp.gov.uk/welfarereform/tpca.pdf

Wilkinson, R. (2005) *The Impact of Inequality: How to Make Sick Societies Healthier*, London: Routledge (see also http://books.guardian.co.uk/reviews/politicsphilosophyandsociety/0,6121,1538844,00.html).

Wilkinson, R. (2007) Personal communication (on an earlier draft of this chapter).

10

Inequalities in premature mortality in Britain: observational study from 1921 to 2007[1]

Thomas, B., Dorling, D. and Davey Smith, G. (2010) 'Inequalities in premature mortality in Britain: observational study from 1921 to 2007', *British Medical Journal*, 23 July.

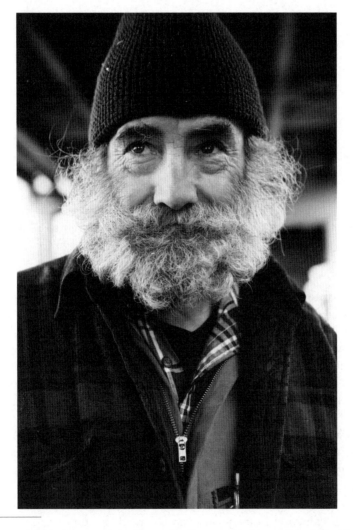

---

[1] Editorial Note: This is the most up-to-date study of geographical inequalities in health undertaken to date. Once full 2011 census data are released during 2013, and the resident population of each area is known, with university students placed at their non-term-time address, it will be possible to update the tables here to 2011, and to make estimates for 2012 and 2013..

What is already known on this topic: Inequalities in mortality reflect inequalities in wealth and rise concurrently. People living in poorer areas have lower life expectancy than people living in less poor areas, and the gap in Britain is wide compared with that in other countries.

What this study adds: The study brings previous research up to date and confirms that inequalities in mortality, when considered by wealth, are still increasing. Although life expectancy for all people is increasing, the gap between the best and worst districts is continuing to increase. Inequality in mortality is now greater than at any time since comparable records began.

Abstract

Objective: To report on the extent of inequality in premature mortality as measured between geographical areas in Britain.

Design: Observational study of routinely collected mortality data and public records. Population subdivided by age, sex, and geographical area (parliamentary constituencies from 1991 to 2007, pre-1974 local authorities over a longer time span).

Setting: Great Britain.

Participants: Entire population aged under 75 from 1990 to 2007, and entire population aged under 65 in the periods 1921–39, 1950–3, 1959–63, 1969–73, and 1981–2007.

Main outcome measure: Relative index of inequality (RII) and ratios of inequality in age-sex standardised mortality ratios under ages 75 and 65. The relative index of inequality is the relative rate of mortality for the hypothetically worst-off compared with the hypothetically best-off person in the population, assuming a linear association between socioeconomic position and risk of mortality. The ratio of inequality is the ratio of the standardised mortality ratio of the most deprived 10% to the least deprived 10%.

Results: When measured by the relative index of inequality, geographical inequalities in age-sex standardised rates of mortality below age 75 have increased every two years from 1990–1 to 2006–7 without exception. Over this period the relative index of inequality increased from 1.61 (95% confidence interval 1.52 to 1.69) in 1990–1 to 2.14 (2.02 to 2.27) in 2006–7. Simple ratios indicated a brief period around 2001 when a small reduction in inequality was recorded, but this was quickly reversed and inequalities up to the age of 75 have now reached the highest levels reported since at least 1990. Similarly, inequalities in mortality ratios under the age of 65 improved slightly in the early years of this century but the latest figures surpass the most extreme previously reported. Comparison of crudely age–sex standardised rates for those below age 65 from historical records showed that geographical inequalities in mortality are higher in the most recent decade than in any similar time period for which records are available since at least 1921.

Conclusions: Inequalities in premature mortality between areas of Britain continued to rise steadily during the first decade of the 21st century. The last time in the long economic record that inequalities were almost as high was in the lead up to the economic crash of 1929 and the economic depression of the 1930s. The economic crash of 2008 might precede even greater inequalities in mortality between areas in Britain.

Introduction

Inequalities in mortality in Britain have persisted over many years. Recent government interventions have aimed to reduce these inequalities but, the evidence suggests, to little effect. The report of the independent inquiry into inequalities in health (Acheson Report)[2] reviewed the situation of health inequalities as they then stood a decade ago and identified policy areas that could enable the government to act to reduce such health inequalities. Several interim progress reports were published by the Department of Health, with a major review published in May 2009.[3]

In early 2010 the latest Marmot review was published.[4] It begins with a misquotation from the poet Pablo Neruda: 'Rise up with me against the organisation of misery.' Although the review contains much useful new evidence and a careful description of the current state of knowledge, its recommendations perhaps fail to live up to its epigram. A particular focus of the review is reflected in its suggestion that: 'If society wishes to have a healthy population, working until 68 years, it is essential to take action to both raise the general level of health and flatten the social gradient.'

Despite government interventions, inequalities in health have not diminished; indeed in some cases the gap might have widened over the past 10 years, reflecting widening inequality in wealth and income over this period. Evidence is currently difficult to interpret, however, as targets have been changing, so have geographical areas for which data are reported.[5] We have therefore extended our previous research on trends in socioeconomic differentials in mortality in Britain (Davey Smith et al. 2002), recalculated standardised mortality ratios for the 1990s in the light of revised population estimates, and carried forward the series to 2007. We have also analysed the longer historical trajectory of mortality inequalities from the 1920s to the present

---

[2] Department of Health (1998) *Independent inquiry into inequalities in health*, London: Stationery Office.
[3] Department of Health. (2009) *Tackling health inequalities: 10 years on*. London: Department of Health.
[4] Marmot, M., Atkinson, T., Bell, J., Black, C., Broadfoot, P., Cumberlege, J., *et al.* (2010) *Fair society, healthy lives: the Marmot Review Executive Summary*. London: Marmot Review Team.
[5] Dorling, D. and Thomas, B. (2009) Geographical inequalities in health over the last century. In: Graham, H, ed. *Understanding health inequalities*, Maidenhead: Open University Press.

day. The data we present are analysed at the geographical level, with areas sorted by various indicators to present a broad perspective on trends in mortality differentials.

Methods

Digital mortality data were supplied with full postcodes for England and Wales by the Office for National Statistics and with postcode sector for Scotland from the General Register Office for Scotland. The postcode information is of the deceased's usual place of residence. We discarded the few records with no postcode (generally of deaths of visitors to Britain) and a few records with no code for cause of death (according to the international classification of diseases). The postcode was used to assign each death to the parliamentary constituency (as constituted in the 2001 general election) in which the deceased lived. Parliamentary constituencies are fairly uniform in population size; part of their design rationale involves an attempt to maximise their homogeneity. The data on deaths were provided for single years and were grouped into two-year aggregations.

At the time of the publication of results from the 1991 census it was generally agreed that the population had been substantially undercounted; this was corrected by researchers at the time, and we used the revised population figures in our previous work (Davey Smith *et al.*, 2002). After the 2001 census, it became apparent that these corrections were themselves incorrect, and further corrections were made.[6] These revised 'estimating with confidence' population figures for the 1991 census were aggregated from 1991 census wards to parliamentary constituencies and interpolated between 1991 and 2000. The mid-year population estimates released by the Office for National Statistics for census area statistics wards for England and Wales and by the General Register Office for Datazones for Scotland were used for the years after 2000; the small area geographical data were aggregated to parliamentary constituencies. As the 2001 census and subsequent midyear population estimates locate students studying away from home at their term-time addresses, we needed to relocate students studying away from home to their home constituencies.[7]

Poverty was indexed by the 2000 Breadline Britain Index.[8] This index measures relative poverty based on a lack of the perceived necessities of life and is widely accepted as a good measure of relative poverty. To avoid circularity we confirmed that the inclusion of any health measures in the index had no material effect on our results (analysis not shown). Parliamentary constituencies were ranked according to this poverty measure and divided into tenths of the population on the basis of this ranking. The tenth below the first decile has the highest poverty and the tenth above the last decile the lowest. We used the same ranking tenths for each of the

[6] Norman, P., Simpson, L., and Sabater, A. (2008) Estimating with confidence and hindsight: new UK small area population estimates for 1991. *Population Space Place*, 14:449-72.
[7] Shaw, M., Thomas, B., Davey Smith, G., and Dorling, D. (2008) *The grim reaper's road map: an atlas of mortality in Britain*. Bristol: The Policy Press.
[8] Dorling, D., Rigby, J., Wheeler, B., Ballas, D., Thomas, B., Fahmy, E., Gordon, D. and Lupton, R. (2007) *Poverty, wealth and place in Britain, 1968 to 2005*, Bristol: The Policy Press.

time periods as the 1991 and 2000 Breadline Britain Indices were closely correlated (analysis not included). We calculated standardised mortality ratios under age 75 for men and women for these tenths by using their overall age specific mortality rates for Britain for the relevant time periods. A standardised mortality ratio of 100 means that there is no difference between the observed and the expected number of deaths in an area, the expectation being based on population size and age/sex structure. A ratio over 100 means that mortality is higher—for example, a ratio of 120 means that mortality is 20% higher than that of the general population.

These two changes (revised population estimates and an updated poverty measure) only minimally influenced the standardised mortality ratios previously published, and all summary statistics such as the relative index of inequality were calculated with the same methods as in our previous work (Davey Smith *et al.*, 2002). Confidence intervals were estimated with standard methods.[9]

Results

Premature death around the millennium

Table 10.1 shows the age and sex standardised mortality ratios for premature death (death below the age of 75) for 1990–2007; an expanded version with all confidence intervals is presented in table A on bmj.com. Table B on bmj.com shows the

Table 10.1: Age and sex standarised mortality ratios (SMRs) and relative index of inequality* (RII) for age 0–74 according to decile of poverty, 1990–2007.

SMR 0-74	1990-01	1992-03	1994-05	1996-07	1998-99	2000-01	2002-03	2004-05	2006-07
Poverty tenth:									
1 (poorest)	129	132	135	137	138	139	138	138	140
2	116	118	118	120	121	119	121	121	123
3	113	115	114	115	115	116	117	117	117
4	105	107	106	108	109	109	107	108	108
5	103	102	102	101	103	103	103	103	104
6	96	94	95	94	95	95	96	95	97
7	91	90	90	90	89	90	90	90	90
8	86	86	85	85	84	84	85	86	84
9	85	83	83	82	81	81	81	81	79
10	80	79	79	78	77	76	76	76	75
Ratio of worst to best	1.61	1.67	1.71	1.76	1.79	1.83	1.82	1.82	1.88
RII	1.61	1.67	1.71	1.81	1.86	1.86	1.90	1.91	2.14

* RII is relative rate of mortality for the hypothetically worst-off compared with the hypothetically best-off person in the population, assuming a linear association between socioeconomic position and mortality risk. Ratio of inequality is ratio of SMR of most deprived 10% to least deprived 10%.

Note: Confidence interval in original paper.

---

[9] Breslow, N. and Day, N.E. (1980) *The analysis of case-control studies*, Lyon: International Agency for Research on Cancer. [Editorial Note: The equations are shown in Chapter 38 of this volume.

population years at risk and number of deaths by tenth of poverty. The worst-off tenth saw a gradual increase in standardised mortality ratio over the time period, while conversely the best-off tenth saw a decrease. The ratio of the worst to best tenths increased over the period, from 1.61 (95% confidence interval 1.61 to 1.62) in 1990–1 to 1.83 (1.82 to 1.83) by 2000–1, levelled off over the next four years, then increased to its maximum of 1.88 (1.87 to 1.88) for 2006–7.

Figure 10.1: Gini coefficient of equivalised inequality in income after tax and before housing costs, 1961 to 2007–08.

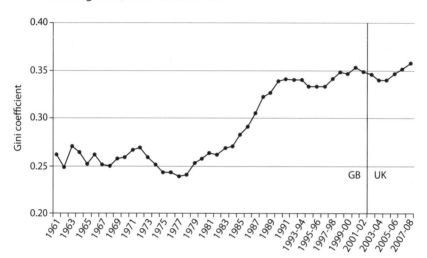

Note: Data are for Great Britain before 2002-03 and for UK subsequently.

The confidence intervals for the standardised mortality ratios are tight because each is based on an underlying population of millions of people over two years. In contrast, the confidence intervals for the relative index of inequality figures are wider because they are based on 641 data points, each point being a parliamentary constituency. This index is the relative rate of mortality for the hypothetically worst-off compared with the hypothetically best-off person in the population, assuming a linear association between socioeconomic position and mortality risk. It has consistently risen over the time period, from 1.61 (1.52 to 1.69) in 1990–1 to 2.14 (2.02 to 2.27) in 2006-7. The increase in the ratio and the relative index of inequality reflects the rising trend (and slight fall in the early 2000s) in income inequality. Figure 10.1 presents time series data on the Gini coefficient of equivalised inequality in income after tax and before housing costs.[10] There is debate as to whether income inequality has recently increased. Barnard states that 'the Gini coefficient for disposable income was almost

---

[10] Institute for Fiscal Studies (2010) Fiscal facts, www.ifs.org.uk/ fiscalFacts

unchanged between 2006/07 and 2007/08',[11] while Brewer *et al* claim that, for the same period, 'income inequality has risen (on most measures) in each of the last three years and is now at its highest level since our comparable time series began in 1961'.[12]

Table C on bmj.com shows equivalent data to table B on bmj.com but for people dying at ages 0–64; table D on bmj.com shows the population years at risk and number of deaths by tenth of poverty. The inequalities are even starker, although the table shows that after increasing inequality to 1998-9, when the relative index of inequality stood at 2.38 (2.24 to 2.52), there was some narrowing until 2004–5 with an index of 2.27 (2.13 to 2.40). The index rose again for the most recent period 2006–7 to 2.38 (2.24 to 2.52) to match the maximum previously recorded, both for inequality ratio (in 2002–3) and by relative index (1998–9). In short, inequalities did fall a fraction in the earliest years of the current century but have since risen back to their previous maximum for people aged under 65 and exceed the previous maximum for those aged up to 74. For those aged under 65, the confidence intervals reported here are wider (the number of deaths involved are lower) and overlap.

Table E on bmj.com shows deaths of those aged 0–64 as a proportion of deaths in the 0–74 age range. Thus in the years 1990 and 1991, around 47% of people dying aged under age 75 in Britain were aged under 65 in the areas with the highest rates of poverty. By the end of the period that proportion had risen to 52%, resulting from a combination of faster falls in mortality from causes more likely to affect older people and because those in the unusually large birth cohort of 1946–7 were only in their mid-40s at the start of the period but in their 60s by the end. In general more of the dead are younger in poorer areas.

The longer historical picture

In previous work, we described standardised mortality ratios for deaths under age 65[13] for the period 1950–92 for areas of Britain. These statistics used only five age bands (age 0, 1–4, 5–14, 15–44, and 45–64) for men and women and were for areas amalgamated from the pre-1974 local authorities. As poverty data were not available for this extended time period, the areas were ranked at each time period by standardised mortality ratios before being grouped by each tenth of the population. Thus these data reflect the maximum geographical inequalities in mortality at each time period. We have now extended this time series back to 1921 and forward to 2007, aggregating the data for the 1920s, 1930s, 1980s, 1990s, and 2000s into approximate decades, and including all other data available for portions of other decades. Table 10.2 shows the standardised mortality ratios, the ratio of worst (highest ratios) to best (lowest ratios) tenths, and the relative index of inequality. The time periods are not

[11] Barnard A. (*2009*) *The effects of taxes and benefits on household income, 2007/8*. Economic Labour Market Review, 3:56-66.

[12] Brewer, M., Muriel, A., Phillips, D. and Sibieta, L. (2009) *Poverty and inequality in the UK*, London: Institute for Fiscal Studies.

[13] Shaw, M., Dorling, D. and Brimblecombe, N. (1998) Changing the map: health in Britain 1951–91. *Sociology of Health and Illness* 20: 694-709.

continuous because of interruptions such as war or the government not collecting the relevant data; nor are the time periods always of equal duration.

Table 10.2: Standarised mortality ratios (SMRs) of decline and relative index of inequality (RII), Britain by area, 1921–2007*.

SMR 0-64	1921-30	1931-39	1950-53	1959-63	1969-73	1981-89	1990-98	1999-2007
Tenth of standardised mortality ratio:								
1 (worst)	138	136	131	136	131	137	149	149
2	122	120	118	123	116	120	123	123
3	113	112	112	117	112	114	114	115
4	108	106	107	111	108	108	108	109
5	104	103	103	105	103	102	99	101
6	97	97	99	97	97	96	94	95
7	90	89	93	91	92	92	91	90
8	83	85	89	88	89	89	86	83
9	78	81	86	83	87	84	78	77
10	72	73	82	77	83	79	73	70
Ratio of worst to best	1.91	1.85	1.60	1.76	1.58	1.74	2.04	2.12
RII	2.50	2.35	1.96	2.25	1.92	2.17	2.64	2.79

* Data series is not continuous, with no data for the 1940s and gaps in mid-'50s, mid-'60s, and from early '70s to early '80s; nor are time periods always of equal duration. For 1980, we used the harmonic mean of decile SMRs for the two periods of which it was composed (1981-5 and 1986-9).

Note: Confidence interval in original paper.

From a ratio of 1.91 at the start of the time period (1921–30), there was a downward trend until around 1960; after this, the ratio decreased to the early 1970s, and since then the trend has been relentlessly upwards with a maximum of 2.12 by the mid-2000s, a ratio higher than at any other decade of the period. The relative index of inequality exhibits the same pattern.

Figure 10.2 shows the gap in life expectancy at birth for 1999-2008 between the local authority with the highest life expectancy and the local authority with the lowest life expectancy for males, females, and all people.[14] Although life expectancy has been increasing for all people over time, it has been increasing faster for the better-off and the gap is now at its widest since 1991.

Discussion

In this long time series (1921–2007) of records of deaths occurring under age 65 and (for historical comparability) age standardised by five broad age groups, we found that inequality in mortality between geographical areas in Britain has been

---

[14] Office for National Statistics (2009) *Correction notice: life expectancy at birth and at age 65 by local areas in the United Kingdom 2006-2008*, www.statistics.gov.uk/downloads/theme_population/LE_UK_2009.xls

Figure 10.2: Difference in life expectancy at birth between the best-off and worst-off districts, 1999–2008.

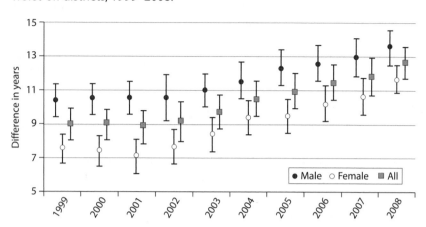

increasing. The continuing rise in the standardised mortality ratio of those living in the areas with the highest tenth of mortality from 1997 onwards suggests that official government policy to reduce inequalities in health has not been successful, at least for the important indicator of premature mortality. The rate at which inequalities in health have continued to rise might seem to have slowed slightly towards the most recent period, but it is important to remember that there are still two years of the 2000s to be included in the series when the data are made available, and some underlying factors such as unemployment have been rising rapidly over the course of those two years; furthermore, in absolute numbers unemployment has increased fastest in the poorest areas.[15]

When considered by tenth of poverty, by the year 2007 for every 100 people under the age of 65 dying in the best-off areas, 199 were dying in the poorest tenth of areas. This is the highest relative inequality recorded since at least 1921. When we looked at people aged under 75, for every 100 people dying in the best-off areas, 188 were dying in the poorest tenth of areas. That is the highest ratio of inequality recorded since at least 1990.

The most informative guide to trends in geographical inequalities in premature mortality remains the relative index of inequality. This compares mortality rates between the poorest and least poor consistently defined groups of parliamentary constituencies in the country, and mortality rates for every constituency contribute to the index, not just the extreme tenths. The relative index of inequality rose quickly by six points from 1990–1 to 1992–3, and then more slowly to stand at 1.86 (1.76 to 1.96) by 1998-9, which held steady until 2000-1 before rising again to 1.91 (1.80 to 2.01) by 2004–5 and then to 2.14 (2.02 to 2.27) by 2006–7. This was the most marked increase recorded over the entire 1990–2007 period. That rise coincided with a rise in child poverty, which had been falling, and official recognition that

---

[15] Dorling, D. (2009) Who will pay the price for the crisis? *Socialist Review*, April.

inequality in income and wealth had also risen[16]—all before the current economic downturn became fully apparent.

The last rapid fall in inequalities in mortality between areas took 21 years, a world war, and introduction of a welfare state and a national health service (between 1929 and 1950–3). Recent research on the immediate aftermath of the 1929–33 crash and depression suggests that in the short term inequalities in mortality between areas rose after the last large economic crash.[17] The longer-term picture suggests that it was only prolonged and enthusiastic state intervention that reduced inequalities in mortality over the 1940–73 period and kept them low for a long time thereafter. These were interventions of the kind that kept the Gini coefficient low until 1978. Similarly, it could be argued that prolonged state disengagement in promoting equality in outcome over the period 1978–2007 allowed inequalities in health between areas of Britain to rise to their current maximum levels.

Strengths and limitations

Although this study was large, population based, and covered a longer time period than other reports, it had several limitations. By considering data aggregated by area we ran the risk of partly invoking the ecological fallacy but avoided the risk run by many studies in health inequalities of invoking the atomistic fallacy.[18] We did not examine the issue of migration, which will have a bearing on the results shown here. Selective out-migration might lead to areas of decreasing relative size and high mortality,[19] but this is an issue for further study. Recent evidence from New Zealand suggests the differential patterns of migration by health status contribute substantially to geographical widening gaps, but such findings are context-specific and might not apply to Britain.[20] We considered only all cause mortality and did not examine the issue of changes in the underlying causes of death. We did this partly because of a paucity of data on cause of death by age, sex, and area for most of the time we considered.

Conclusions and policy implications

Social inequalities in mortality rates are influenced by complex and long term processes. They reflect the outcome of socially patterned exposures in early life and the cumulative effect of experiences in adult life (Davey Smith, 2007). Recent

---

[16] Elliot, L. and Curtis, P. (2009) UK's income gap widest since 60s: Labour admits child poverty failure, incomes of poorest fall, *Guardian* Newspaper, 8 May.

[17] Dorling, D. and Thomas, B. (2009) Geographical inequalities in health over the last century. In: Graham, H., ed. *Understanding health inequalities*. Open University Press.

[18] Tunstall, H.V. Z., Shaw, M. and Dorling, D. (2004) Places and health, *Journal of Epidemiology Community Health*, 58:6-10.

[19] Davey Smith, G., Shaw, M. and Dorling, D. (1998) Shrinking areas and mortality, *Lancet*, 352:1139-40.

[20] Pearce J. R. and Dorling, D. (2010) The influence of selective migration patterns among smokers and nonsmokers on geographical inequalities in health, *Annals of the Association of American Geographers*, 100, 2, 393-409.

changes in social and fiscal policy and their consequences cannot be expected to eradicate such inequalities. They can, however, be judged with respect to their predicted effect on social inequality in the short and long term, and from varying perspectives surprisingly little has been done to alter the fundamental structures of social inequality in the UK over the past decade (Hills, Sefton and Stewart, 2009; Goldthorpe, 2009). Furthermore, over the next decade a combination of knock-on effects of the current downturn and relaxation of existent controls over tendencies for economic inequalities to rise will probably accelerate, rather than attenuate, the observed increases in inequalities in mortality. In this light the comprehensive but diffuse approaches in official responses to health inequalities are inadequate (Global Health Equity Group, 2010).

By treating the undoubted multidimensional contributors to health inequalities as though they act at the same level and by failing to prioritise the need to reduce the fundamental drivers of social inequality, the government's commitments to reduce inequalities in mortality have been largely ineffective, as predicted when the first such document, the Acheson report, was released (Davey Smith, Morris and Shaw, 1998).

This paper is dedicated to the memory of Jerry Morris, a lifelong advocate of serious efforts to reduce inequalities in health.

References

Davey Smith, G. (2007) Boyd Orr Lecture: Life-course approaches to inequalities in adult chronic disease risk, *Proceedings of the Nutrition Society*, 66, 216–236.

Davey Smith, G., Dorling, D., Mitchell, R. and Shaw, M. (2002) Health inequalities in Britain: continuing increases up to the end of the 20th century. *Journal of Epidemiology and Community Health* 56: 434-5.

Davey Smith, G., Morris, J.N. and Shaw, M. (1998) The independent inquiry into inequalities in health, *BMJ* 317:1465-6.

Goldthorpe, J.H. (2009) Analysing social inequality: a critique of two recent contributions from economics and epidemiology, *European Sociology Review*, doi:10.1093/esr/jcp046

Global Health Equity Group (2010) www.ucl.ac.uk/gheg/marmotreview/Documents.

Hills, J., Sefton, T. and Stewart, K. (2009, eds.) *Towards a more equal society?*, Bristol: The Policy Press.

SECTION III
Medicine and politics

11

Medicine is a social science, and politics is nothing else but medicine on a large scale

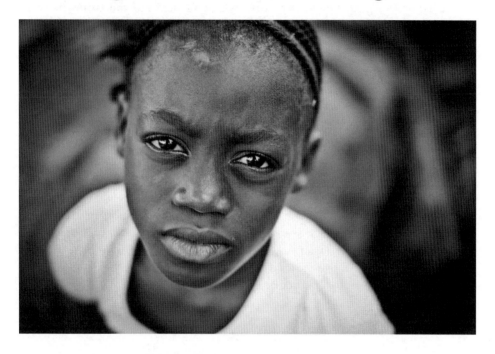

Evidence that 'the most powerful determinants of health in modern populations are to be found in social, economic, and cultural circumstances' (Blane et al, 1996) comes from a wide range of sources and is also, to some extent, acknowledged by Government (Townsend and Davidson, 1992; Social Exclusion Unit, 1998; Department of Health [DH], 1992; Acheson, 1998; Wanless, 2004). Yet differences in health experiences between areas and social groups (socio-economic, ethnic and gender) remain.... How these inequalities in health are approached by society is highly political and ideological: are health inequalities to be accepted as 'natural' and inevitable results of individual differences both in respect of genetics and the silent hand of the economic market; or are they abhorrences that need to be tackled by a modern state and a humane society? (Bambra et al, 2008)

There is so much written on medicine and politics that it can easily overwhelm – Rudolf Carl Virchow's quote,[1] the title of this chapter, is often repeated. In Britain the six reports referred to in Clare Bambra's (and colleagues') statement (above) give a summary that spans the field, from the work of David Blane and his colleagues, to Peter Townsend and Nick Davidson's Penguin edition of the Black Report, to various reports of government departments and agencies, to the work of recent chief medical officers such as Donald Acheson and even of bankers such as Derek Wanless. Wanless, who was commissioned by Gordon Brown to give the view of a financier, wrote a report entitled *Securing good health for the whole population*, which, among other things, recommended that: '*HM Treasury should produce a framework for the use of economic instruments to guide government interventions in relation to public health*' (Wanless, 2004, p 184).

There is an alternative way to frame thinking about how medicine and politics are linked, other than through following recent literature. This is to begin to routinely recognise politics and health in what you see in everyday life. You can do this even as you check your emails in the morning. The university I work in regularly sends emails with details of the deaths of members of staff, both current and retired. These list the post they held and the department they worked in. Almost invariably you read every notice even though you are very unlikely to have ever met the person named. Almost invariably (again) the professors live the longest and the cleaners live the shortest lives. All that varies is where the funeral is to be held and whether money should be given to a particular charity. Here is one:

> *The Vice-Chancellor regrets to announce the death of*
> Mrs XXXXXX XXXXXXX
> *Cleaner in the Department of Estates and Facilities*
> *Management and a member of staff from 1999*
> *Aged 59 years*
> *which occurred on 8 January 2012*
> *The funeral has already taken place*

Very shortly after that brief 42-word announcement was posted, another mass email to all staff was sent. It included over 500 words announcing the appointment of a new member of the senior management team of the university. I often wonder if, rather like the ranking of items on deaths on the evening news according to how remote the country is, the number of words used in official declarations is in inverse proportion to the officially perceived importance of the event. A minor bureaucrat appointed, in his or her 40s, receives almost ten times the wordage befitting a 59-year-old cleaner's death. All this sends out messages, about how much people are

---

[1] The original was in German. In English: '*Medicine is a social science, and politics is nothing else but medicine on a large scale. Medicine, as a social science, as the science of human beings, has the obligation to point out problems and to attempt their theoretical solution: the politician, the practical anthropologist, must find the means for their actual solution…. The physicians are the natural attorneys of the poor, and social problems fall to a large extent within their jurisdiction*' (http://en.wikipedia.org/wiki/Rudolf_Virchow#Political_career).

worth, about when they are expected to die, about how shocked we are, or should be, or are not.

A few months earlier the following 220-word letter was sent to members of the House of Lords. Five times as many words as the notice of the cleaner's death, less than half as many as the celebration of the bureaucrat's appointment. I reproduce it below to illustrate contemporary medicine on a large scale:

Addressed to individual members of the House of Lords

We write as public health doctors and specialists from within the NHS, academia and elsewhere to express our concerns about the Health and Social Care Bill.

The Bill will do irreparable harm to the NHS, to individual patients and to society as a whole. It ushers in a significantly heightened degree of commercialisation and marketisation that will lead to the harmful fragmentation of patient care; aggravate risks to individual patient safety; erode medical ethics and trust within the health system; widen health inequalities; waste much money on attempts to regulate and manage competition; and undermine the ability of the health system to respond effectively and efficiently to communicable disease outbreaks and other public health emergencies.

While we welcome the emphasis placed on establishing a closer working relationship between public health and local government, the proposed reforms as a whole will disrupt, fragment and weaken the country's public health capabilities.

The government claims that the reforms have the backing of the health professions. They do not.

Neither do they have the general support of the public.

It is our professional judgement that the Health and Social Care Bill will erode the NHS's ethical and cooperative foundations and that it will not deliver efficiency, quality, fairness or choice. We therefore request that you reject passage of the Health and Social Care Bill.

Yours sincerely,

Signed by 77 public health doctors and specialists in the NHS, and including eight professors.

Despite the letter being short, to the point and signed by many people, one signatory in particular was singled out for censure, Professor John Ashton, Joint Director of Public Health for NHS Cumbria.

Shortly after publication of the above text Professor Ashton received a letter warning him that under the NHS Code of Conduct it was *'inappropriate for individuals to raise personal concerns about the proposed Government reforms'*. It added that he was required to attend a meeting with the NHS Cumbria's Chief Executive, Sue Page, to explain and account for his recent actions. Professor Ashton suspected the order to write the letter had come '... *from the office of Health Secretary Andrew Lansley*' (McGowan, 2012). The Health Secretary insisted he knew nothing about that specific letter, but did not deny he had given more general instructions that resulted in that letter being sent (Williams, 2012).

Geography broadens the mind

A month after the letter to individual members of the House of Lords was written, I was with students on a geography fieldtrip in Athens. It was early November 2011. Again, just like the routine email about the cleaner's untimely death, everyday events appeared far more telling than much current writing in academia, or even letters of protest that were being written by one set of professionals to be read by a set of Lords, Ladies, Baronesses and Barons. Here is what I saw:

After the cuts[2]

I travelled into the city after the cuts had been made. There were tourists on the train and people from other countries visiting their relatives. "What can I say?" the man opposite me shrugged, who was travelling from Germany to visit his daughter. "She fell in love, she's settled here now, it's a pity but she's still in love and has children, they speak the language, this is their home now."

The city was quiet, much quieter than I had seen it before. Last year I had seen people searching in bins for food for the first time here. They were probably foreigners. The foreigners always lose out first. However, this year there were far fewer visitors, far less food in the bins, this year was very different. I didn't see anyone searching in bins. Instead what I saw, all the time, was begging.

There was begging in the streets, begging on the underground, begging quietly in corners, begging a bit more forcibly, people standing in front of me for a minute just looking in my eyes. Not the kind of begging I was used to. People begging while breastfeeding a baby. Not that fake begging with babies I had grown used to, I could tell by her eyes that she needed the money.

People were giving money. It was mostly the old people who gave, and they mostly gave the smallest of coins so those who were begging had to keep on begging, all day, just to get enough for a small meal. It was mostly older people giving to younger people and you knew that the older ones did not really have the money, that they would go hungry and cold for giving it.

---

[2] http://falseeconomy.org.uk/blog/this-is-what-austerity-looks-like, first posted as Dorling, D. (2011) 'This is what austerity looks like', False Economy Website Comment, 15 November 2011.

The begging look was not just on the streets. Shopkeepers were sitting behind their glass fronts willing the few tourists there were to come into their premises. Most shops were empty almost all of the time but what else to do but sit and wait? There is no other way. Restaurants, even in what were the busiest of places, were more than half empty. Again it is the tourists who have money and there are not enough of them. Locals don't appear to eat out much anymore.

The gas is being turned off in many apartment blocks. If you have some savings you can pay to run an electric heater. It costs more, but this situation is not about efficiency, it is about the money running dry. When there are strikes they are no longer about people wanting more, but about people demanding to be paid for the work they have done. They blockade until they are paid.

Every day you hear stories of people taking what money they have out of the country, to somewhere safer. Every day you feel that it is all spiralling down a little further, that more of the young people who can are leaving, that there is less and less to go round and for every note that isn't spent, the spending of another person who would have got that note also falls. People become more careful. Prices of what there is rise, rents don't fall as much as earnings, more and more are made homeless.

And what do the people say? They say "Go back and tell them that we are not lazy, that we can work hard," but many don't say much at all, they just look haggard and tired. Having the hope slowly kicked out of you by a multitude of events at first makes you angry, then you become resigned and next you become scared. What you thought could never happen is happening.

Athens, November 2011

Elitism and lack of imagination

It can be difficult to reconcile what you see on the streets with what you may read in the library in journals and in textbooks. Often such publications appear to be describing a very different planet simply because politics separates people so much. Almost a decade ago a debate was held in the pages of an elite but rather obscure medical journal, *QJM: An International Journal of Medicine, 'Published on behalf of the Association of Physicians'*. This is an association that on its homepage greets visitors with an announcement of which of its members received knighthoods during the year (see Figure 11.1).

The opening shot in the debate was a paper entitled 'The politics of medicine' (Daniels, 2003) which began with following words:

Figure 11.1: Medicine and politics

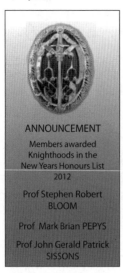

ANNOUNCEMENT

Members awarded
Knighthoods in the
New Years Honours List
2012

Prof Stephen Robert
BLOOM

Prof Mark Brian PEPYS

Prof John Gerald Patrick
SISSONS

Source: Redrawn from http://theassociationof physicians.co.uk/forum/ wp-content/uploads/ 2012/01/announcement -full1.jpg

Medicine and politics are inextricably intertwined, and yet they are very different enterprises. Political conditions can have a dramatic effect upon life expectancy: famine, for example, is now believed to occur only in conditions where there are few freedoms, including that of information.

The first reference given was to the work of Amartya Sen (on famine). It is now commonly understood (outside of this kind of medicine) that it was not lack of information that caused the famines so much as the misuse of power. Sen's work showed that there was a particular misuse by the British in India. However, most physicians reading the article were unlikely to spot the sleight of hand with which it began. The paper is worth reading, particularly for its use of many Latin phrases. Furthermore the author of this misleading opening shot went on to suggest that:

The pronouncements of the major medical journals on broad political matters are inclined to be naive, and often do not seem to recognize that other points of view are possible. Equality is almost always treated as if it were unequivocally a benefit.... Civilization is not reducible to justice, and is ultimately more valuable than justice.

By 'civilization', I take the writer as appearing to mean *'the kinds of things I like'*, things that appear to include having a sense of superiority over others and thinking he deserves more.

The first reply to be reproduced within the journal came quickly (Barr *et al*, 2004). Its first two sentences read:

In a recent QJM editorial, Daniels began by stating that medicine and politics are inextricably intertwined, yet concluded that medical journals should publish less 'political; material in favour of a more technical agenda. If journals adopt this approach, they are failing doctors, patients and wider society.

More of this rebuttal is worth quoting in some detail:

Many of the issues that influence both health and the practice of medicine are deemed political; it is therefore appropriate for medical journals to inform health professionals about these issues.

Even the best evidence-based technical medical intervention will be unsuccessful if the political solutions that allow it to be implemented are not identified. Jones et al estimate that the implementation of a limited range of interventions could prevent 63% of the

worldwide 10 million deaths per year in the under-5 age group. The interventions considered in this analysis were selected based on their evidence and feasibility for high coverage in low-income settings. If the objective is to improve global health, we have to look beyond the randomized control trial to what is really impeding progress, even if this leads us into slightly less comfortable 'political' areas.

Technical matters are far from being a refuge from politics. Even the most seemingly apolitical and technical medical article profoundly reflects its political environment. As Taracena states, 'every medical article published is the culmination of a long journey that started from a political decision: devoting resources to medical care and research'. For example, the current emphasis on clinical trials in journals reflects the large input of funding into such research by pharmaceutical companies, rather than priority setting based on burden of disease or cost-effective analysis. Indeed, only 10% of the US$70 billion spent on health research and development each year is targeted on the diseases that account for 90% of the global burden of disease – a 10/90 research gap.

The reply below was received in turn (Jones, 2004), quoting in this case from Le Fanu:

… absolute poverty, which may be associated with an inadequate diet, overcrowding, poor hygiene and lack of protection from the elements, can harm the human organism and cause disease, but he emphasizes that relative poverty, the type of poverty that exists in the UK, is an unlikely cause of disease.

This was bad timing – in the same year, *Status syndrome* was published (written by Michael Marmot), which is best remembered for explaining how relative poverty can cause disease. In a sentence it demonstrated that: *'Stress thrills the rich, but kills the poor'* (Kohn, 2004).

Today, almost a decade on, it is widely acknowledged that politics plays a crucial role in medicine. The first chapter that follows in this section, Chapter 12, briefly discusses how better to explain what you lose in terms of life expectancy when smoking a single cigarette. In trying to popularise the statistics it equates the loss to, among other things, the time it takes to engage in *'fairly frantic sexual intercourse'*. That article, published in 2000, was just one of hundreds of thousands of pieces that led towards the political decision in favour of the banning of smoking in enclosed public places. Today, in 2012, even Coalition government politicians are now advocating that cigarettes should be sold only in plain packets with almost no advertising allowed. The tobacco companies are claiming that this infringes the 'property rights' of their packaging, including, of course, all those sexually suggestive images of 'Marlborough man' and earlier images of women toying with cigarettes. Sex, death and politics have always been closely linked. They continue to be.

Take, for instance, a recent article on the role of politics and public acceptance in introducing human papilloma virus (HPV) vaccines in Canada (Mishra and Graham, 2012). In short, the article discusses the recommendation of vaccination for Grade 7 (ages 11 and 12) girls, and the criticism that followed its speed of rollout in high schools, which was followed by further controversy concerning the making of HPV immunisation mandatory in schools. This particular political reception of HPV vaccines has resulted from a particular convergence of scientific, marketing, healthcare policy, media and social discourses, which was, it is suggested by Mishra and Graham, further complicated by the fragmentation of decision making between parents and their adolescent children regarding immunisation.

Where public health messages had framed HPV immunisation as empowering young girls in the prevention of cervical cancer, this had largely neglected the role HPV vaccines could play in preventing penile, oral and anal cancers, and consequently it became seen as being a 'girl vaccine', and hence one which omits young boys from discussions about immunisation. These messages, it is claimed, sideline the male risks of HPV exposure and help to perpetuate sexist ideas about female vulnerability and sexual behaviour, while creating a politically and publicly acceptable discourse that focuses on prevention of cancer and obscures any discussion about sex:

> *The HPV's early identification as a girl vaccine depended on a moral sanitisation of the vaccine. This made it more acceptable during its initial introduction but distanced it from clinical and epidemiological realities. Creating a politically safe and palatable message for a receptive and desirable market trumps the scientific and clinical facts. In contemporary societies people are expected to proactively acquire and interpret knowledge.... But when increased access to knowledge may enhance anxiety and scepticism, or threaten acceptable norms, it may be kept silent.* (Mishra and Graham, 2012, p 66)

Politics runs throughout medicine. This can be seen in how Members of Parliament (MPs) attempt to bully health researchers (see Chapter 13 below), and in how governments deliberately release unfavourable health reports when Ministers are on holiday and their deputies are unavailable. They do this to try to reduce media coverage (see Chapter 14). It can be seen within all the Machiavellian attempts to coerce the sick to work when they are unable to work or there is no suitable work for them, attempts that are dressed up as welfare reform (see Chapter 15). It is even possible to claim that had the last Labour government been a little more successful in its health policies, the outcome of the last general election could have been different. A handful more Labour seats and the UK would have had a Lib–Lab Coalition (see Chapter 16). As it was, because of a few votes, or lack of them, in a few marginal seats, what has occurred from June 2010 onwards has been far more severe public service cuts than would have likely been the case otherwise (see Chapter 17). The country had become politically polarised along geographical lines in a way that it is hard to find previous parallels for (see Chapter 18). Given all this, it is hardly surprising to find all kinds of inequalities increasing.

Coalition policies and social inequalities[3]

In the year following May 2010 the new Coalition government introduced a series of policies and reviews that have resulted in increasing key inequalities, because, like many of their New Labour predecessors, the majority of the Coalition members believe that many social inequalities cannot be greatly reduced.

Just before the 2010 General Election Liberal Democrat leader Nick Clegg complained that the gap between the mean average incomes of the richest fifth as compared to the poorest fifth in the UK had risen from 6.9 times in 1997 to approach 7.2 times as much towards the end of Labour's 13 years in power. This shift took the UK one quarter of the way towards becoming as unequal in income as the world's most unequal large affluent country, the US. And within the course of just 18 months the Emergency Budget (22 June 2010), the March 2011 Budget and the Comprehensive Spending Review (November 2011) combined had moved the UK further towards becoming the most unequal affluent nation.

The International Monetary Fund (IMF) estimates that the current plans of the Chancellor of the Exchequer, George Osborne, for cuts to public spending will result, by 2015, in the UK spending a lower proportion of its GDP (gross domestic product) on public goods than any comparable European country and, for the first time since records began, a lower proportion through government expenditure than is spent in the US. Far-right members of the Republican Party (and Tea Party activists) in the US have started to single out the UK as a country they would like to emulate.

A year into the Coalition government and, by income ratio, the UK remains the fourth most unequal of the 25 richest countries in the world. Within the UK, inequalities in income and wealth rose during 2010 as the rich got richer and the poor got poorer. But why exactly did this inequality arise, and why did New Labour mostly fail to reduce social inequalities?

Just before the May 2010 General Election I wrote *Injustice* (Dorling, 2010), an academic book that suggested that the five social evils identified by Beveridge at the dawn of the British welfare state – ignorance, want, idleness, squalor and disease – were taking new forms, with social injustices now being recreated, renewed and supported by five new sets of 'unjust' beliefs. These beliefs are that elitism is efficient, exclusion is necessary, prejudice is natural, greed is good and despair is inevitable.

In just the first 18 months following May 2010 the Coalition government advanced many policies that further demonstrate that these beliefs are widely held. The 'unjust' beliefs necessary to maintain inequality have thus persisted into 2010 and beyond, and are now independently being recognised by popular political commentators rather than solely being the subject for 'quieter' academic study. Examples of their continued relevance to British life include:

---

[3] A slightly differently worded version of this section of the chapter first appeared as: Dorling, D. (2011) 'Government policies have increased social inequalities in the past year', Compass website commentary, 18 April (http://is.gd/gNjmwB).

- *Elitism is efficient:* the 2010 Browne review of higher education[4] recommended limitless 'market' fees for higher education. A tripling of the annual fees for university tuition was duly announced by the Coalition government in autumn 2010, meaning that higher education in Britain has become the most expensive and hence will likely soon be the most elitist in Europe. It is possible that many courses will become even more expensive than the most privatised US higher education. The Coalition also largely abolished the Educational Maintenance Allowance, which has consequently dissuaded many young people from disadvantaged backgrounds from staying on at school, and will further impoverish many of those who do stay on. University admissions in England fell in September 2012.
- *Exclusion is necessary:* Frank Field's independent review of child poverty,[5] which started in June 2010, has poured scorn on the use of European-wide definitions of child poverty rather than trying to solve the problem of poverty. Field suggested redefining the problem, saying that there would always be many people living on less than 60 per cent of median incomes and that could not be avoided. At the same time, the top of the income scale has seen the return of bankers' bonuses, just as plans were being made to cut benefits. Both the excessive pay and the cuts to the incomes of the poorest were presented as 'necessary', and the failure to enact banking reform has been intricately linked with the failure to reduce poverty. What Field appeared not to understand is that if a few people are paid excessively, then there is less to go around for the millions who live on very little.
- *Prejudice is natural:* everyone in an organisation deserves to be valued, and to blatantly not do so is prejudice. Will Hutton's independent review of the pay divide,[6] commissioned by the Coalition government, ignored progressive suggestions. These included proposing the exclusion from public sector contracts of those private sector companies that exceed a 20:1 income ratio between the highest and lowest paid. Allowing the public and private sector firms that take public sector contracts to pay a few people very highly will ensure that youth unemployment will continue to rise. The interim report[7] initially implied that public sector organisations should be constrained to not exceed this 20:1 ratio, but the notes at the back of the report suggest excluding anyone from the calculation not deemed to be 'core staff'. The final report, published in March, failed even to make this watered-down recommendation to curtail top pay. The review, in effect, supported the status quo of excessive inequality in pay.
- *Greed is good:* in 2010 the wealthiest people in Britain, as revealed in *The Sunday Times* Rich List, saw their greatest ever annual gains in wealth, a yearly rise of

---

[4] *Securing a sustainable future for higher education*, published on 12 October 2010. The National Archives copy can be found at http://webarchive.nationalarchives.gov.uk/+/hereview.independent.gov.uk/hereview/

[5] *The foundation years: Preventing poor children becoming poor adults*, published in December 2010. As of July 2012 a copy could be found at www.nfm.org.uk/news/77-family-policy/486-frank-field-final-independent-report-on-poverty-and-life-chances

[6] *Hutton review of fair pay in the public sector*, published in March 2011. As of July 2012 a copy could be found at www.hm-treasury.gov.uk/indreview_willhutton_easyread.htm

[7] A better document than the final report: www.hm-treasury.gov.uk/indreview_willhutton_interim.htm

29.9 per cent, to stand at £335.5 billion shared between the 1,000 wealthiest people in Britain. Their wealth rose again by 25 per cent in 2011 to reach almost £400 billion before rising again to over £412.8 billion in 2012. At the same time, the number of billionaires in the UK had increased by March 2011 by 10.4 per cent, to stand at 32, and by 15.6 per cent in the year to March 2012 to stand at 37 despite the country becoming much poorer overall as GNP (gross national product) fell in both 2011 and early 2012 (Prince, 2012). The very rich and super rich are taking more of Britain's shrinking share of world income. It would be naive to think that that can happen without a framework that condones it.

- *Despair is inevitable:* Sir Michael Marmot's[8] review of health inequalities (Marmot, 2010), although providing and promoting again in repackaged form a great deal of the evidence as to how great health inequalities in Britain are, and how they have risen so much in recent decades, failed to focus on the need to consider the excesses at the top end of the social hierarchy (Pickett and Dorling, 2010). It concentrated too much on material deprivation at the bottom. Since 2011, more evidence has emerged of the harm caused as the very rich are pulling away from the rich, and the rich are pulling away from the merely affluent. The affluent see the gap growing between them and people on average incomes (average incomes which in the UK recently began to fall), and those on average incomes have begun to fear even more falling behind further as the greatest cuts of all have been made to the incomes of the poorest tenth. This results in many people suffering more and more from stress due to growing financial inequalities, but the most common response to this remains, 'Bad luck, that's life'.

Despite rhetoric about a fairer society, these examples show that Coalition government policies are creating anything but fairness, which is why inequalities and injustice are currently growing. What is clear is that much that is currently wrong is viewed as either unavoidable or justifiable. What must change are the beliefs that end up seeing growing inequalities as inevitable, or, at the misguided extreme, as beneficial.

References

Acheson, D. (1998) *Independent inquiry into inequalities in health*, London: The Stationery Office.

Bambra, C., Smith, K. and Kennedy, L. (2008) 'Politics and health', in J. Naidoo and J. Wills (eds) *Health studies*, London: Palgrave Macmillan, pp 257-86.

Barr, D. *et al* (2004) 'Politics and health', *Quarterly Journal of Medicine*, vol 97, no 2, pp 61-2.

Blane, D., Brunner, E. and Wilkinson, R. (eds) (1996) *Health and social organization: Towards a health policy for the twenty-first century*, London: Routledge.

---

[8] The same person whose seminal book *The status syndrome* (Marmot, 2004) is referred to above. See www.instituteofhealthequity.org/projects/fair-society-healthy-lives-the-marmot-review. For the latest turn on this issue at the time of writing, see Kivimäki *et al* (2012).

Daniels, A. (2003) 'The politics of medicine', *Quarterly Journal of Medicine*, vol 96, pp 695-7.

DH (Department of Health) (1992) *The health of the nation: A strategy for health in England*, London: HMSO.

Dorling, D. (2010) *Injustice: Why social inequality persists*, Bristol: The Policy Press.

Jones, E.A. (2004) 'Technical medical interventions and the health of populations', *Quarterly Journal of Medicine*, vol 97, no 5, p 309.

Kivimäki, M. *et al* (2012) 'Job strain as a risk factor for coronary heart disease: a collaborative meta-analysis of individual participant data', *The Lancet*, 14 September, doi: 10-1016/S0140-6736.

Kohn, M. (2004) 'Stress thrills the rich, but kills the poor', *The Independent*, 18 June (www.independent.co.uk/arts-entertainment/books/reviews/status-syndrome-by-michael-marmot-6167269.html).

McGowan, P. (2012) 'Cumbria's health boss told off for having an opinion', *Carlisle News and Star*, 22 February (www.newsandstar.co.uk/news/cumbria-s-health-boss-told-off-for-having-an-opinion-1.927427?referrerPath=news).

Marmot, M. (2004) *The status syndrome: How social standing affects our health and longevity*, New York: Times Books.

Marmot, M. (2010) *Fair society, healthy lives, The Marmot Review*, London: The Marmot Review.

Mishra, A. and Graham, J.E. (2012) 'Risk, choice and the "girl vaccine": unpacking human papillomavirus (HPV) immunisation', *Health, Risk and Society*, vol 14, no 1, pp 57-69.

Pickett, K. and Dorling, D. (2010) 'Against the organisation of misery? The Marmot Review of Health Inequalities', *Social Science & Medicine*, vol 71, pp 1231-3.

Prince, R. (2012) 'Forbes list: J.K. Rowling fortune under vanishing spell', *The Telegraph*, 7 March (www.telegraph.co.uk/culture/books/booknews/9129981/Forbes-list-JK-Rowling-fortune-under-vanishing-spell.html).

Social Exclusion Unit (1998) *Bringing Britain together: A national strategy for neighbourhood renewal*, London: The Stationery Office.

Townsend, P. and Davidson, N. (1992) 'The Black Report', in P. Townsend and N. Davidson (eds) *Inequalities in health*, London: Penguin.

Wanless, D. (2004) *Securing good health for the whole population*, London: The Stationery Office (http://webarchive.nationalarchives.gov.uk/+/http://www.hm-treasury.gov.uk/media/9/E/Wanless04_ch9.pdf).

Williams, L. (2012) 'Liverpool doctor John Ashton "outraged" by disciplinary hearing over Health Bill criticism', *Liverpool Echo*, 22 February (www.liverpoolecho.co.uk/liverpool-news/local-news/2012/02/22/liverpool-doctor-john-ashton-outraged-by-disciplinary-hearing-over-health-bill-criticism-100252-30387184).

12

Time for a smoke: one cigarette is equivalent to 11 minutes of life expectancy[1]

Shaw, M., Mitchell, R. and Dorling, D. (2000) 'Time for a smoke: one cigarette is equivalent to 11 minutes of life expectancy', *British Medical Journal*, vol 320, p 53.

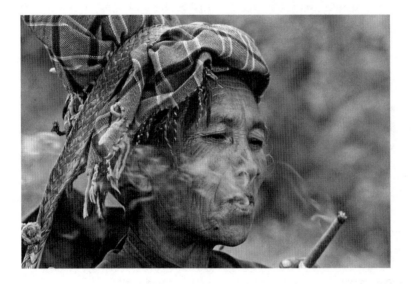

Editor—Studies investigating the impact on mortality of socioeconomic and lifestyle factors such as smoking tend to report death rates, death rate ratios, odds ratios, or the chances of smokers reaching different ages. These findings may also be converted into differences in life expectancy. We estimated how much life is lost in smoking one cigarette.

Our calculation is for men only and based on the difference in life expectancy between male smokers and non-smokers and an estimate of the total number of cigarettes a regular male smoker might consume in his lifetime. We derived the difference in life expectancy for smokers and non-smokers by using mortality ratios from the study of Doll *et al* of 34,000 male doctors over 40 years.[2] The relative death rates of smokers compared with non-smokers were threefold for men aged 45–64 and twofold for those

---

[1] Letter written jointly with Mary Shaw and Richard Mitchell, who worked at the University of Bristol. Competing interests in 2000: Drs Shaw and Mitchell are non-smokers. Dr Dorling is a smoker (20 cigarettes a day).
[2] Doll, R., Peto, R., Wheatley, K., Gray, R. and Sutherland, I. (1994) Mortality in relation to smoking: 40 years' observations on male British doctors, *British Medical Journal*, 309, 901–11.

aged 65-84, as corroborated elsewhere.[3] Average life expectancy from birth for the whole population or subgroups can be derived from life tables. Applying the rates of Doll *et al* to the latest interim life tables for men in England and Wales, with adjustment for the proportion of smokers and non-smokers in each five-year age group,[4] we found a difference in life expectancy between smokers and non-smokers of 6.5 years.

We used the proportion of smokers by age group, the median age of starting smoking, and the average number of cigarettes smoked per week in the 1996 general household survey.[5] We calculated that if a man smokes the average number of cigarettes a year (5,772) from the median starting age of 17 until his death at the age of 71 he will consume a total of 311,688 cigarettes in his lifetime.

If we then assume that each cigarette makes the same contribution to his death, each cigarette has cost him, on average, 11 minutes of life: 6.5 years = 2,374 days, 56,976 hours, or 3,418,560 minutes; 5,772 cigarettes per year for 54 years = 311,688 cigarettes; 3,418,560/311,688 = 11 minutes per cigarette.

This calculation is admittedly crude—it relies on averages, assumes that the health effects of smoking are evenly spread throughout a smoker's lifetime, presupposes that the number of cigarettes smoked throughout a lifetime is constant, and ignores the difficulties in classifying people as either lifetime smokers or non-smokers.[6] However, it shows the high cost of smoking in a way that everyone can understand.

The first day of the year is traditionally a time when many smokers try to stop, and on 1 January 2000 a record number might be expected to try to start the new millennium more healthily. The fact that each cigarette they smoke reduces their life by 11 minutes may spur them on. Table 12.1 shows some better uses for the time they save.

Table 12.1: Opportunities gained in stopping smoking by amount smoked.

Amount smoked	Life lost	Opportunity gain
One cigarette	11 minutes	Telephone call to friend; read of newspaper; brisk walk; or fairly frantic sexual intercourse
Pack of 20 cigarettes	3 hours 40 minutes	Long film (for example, Titanic); two football matches; one shopping trip; Eurostar journey from London to Paris, including visit to cafe; running in London marathon; or tantric sex
Carton of 200 cigarettes	1.5 days	Visit to friends or family; one very serious shopping trip; Wagner opera; flying round the world; or romantic night away

[3] Phillips, A.N., Wannamethee, S.G., Walker, M., Thomson, A. and Davey Smith, G. (1996) Life expectancy in men who have never smoked and those who have smoked continuously: 15 year follow up of large cohort of middle aged British men, *British Medical Journal*, 313, 907-8.

[4] Office for National Statistics (1997) *Mortality statistics: general* (Series DH1 No 30), London: Stationery Office.

[5] Office for National Statistics (1996) *General household survey: living in Britain*, London: Stationery Office.

[6] Suidicani, P., Hein, H.O. and Gyntelberg, F. (1997) Mortality and morbidity of potentially misclassified smokers, *International Journal of Epidemiology*, 26:321-7.

13

Private finance: Select Committee's report used parliamentary privilege unacceptable[1]

Macfarlane, A., Heyman, B., Dorling, D. *et al*, Letter to *British Medical Journal* (2002) vol 324, p 1584.

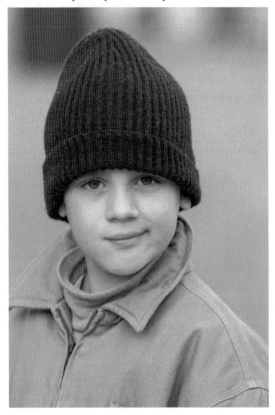

[1] Letter signed by Alison Macfarlane (City University), Bob Heyman (City University), Daniel Dorling (University of Leeds), Dave Gordon (University of Bristol), George Davey Smith (University of Bristol), Helen Dolk (University of Ulster), Helen Roberts (City University), Ian Basnett (consultant in public health), Ian Roberts (London School of Hygiene and Tropical Medicine), Jane Lewis (University of Oxford), Jennie Popay (University of Lancaster), Martin McKee (London School of Hygiene and Tropical Medicine), Miranda Mugford (University of East Anglia), Rodney Barker (London School of Economics and Political Science), Rosalind Raine (London School of Hygiene and Tropical Medicine), Sally Baldwin (University of York), Sally Glen (City University), Stephen Platt (University of Edinburgh) and Trevor Sheldon (University of York). The letter was written in response to the letter shown in Figure 13.1

Editor—We are deeply concerned at the misrepresentation in the House of Commons Select Committee on Health's report, *The Role of the Private Sector in the NHS*[2], of evidence critical of the private finance initiative (PFI) given by University College London's Health Policy and Health Services Research Unit.

We believe that the Committee's criticism of research by the Unit is an unacceptable use of parliamentary privilege to attack academic scholarship. Paragraphs 65 to 69 of the report give an inaccurate account of statements made in evidence and in published research. In particular, they misrepresent evidence that the unit gave to the Committee and allege that the Unit's research was unsound without providing any evidence of this.

This will undoubtedly deter other researchers from acting as expert witnesses to select committees in the future, especially if their findings do not accord with prevailing government policies.

It is important that parliamentary select committees take evidence from witnesses with a wide range of views and examine them critically and robustly in relation to government policies. Contrary to the comments made in the report, the Unit's published research on public health and the private finance initiative is respected both internationally and nationally.

We call on the House of Commons Health Committee to withdraw these unsubstantiated comments[3] and urge others who support fair reporting and use of evidence given to select committees to reinforce this request. This can be done by writing to the House of Commons Health Committee, House of Commons, London SW1A 0AA or emailing the committee at healthcom@ parliament.uk

---

[2] House of Commons Health Committee (2002) *The role of the private sector in the NHS.* HC 308-I. London: The Stationery Office
[3] Editorial Note: See Figure 13.1.

Figure 13.1: Letter published on the BMJ website, 23 May 2002

Sir,

The issue of 18 May (2002;324) contained an interesting juxtaposition of information. There was a repeat of Allyson Pollock's arguments against the Private Finance Initiative (PFI), a news item on PFI and a report on the House of Commons Select Committee on Health's "Inquiry into the Role of the Private Sector in the NHS". It would have been helpful if these items had been "joined up" and if the Select Committee's report had been given greater attention.

The Select Committee "were unimpressed with much of the University College London's Health Policy and Health Services Research Unit's (HPHSRU) research and its arguments against the Private Finance Initiative". Yet the BMJ has based its debate on PFI almost exclusively around articles by this Unit. The Committee made several comments about Prof. Pollock's evidence (paras 65-69) and commented that "This has raised serious questions about the HPHSRU's ability to analyse rationally the finances of the NHS". Most significantly the Select Committee said: "We found the lack of sound analysis from the HPHSRU additionally worrying because it has been the source of advice for many groups including unions and professional associations, all of whom have used parts of the Unit's work as a justification for their antagonistic attitudes towards the private sector."

The Select Committee found that "PFI is still being blamed for numerous ills not directly related to it whereas the many benefits ascribed to PFI have yet to be proved. The time has come for a more rational and objective debate…." They also concluded: "Similarly some of the antagonistic extreme views that are put forward by the HPHSRU and by other organisations have not helped to promote a sensible and mature debate about what is best for patients and staff in the NHS."

Surely it is now time for the BMJ (and the BMA) to move on from its blind antagonism to PFI. It should be more critical of the evidence it presents in its articles and engage rationally in the debate. Ultimately it is likely that PFI is neither as bad nor as good as the extremists present. In the meantime we are being distracted from identifying and debating the real health questions that lie beyond arguments about how new hospitals are funded.

We need to consider what priorities drive us to spend so much of our NHS resources on hospital buildings and are those priorities right. We need to ask is it right that our obsession with counting acute beds is blinding us to the health problems that cannot be solved by a hospital bed. We need to think about how, in the 21st century, we deliver health care (and even health!) outside hospitals. We need to look at how we develop capacity to manage illness in a whole systems way as advocated by the National Beds Inquiry [1] and, more importantly, how we incorporate acute hospital planning into a holistic approach to health planning and development as set out by the Kings Fund [2]. That is where the real questions are and, in the end, that is where the best interests of patients lie.

Brian McCloskey

Professor of Public Health

University College Worcester

Email: B.McCloskey@worc.ac.uk

Competing interests: as before - I instigated the review of services in Kidderminster that eventually involved Worcestershire's new PFI
[1] Department of Health. Shaping the future NHS: long term planning for hospitals and related services. Consultation document on the findings of The National Beds Inquiry. London: Department of Health, 2000
[2] Appleby J, Harrison A. Health Care UK 2000: Autumn Issue - The King's Fund Review of health policy. King's Fund, London; 2000. ISBN 1857174143

Source: http://www.bmj.com/content/324/7347/1178.1?tab=responses

14

Government cover-ups: Labour's 'Black Report' moment[1]

Shaw, M., Dorling, D., Mitchell, R. and Davey Smith, G. (2005) Letter to *British Medical Journal*, vol 331, p 575

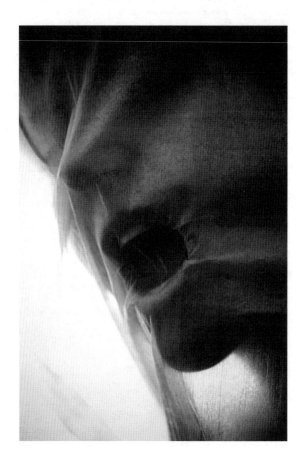

---

[1] This letter, first published on-line as a rapid response, was originally submitted to the *BMJ* as an editorial co-authored with Mary Shaw, Richard Mitchell, and George Davey Smith.

Editor—The release of the government's latest report on health inequalities on 11 August was curious.[2] Reminiscent of the covert release of the Black report on August bank holiday in 1980, the report appeared when the minister for public health was on holiday and her deputy unavailable[3].

Personal trainers

In July 2003 the government stated that there would be an annual report from the Department of Health on health inequality indicators related to the health inequality targets. Nothing appeared for more than two years, although the data that were eventually released had been available for some time,[4] and when they did appear it was, conveniently, after the election. Even stranger, the press release for the latest report deflected attention from the key finding of widening inequalities in life expectancy and infant mortality by headlining the 12 '*early adopter sites*' with their '*health trainers*'. The minister said, '*Many people have difficulty in changing to a healthier way of life… Health trainers are one of the many initiatives in the white paper which will help narrow this gap by supporting people to make healthier choices in their daily lives.*'[5]

To Labour traditionalists, opposed to victim-blaming approaches to health promotion, this may have triggered memories of Conservative minister Edwina Currie admonishing the poor to buy cheap but healthy food. To New Labour, however, it may be grist to the mill.

Shifting goal posts

The circumstances of the release of the report should not be allowed to detract from its main message—that health inequalities, as measured by both spatial differences in life expectancy and socioeconomic differences in infant mortality, have widened. The latest data for life expectancy (2001-3) show that the gap between England as a whole and the fifth of local authorities with the lowest life expectancy has increased, by 2% for males and by 5% for females.

---

[2] Department of Health (2005) *Tackling health inequalities: status report on the programme for action*. www.dh.gov.uk/PublicationsAndStatistics/Publications/PublicationsPolicyAndGuidance/PublicationsPolicyAndGuidanceArticle/fs/en?CONTENT_ID=4117696&chk=OXFbWI (accessed 1 Sep 2005).

[3] Dyer, O. (2005) Disparities in health widen between rich and poor in England, *British Medical Journal*, 331, 419 (20-27 August).

[4] Shaw, M., Dorling, D., Gordon, D. and Davey Smith, G. (2005) Health inequalities and New Labour: how the promises compare with real progress. *British Medical Journal*, 330, 1016-21.

[5] Department of Health (2005) Health trainers for disadvantaged areas. Press release, 11 Aug 2005. (2005/0285.) www.dh.gov.uk/PublicationsAndStatistics/PressReleases/PressReleases Notices/fs/en?CONTENT_ID=4117720&chk=j8T/Dk (accessed 1 Sep 2005).

The assessment of trends in health inequalities has not been helped by targets that have had their spatial and social units altered, start dates shifted, and measures changed repeatedly in their short lives. The life expectancy target first mentioned health authorities (which were soon abolished), then the fifth of local authorities with the lowest life expectancy, and now a 'spearhead' group. Curiously, the 12 early adopter sites with their health trainers overlap with (but are not exclusively drawn from) the spearhead group. The spearhead group will (for now) be used to measure progress towards the life expectancy target.

The infant mortality target has likewise been reformulated, as the official measure of social class has changed. Moreover, neither of the targets is a true health inequalities target as they compare the worst-off groups with the average for the population as a whole rather than considering the entire distribution. Indeed, the rapid moving of goal posts seems to have confused the drafters of this report, with 2001, 2002, and 2003 all being described as start dates. In fact, New Labour's health inequality targets were announced in July 2000 in the NHS plan and formalised in February 2001.[6, 7]

Widening inequalities

In opposition Labour consistently promised to implement the recommendations of the Black report and was incensed by the attempt to cover it up 25 years ago, as well as by the similar attempt to suppress the impact of the follow-up report in 1987.[8]

The hushed up release of this report raises fears that the bold statements and unprecedented promises of Labour's first years in power—for example, the pledge to eradicate child poverty within a generation—have now been wholly over-taken by the individualistic rhetoric of behavioural prevention and 'choosing health' and its three principles of 'informed choice, personalisation, and working together'. The linking of the adverse trends in health inequalities with the introduction of health trainers is a prime example of this.

Although the proportion of children living in low income households is a national indicator, the report nowhere mentions measuring, let alone directly tackling, the static or widening inequalities in income and wealth that New Labour has presided over, widening housing wealth inequalities being a prime example.[9] Perhaps rather than focusing on changing the health choices of

[6] Department of Health (2000) *The NHS plan: a plan for investment, a plan for reform*. London: HMSO.
[7] Department of Health (revised 2002) Health inequalities—national targets on infant mortality and life expectancy—technical briefing, www.dh.gov.uk/assetRoot/04/07/78/96/04077896.pdf (accessed 1 Sep 2005).
[8] Berridge, V. (2002,ed) The Black report and the health divide, *Contemporary British History*, 16, 131-71.
[9] Shelter (2005) *The great divide: an analysis of housing inequality*. London: Shelter.

millions of people the government should think more about a healthier way to govern and at last choose to use the tax and benefit systems to kerb growing social inequalities in income and wealth.

Note

The complete version of this letter was available at http://bmj.bmjjournals.com/cgi/eletters/331/7514/419#115362 [but can now be found at: www.dannydorling.org/?page_id=451].

Addendum

The Government Minister Caroline Flint replied on 9 September,[10] presumably after returning from holiday (she didn't explain where she had been in August). She said:

> *We are determined to reduce health inequalities. The report showed that we are moving in the right direction and highlighted the further work that needs to be done.... However, the report's data dated back to 2003. Last November, we published the Choosing Health White Paper aimed at improving health and tackling health inequalities. Health trainers are one of many initiatives in Choosing Health which will help narrow the inequalities gap by helping people to make healthier choices in their daily lives. Infant mortality rates, a key indicator of health inequalities, have fallen in the 'routine and manual' group as well as the total population. Government action including Sure Start, better neonatal services, stop smoking services, breastfeeding campaigns are all having an impact. Progress is slower in more disadvantaged areas which is why spearhead primary care trusts are piloting many of the key Choosing Health recommendations, including health trainers, in those areas. Health inequalities are and will continue to be a Government priority.*

Health inequalities rose for at least the next five years.

---

[10] Flint, C. (2005) Health Inequalities, rapid response, BMJ website – available at: http://www.bmj.com/content/331/7516/575.1fiab=responses [as of 28 May 2012].

15

Putting the sick to work: the real Mental Health Bill

Extract from Dorling, D. (2007) 'Guest Editorial: The real Mental Health Bill',
Journal of Public Mental Health vol 6, no 3, pp 6-13.

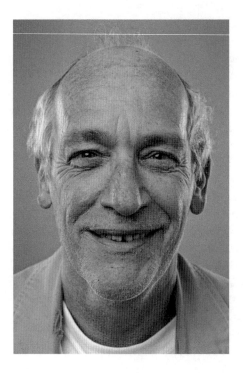

What follows is a tale from the arcane workings of government in Britain. It has ,
nonetheless, wider implications for how people and mental health are viewed more
widely; how international consultancy, insurance, technology and pharmaceutical
firms gain influence in determining the crucial detail of public policy; and how,
despite all the consultation that is said to occur, the key decisions are quietly made
long before the debate occurs. My basic claim is that in Britain the real Mental
Health Bill is the new Welfare Reform Bill.

In November 2006, the Mental Health Bill was introduced to the House of
Lords by Lord Warner, the now retired Minister of Health. [As I wrote the editorial
this chapter is based on, the Bill was slowly working its way through a Committee
stage of the House of Commons. Almost endless questions were being asked] about
when and where folk can be deprived of their liberty; for what exactly; and then,
if they are so deprived, what rights ought they to be left with, and ought they to

pay the costs of their own accommodation if so imprisoned. This was the Mental Health Bill of the 2006–2007 session of parliament. It is important to point out these dates, since reading the details of the debate between committee members – especially the Dickensian penny-pinching – it becomes hard to tell the century in which they are talking. Readers of *Hansard* are given a clue when the chairman reprimands committee members, like naughty school children, for texting on their mobile phones in his sight (Cook, 2007).

Depriving individuals of their liberties of course requires serious debate and Members of Parliament should be paying attention through such deliberations, but what was introduced by Lord Warner in November 2006 was not, however, the real Mental Health Bill. That is yet to come.… For while the Commons was debating their Lordships' Bill [on the mental capacity and serious medical treatment of the populous, another debate was being held more quietly, but not in silence, in a hall elsewhere in Westminster, and also further a field in 'cyberspace'].

Jim Murphy, Minister for Work in early 2007 (and at the other end of the demographic to Lord Warner) had recently been agonising over those too ill to work. To demonstrate his transparency and his fluency with new technology he went one step further than texting and had an official blog. Very few people commented on his blog, but a couple of weeks before Lord Warner in the Lords introduced his Bill, Jim raised the issue of how Personal Capability Assessment (PCA) reviews were too weighted, in his mind, towards those with physically disabilities. More ought to be done, in particular, to steer those with mental health problems back to work, using his department's army of private physicians – outsourced though Atos Origin, the international information technology services company – employed to raise the sick to their feet and set them to their labours. The first response to this news was a comment posted four days later:

> *I found the assessment very hard – I'm bipolar, and yet the doctor had out-of-date notes – and was arguing with me about things like what my disability really was, and eventually told me that all I needed to do was go onto medication and then I'd 'function normally'. As someone that's spent most of her life working hard to stay off of medication, I thought this was a very mean and out of line thing to say. As it turns out, I'm still considered unable to work, but those interviews really are terrifying, something I'd like to see addressed. Y'can't really go in there and show your best if the place scares you into your worst.* (Anon, 2006)

Jim was reassuring in his reply: '*Nobody should have to put up with a scary experience when they attend an examination*', he said. In the brave new world of the internet, patients can easily come to believe that they really are having a discussion with a government minister. [Quite what their physician will make of this tale is hard to imagine.] Is talking to ministers in cyberspace akin to hearing voices in past times? A dozen days later a second comment to Jim's posting came: '*Very interesting and beautiful site. It is a lot of ful [sic] information. Thanks.*' It received no reply from the minister. The third comment a couple of days later again was from a person who wanted to work but found gaining work difficult because of their irregular – and hence perceived as not dependable – employment history. Jim suggested they consult the Disability Discrimination Act and perhaps try out his department's Job Introduction Scheme.

Jim's heart was in the right place, but did he pause to wonder why so many now find themselves in this position? Hundreds of thousands of people have not worked for more than two years because of mental health problems; indeed they form the majority of the more than two million people who survive through receiving Incapacity Benefit (Freud, 2007, page 4, Figure 2 and PFMHTWG, 2006, page 8).

... Jim's heart hardened a month later, however, when the fourth and final respondent to his blog wrote the following and received a frosty response (the first part of which presumably relates to part of the comment edited out of the website):

> *I also have problems with my mental health and feel there is a lack of empathy all round including people who deal with benefit claims. How are we expected to go back to an employer with a problem when your confidence gets constantly knocked by the people who are actually supposed to be helping you in the first place i.e. jobcentre staff and there [sic] call centre staff. They are implicitly rude and condescending and don't want you on the phone or at there [sic] desk and will tell you anything to get rid of you. The answer to the problem of getting people with mental health issues back to work is simple. Retrain government jobcentre staff to be more approachable and all round nicer people then maybe we will find the confidence to ask for help and look for jobs!!!"*

Jim Murphy responded:

> *... I don't agree that child poverty will get worse. We're providing more help to families who need it most, and more work opportunities for those who can work (as well as support for those who can't) and this is all contributing to our aim of halving child poverty by 2010 and eradicating it by 2020.*
>
> *I recognise that some people may regard the money we spend on cutting benefit fraud as a waste but Income Support and Jobseeker's Allowance fraud has reduced by around two thirds in comparison to 1997/98. The advertising campaigns also help to raise public awareness of benefit fraud and reinforce that benefit theft is wrong and socially unacceptable.*

Three months later Jim's department admitted that child poverty had risen. And with that the comments ended (or were blocked – in cyberspace you never know which).

And that may well have been the extent of the consultation on the minister's acceptance of the Physical Function and Mental Health Technical Working Group's (PFMHTWG, 2006) *Report on the Transformation of the Personal Capability Assessment of the Department for Work and Pensions*. If you have read this far I'm assuming you are interested in what was actually being suggested. So just what did this snappily titled report suggest (and Jim, as he announced on his blog in October 2006, accept)? And who produced it?

The remit of the Department for Work and Pensions working groups included, especially in relation to those with mental health problems, '*accurately identify[ing] those who in spite of their condition are fit to continue to work*' (page 2). They did this by attempting to assess the level of functional limitation at which it is unreasonable to require a person to engage in work....

The mental function part of the assessment currently involves a series of yes/no answers to questions concerning a claimant's ability to cope with pressure, complete tasks, interact with others, and generally get through the day. This is thought by the PFMHTWG groups to be too crude. In addition, just to confuse, the current system treats as 15, not 12, the sum of a mental health score of 6 and a physical health score of 6. The person who came up with that clearly had a mathematician's sense of humour or enjoys confusing people who claim benefits (because they are too ill to work). (For those who enjoy non-Euclidean mathematics 6+6=15 is 2+2=5 three times over.) Directly after imparting these details regarding their weird mathematics the technical working groups blandly report that: '*To date the PCA remains the best assessment of its type in the world*' (page 8). Yes, they really do have a sense of humour! More seriously, however, they do in the same paragraph acknowledge that the Disability Discrimination Act has altered the landscape requiring employers to make reasonable adjustments to enable people with disabilities to work. Although the British government appears more interested in compulsion than freedom, it is important to note that most people who cannot work because of illness would like to work – but in the right conditions.

...

It is worth repeating that any of us, or our children, friends or family, could find ourselves in years to come being take step by step through the new system, by an Atos Origin physician whose first responsibilities are to the shareholders of the private firm who employs him or her.

It is said that the new-style PCA will attempt to be positive, exploring claimants' motivations, aspirations, self-confidence and whether their current medication (if they are on any) has detrimental effects and what could be done about that – but it is all focused on the individual. The problem of lack of work in Britain is not the problem of individuals, of those currently outside of the workplace, but of the lack of a supply of suitable work, just as with education, housing and health care and opportunity (Dorling, 2006). In the past when there was more enjoyable (or at least not such demeaning) work, and more work of the right kind at the right time, far more people suffering a variety of mental health problems worked (see Beatty *et al*, 2007, and much of their work that precedes this publication).

It would be wrong to think that those making the new PCA assessments, to be carried out by trained healthcare professionals, will have *only* the financial health of their employers' shareholders at heart. Their employers will be paid by the DWP and so they will also have the ministry's interests and rules at heart (or at least in their heads). Those rules include the requirement that trained healthcare professionals will not discuss their reports with those they are reporting on. That would be far too time-consuming. And, after all, the reports are the property of DWP. Instead they will pass them on – presumably to medically untrained personal advisors who will discuss them with the claimants. The PCA reports will also be given to '*private and voluntary sector providers of condition management programmes, and to the person's GP*' (PFMHTWG, 2006, p 19). Later in the report it says that passing on to the GP might be with the claimant's consent. No comment is made as to whether claimants assessed as mentally ill will have any opportunity to give their consent before their details are passed on to the arms-length condition management programme provider.

Feelings such as being powerless; that others do not have your interests at heart; that you have little control over your future; that you should be anxious and that you are inadequate; should be pessimistic and your opinions and you are not worth much – all these may well result from the process that the introduction of the arms-length management programme provides. Without an understanding of why there has been such a great rise in the numbers of people with mental health problems unable to work, this process could well add to the burden of such illness.

The report makes no comment as to what level of support people should be able to expect at work to help them back to work other than implying that all that can be expected is that which a '*reasonable employer would be expected to provide to any person in employment*' (page 23). No special treatment apparently. With luck, and – as such unthinking ambivalence is at odds with other legislation – with hope, some of the piloting will soften the edges of the recommendations. However, at the heart of this official thinking is a very individualist view of society made up of autonomous people, some of whom are problems. For me, it is because their basic view of society is wrong that their policies will not work. We should be looking first at how the way we now organise ourselves makes so many of us ill. But we don't and that is the first of our collective mistakes with the real Mental Health Bill. So who is making these mistakes?

As to the producers of the PFMHTWG report, membership of the working groups reflected, we are told, a wide range of expertise in relevant fields, although none of the authors are named up front other than the chair, the head of the DWP Health and Benefits Division herself. (Rather like MI5 now naming 'M', it appears that the moniker of the head of Health and Benefits can also now be spoken although, just as with M, no pictures are provided.) The other members of the group apparently worked closely with stakeholders although they only consulted in a limited way with 'service users'. An annex lists who these group members were. Several are associated with private providers or insurers (including a representative of Atos Origin, which currently profits from carrying out DWP assessments). Apparently, whenever the PFMHTWG felt they were not fully equipped to do the job, other experts were quickly co-opted to bring the necessary skills. And the purpose of the PFMHTWG is indeed to lay the groundwork for 'a product' available for the Welfare Reform Bill, and for the passage of secondary legislation through Parliament (page 5). The Welfare Reform Bill was given Royal Assent on 3 May 2007.

For the architects of the Welfare Reform Bill, the real Mental Health Bill, there is much more work to be done, but, as is increasingly the case with reports such as that of the PFMHTWG, clues are given in their future work remit as to what the answers will be: *'to validate it as a fairer, more robust, and more accurate assessment of benefit entitlement'*. And, no, I didn't make that up (see page 6), they really do say what the findings of a future validation study will be even before they commission that study! ... And how did the democratically elected Member of Parliament and the responsible government Minister report on the ascendancy of his Bill into law when communicating to the masses via his blog:

> *The main change I mentioned will be the introduction of the Employment and Support Allowance which will replace Incapacity Benefit and Income Support based on incapacity or disability next year. This will bring to life a fundamental change in the welfare state that we have been talking about on this blog in some detail, namely the move towards your ability to work, not your incapacity to work.*
>
> *The new Personal Capability Assessment will mean this approach is embedded into the system and I think we can look forward to more people getting better, targeted help in getting them back to work.*
>
> *For the majority of people, this will mean additional responsibilities to be actively preparing or looking for work.*

(www.dwp.gov.uk/welfarereform/blog/ – 4 May 2007)

[As I first wrote these words, 17 days after 4 May 2007, not a single loyal subject had hit the *'to comment'* button and responded.]

...

Addendum

Five years and one month later the web page refereed to above states:

> *Sorry, that page has been archived*

Click on the archive link and you can read:

> *Following the Cabinet re-shuffle Jim Murphy has moved on to take up the post of Minister of State at the Foreign and Commonwealth Office. The Welfare Reform blog is now closed to new posts but you can still read old ones.*

All the comments I refer to above appear to have been deleted.

Maybe, in some institution somewhere, an anonymous person is trying to explain to the authorities that they are not mad and that they really did have a conversation through his blog with the Minister, Jim Murphy, before he moved on to become 'Minister of State at the Foreign and Commonwealth Office'. They find the archived website but their comments about being bipolar have been deleted. *'He really did reply to me,'* they protest, but no one believes them. They just tick 'My mental problems impair my ability to communicate with other people' on the new Mental Health Assessment scoring sheet (see Figure 15.1).

Figure 15.1: The Mental Health Assessment – Descriptors and scores

The mental health assessment is a separate part of the Personal Capability Assessment. Like the physical assessment it involves scoring points from descriptors but you are not shown or directed to address these on the questionnaire. Even if you are asked to attend at a medical examination you will still not be directly asked about all the descriptors shown below. Which descriptors are satisfied and how many points you score will be based on the opinion of the doctor at the examination, together with any other evidence available, such as the details you give on the form and notes from your GP or anyone else helping you. The descriptors are divided into four main areas of difficulties that you may have. Points can be scored and added together from any of the areas and questions shown below.

Descriptors	Points
Completion of tasks	
I cannot answer the telephone and reliably take a message	2
I often sit for hours doing nothing	2
I cannot concentrate to read a magazine article or follow a radio or television programme	1
I cannot use a telephone book or other directory to find a number	1
My mental condition prevents me from undertaking leisure activities that I previously enjoyed	1
I overlook or forget the risk posed by domestic appliances or other common hazards due to poor concentration	1
Agitation, confusion or forgetfulness has resulted in my having potentially dangerous accidents in the 3 months before the day the benefit is claimed for	1
My concentration can only be sustained by prompting	1
Daily living	
I need encouragement to get up and dress	2
I need alcohol before midday	2
I am frequently distressed at some time of the day due to fluctuation of mood	1
I do not care about my appearance and living conditions	1
Sleep problems interfere with my daytime activities	1
Coping with pressure	
Mental stress was a factor in making me stop work	2
I frequently feel scared or panicky for no obvious reason	2
I avoid carrying out routine activities because I am convinced they will prove too tiring or stressful	1
I am unable to cope with changes in my daily routine	1
I frequently find there are so many things to do that I give up because of fatigue, apathy or disinterest	1
I am scared or anxious that work would bring back or worsen my illness	1
Interaction with other people	
I cannot look after myself without help from others	2
I get upset by ordinary events and this results in disruptive behavioural problems	2
My mental problems impair my ability to communicate with other people	2
I get irritated by things that would not have bothered me before I became ill	1
I prefer to be left alone for 6 hours or more each day	1
I am too frightened to go out alone	1

Source: http://www.tameside.gov.uk/benefits/capabilityassessment

[Editorial Note: This was the point-scoring system as of October 2010, which citizens of Tameside borough were being advised of through this website (still available in September 2012). The points system have been changed. There are many websites offering advice to mentally ill people on this. Increasing numbers of these sites are trying to charge for the information they give. People who become 'panicky for no obvious reason' can be easy prey.]

References

Anon (2006) Comment 1, Welfare reform blog, http://www.dwp.gov.uk/welfarereform/blog/index.php/2006/10/19/mental-health-action/#comments

Beatty, C., Fothergill, S., Gore, T., and Powell, R. (2007) *The real level of unemployment*, Report, Sheffield: CRESR, http://www.shu.ac.uk/cresr/downloads/publications/The%20Real%20Level%20of%20Unemployment%202007-.pdf

CCJS (Centre for Crime and Justice Studies) (2007) *History of the CJS*, http://www.kcl.ac.uk/depsta/rel/ccjs/history.html

Cook, F. (2007) *Public Bill Committee, Mental Health Bill*, Afternoon session, Tuesday, 15 May, end of col 416, http://www.publications.parliament.uk/pa/cm200607/cmpublic/mental/070515/pm/70515s01.htm

Dorling, D. (2006) Inequalities in Britain 1997-2006: The dream that turned pear-shaped, *Local Economy*, 21(4) 353–361, http://sasi.group.shef.ac.uk/publications/2006/dorling_inequalityinBritain1997_corrected.pdf

Dumit, J. (2005) The depsychiatrisation of mental illness, *Journal of Public Mental Health*, 4, 3, 8-13.

Elliott, L. and Atkinson, D. (2007) *Fantasy island*, London: Constable and Robinson. For a long extract of the book see: http://books.guardian.co.uk/extracts/story/0,,2082838,00.html

Engel, N. (2007), MP for North East Derbyshire, contribution to Westminster Hall debate on the Government Employment Strategy, Thursday, 17 May, Hansard: col 341WH, http://www.publications.parliament.uk/pa/cm200607/cmhansrd/cm070517/halltext/70517h0003.htm

Freud D. (2007) *Reducing dependency, increasing opportunity: options for the future of welfare to work, An independent report to the Department for Work and Pensions*, London: Department for Work and Pensions.

PFMHTWG (Physical Function and Mental Health Technical Working Groups) (2006) *Transformation of the Personal Capability Assessment*, Department for Work and Pensions, September, http://www.dwp.gov.uk/welfarereform/tpca.pdf

Wilkinson, R. (2005) *The impact of inequality: How to make sick societies healthier*, London: Routledge. See also http://books.guardian.co.uk/reviews/politicsphilosophyandsociety/0,6121,1538844,00.html

16

Losing votes and voters: would action on inequality have saved New Labour?[1]

McCartney, G., Collins, C. and Dorling, D. (2010) 'Observation: Would action on health inequalities have saved New Labour?', *British Medical Journal*, 23 June, vol 340, p 1388.

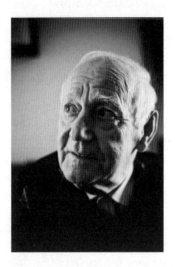

Had Labour narrowed the mortality gap, the current parliament might have looked different

Inequality in health is among the factors that could have made a crucial difference in this year's UK general election. How? We know that the gap in life expectancy between the worst and best local authorities grew in the 10 years after New Labour was elected in 1997. The effects of this inequality have not been politically neutral. In the areas that tend to elect Labour party representatives people are likely to die relatively young, and in the areas that tend to elect Conservative party representatives people tend to live longer.

Taking older voters at previous elections from 1997, 2001, and 2005, we can confidently say that a higher proportion of those who voted Conservative than of Labour voters were still around to do so again in 2010. The great irony is, of course, that this growth in health inequality is now part of the legacy of the longest ever period of Labour government.

---

[1] Editorial Note: It is still possible that the action Labour did take will have an effect on reducing future premature deaths among its voters and perhaps that may tip the balance in future elections.

The quotation 'Vote early—and vote often' has been attributed to Chicago politics. However, an interpretation of the saying can perhaps help cast some light on the recent UK general election result and the subsequent emergence of the Conservative–Liberal Democrat coalition.

New Labour was elected in 1997 on a manifesto that included tackling the underlying causes of bad health and reducing health inequalities. Frank Dobson, as the government's first health secretary, wanted to establish the basis for the future use of the slogan 'vote Labour, live longer'.

After 13 years in government Labour has lost power. The election produced a 'hung parliament'. Theoretically 326 seats are required for a parliamentary majority, though in practice fewer would have been workable. With 258 seats Labour could not quite, even with the support of the 57 Liberal Democrats, come close enough to the required figure. The Tories failed to win an outright majority because their vote rose by most in seats that they already held. But with 306 seats a coalition with the Liberal Democrats became possible.

With such a finely balanced result, anything that could meaningfully have influenced where and how votes were cast in the election could be advocated as tipping the balance of power. One such thing is a continuing inequality in terms of the opportunity that certain people, in certain places, with certain political dispositions get to 'vote often'—not in the literal sense of frequency of voting but in terms of the number of opportunities to vote across their lifetimes.

National statistics show that the gap in life expectancy between the worst and best local authorities in the United Kingdom grew from under nine years in 1997 to almost 13 years by 2007. This suggests that during the period of the New Labour government the 'political participation expectancy gap' between these local authority areas grew— because of differences in mortality—from roughly two to three general elections.

The effects of this inequality, as indicated above, have not been politically neutral. Those politically disposed to the Tories have tended to benefit from it. In relation to Dobson's slogan, we might say that those who voted Labour before 2010 did tend to live a bit longer but that those who voted Conservative tended to live rather longer still—and vote more often.

Mass electoral participation is, in historical terms, a relatively recent phenomenon in the United Kingdom. It was not until 1928 that the suffrage, or 'right to vote', was secured for virtually all adults over 21. Without this progress it would have been hard to have imagined the 1945 Labour landslide that helped usher in the NHS. Even given that, the post-1945 intake of members of parliament showed inequalities in mortality reflecting the communities from which they were drawn.

The hope invested in voting among many of today's 'socially excluded' communities is rather lower than that of their 'politically excluded' forebears. In such areas the proportion of people using their vote has fallen precipitously, representing a further loss in terms of the number of Labour votes. When asked, people who abstain say they would be much more likely to vote Labour than Conservative.

Abstention reflects a feeling that voting matters less and doesn't change anything very much. This is a feeling that is backed by some fairly compelling arguments and evidence about the operation of our democracy in recent decades. Democratic institutions in Britain have seemed, in recent years, increasingly to separate people from, rather than connect them to, the operation of power.

However, as this most recent election has shown in its own very particular way, the securing of a parliamentary majority remains crucial to the operation of this 'democracy'. Voting does matter. The parties were aware of the demographics. In the marginal constituencies in particular, their backers' resources were expended to maximise their vote. And the legacy of New Labour was such that the Tories had many more of their older voters still around to mobilise.

Had it narrowed rather than widened the mortality gap in the UK during its term of government, the balance of the current parliament might have been a bit different—perhaps different enough to have facilitated a coalition that would have seen Labour retain its Downing Street presence[2].

Figure 16.1: Ministers' Mortality League Table, 1997–2010.

Minister	Status	Constituency	Excess deaths	
Donald DEWAR	Secretary of State for Scotland	Glasgow Anniesland		2496
Clare SHORT	Secretary of State for International Development	Birmingham Ladywood		1729
Frank DOBSON	Secretary of State for Health	Holborn & St Pancras		1547
George ROBERTSON	Secretary of State for Defence	Hamilton South		1014
Jack STRAW	Secretary of State for the Home Department	Blackburn		936
Nick BROWN	became Minister for Agriculture, Fisheries and Farming	Newcastle East & Wallsend		832
Alistair DARLING	Secretary of State for Social Security	Edinburgh Central		819
John PRESCOTT	Deputy Prime Minister	Hull East		793
Chris SMITH	Secretary of State for Culture, Media and Sport	Islington South & Finsbury		728
David BLUNKETT	Secretary of State for Education and Employment	Sheffield Brightside		637
Mo MOWLAM	Secretary of State for Northern Ireland	Redcar		572
Alun MICHAEL	became Secretary of State for Wales	Cardiff South & Penarth		507
Alan MILBURN	became Chief Secretary to the Treasury	Darlington		481
Stephen BYERS	became Secretary of State for Trade and Industry	North Tyneside		429
Tony BLAIR	Prime Minister	Sedgefield		416
Gordon BROWN	Chancellor	Dunfermline East		325
Robin COOK	Foreign Secretary	Livingston		312
Margaret BECKETT	became Leader of the House	Derby South		299
Jack CUNNINGHAM	became Minister for the Cabinet Office	Copeland		234
Ann TAYLOR	became Chief Whip	Dewsbury		104

Note: Excess deaths aged under 65 attributable to not reducing inequalities in health.

Also deceased – Donald Dewar, Mo Mowlam and Robin Cook.

Source: Table 7a of Dorling, D. (1998) Whose voters suffer if inequalities in health remain? *Journal of Contemporary Health*, 7, 50-54. (Revised on 8 February 1999 – cabinet posts as of that date).

[2] Editorial Note: Figure 16.1 was not included in the original article. It is reproduced here from an old table (shown in a new form) listing how many voters were lost due to premature deaths under the age of 65 that would not have occurred had New Labour achieved the reduction in health inequalities its Government had promised. These losses are just for Cabinet members' seats for the period 1997–2010 for the Cabinet Ministers in office in 1999. Note that three of the 20 Cabinet members (15%) had themselves died by 2005.

17

Mapping inequalities in Britain[1]

Dorling, D. and Thomas, B. (2011) 'Mapping inequalities in Britain', *Sociology Review*, vol 21, no 1, pp 15-19.

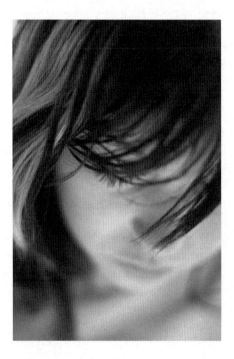

This paper draws on three of the key topics we discuss in our latest atlas, *Bankrupt Britain: An atlas of social change* (Dorling and Thomas 2011).

Public sector cuts: local and national implications

In June 2010 the Department for Communities and Local Government published what is likely to become one of the most infamous documents of the economic recession, titled *Local government contribution to efficiencies in 2010/11* (DCLG 2010). This document set out what many have argued are some of the most unfairly distributed cuts ever to be imposed on local government in England. The poor and the poorest areas of the country appeared to have been targeted to receive the deepest and most sustained cuts. This mirrored the effects of the national budget of that month that was also found, on examination by the Institute for Fiscal Studies

---

[1] Written with Bethan Thomas for a magazine aimed at A level students.

(2010), to be highly regressive (taking more from the poor as a proportion of their income than from the rich). It may well not have been a coincidence that almost all of the areas to suffer the greatest service cuts contained a large majority of people who had voted against the two parties that had come to form the new coalition government.

Figure 17.1a shows where from April 2011 the main cuts will hit most, least, and not at all. These are the first relatively modest local government cuts, of 'just' £6 billion. However, not a penny of that £6 billion is to be saved by the citizens of generally well-heeled districts such as Chiltern, South Bucks, most of Devon, Christchurch, most of Dorset, Cheltenham, the Cotswolds, Winchester, Broxbourne, most of Hertfordshire, Tunbridge Wells, Harrogate, most of Oxfordshire (but not Oxford), all of Surrey, the Malvern Hills and another hundred or so generally 'leafy' and mostly 'Tory' or 'Liberal Democrat' areas. Some of the counties these districts lie in will see cuts, but all of less than 0.9% and some as small as 0.6% of their budgets. The smallest reported cut of all, of just 0.1%, will be to the budget of the Corporation of the City of London.

It is mostly in the North and in cities where the local cuts in government spending from April 2011 onwards will be greatest, initially reducing budgets by 1% and 2%, in places like: Sheffield, Barnsley, Bradford, Bolton, Corby, Kingston upon Hull, Gateshead, Stoke-on-Trent, Sunderland, Salford, Nottingham, Stockton-on-Tees, Hartlepool, Doncaster, Redcar & Cleveland, Liverpool, Knowsley, Middlesbrough, St Helens, Blackpool, Barrow-in-Furness, Bolsover, Hastings and Burnley, and in a couple of dozen similar areas. Anyone with a rudimentary knowledge of English electoral geography knows that the map resembles, more than anything else, a map of where people are poor, and where most abstain at general elections or vote Labour.

The public sector is proportionately larger in poorer areas than in rich areas as poorer areas have more need of social workers, housing officers and so on. Figure 17.1b shows the proportion of people aged 16–64 in each district of Britain who are in employment, and who are working in public administration, education and health (a few of the education and health workers will be employed in the private sector). The proportions of people employed in the public sector are highest in Richmondshire with the army base in Catterick (46% of local workers are state employed), in the Scottish islands of Eilean Siar (where a small population requires 43% state employment) and in Oxford (dominated by universities and hospitals, just under 43%). The lowest proportions are in generally well-off, not-too-isolated rural areas, such as Tamworth (15%), Maldon (17%), North Warwickshire (18%) and Melton (19%), and also in Kensington & Chelsea (19%).

The final map in this section, Figure 17.1c shows the unemployment that would result from massive cuts of a quarter of all public sector jobs. It is drawn by taking current unemployment rates and adding to those a quarter of the public sector workforce. This assumes that all those laid off do not get other work or retire or move, but also that their unemployment does not result in knock-on rises in joblessness in their local areas as local services, shops, cafes and amenities (that public sector workers could once afford) close down. Some 407,000 employees, almost 5% of

Figure 17.1: **(a)** 2010-11 reduction in main revenue grant allocations (%), local authorities, England. **(b)** 2009 proportion of employees in the public sector (%), local authories, Britain. **(c)** Projection of unemployment rates given a 25% cut in public sector employment, local authorities, Britain.

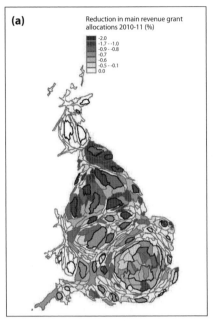

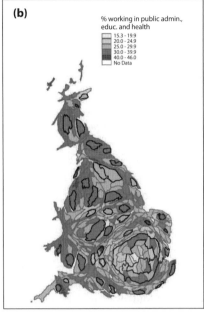

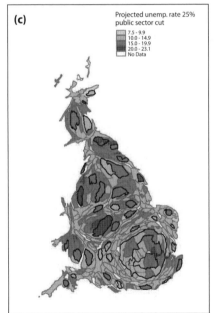

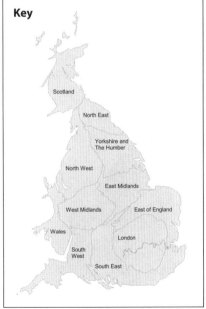

Source: Dorling and Thomas, 2011.

the entire public sector workforce, work in just four cities and make up just under a third of all employees there: Birmingham (36% of employees), Sheffield (35%), Glasgow (34%) and Leeds (27%). However, these are dwarfed by the public sector workforce of London at 990,000 workers (a 27% share of the workforce).

We have already seen that the cuts are not to be evenly spread across the country, so Figure 17.1c may well overestimate the effects of cuts in the South, and underestimate them in the North.

Legalising tax evasion on inheritance

Most people believe in obeying the law, in following social norms, and think that citizens have a moral duty to pay tax. Tax provides the funding that the state requires to run government, to prevent people starving, to give all an education and a health service. It is said to be the money that stops us descending into anarchy and helps to create the society in which we live. A few other people quite like the idea of anarchy (they are called anarchists) but they have rarely lived under such a system. When businesses do not pay their full taxes they secure an unfair advantage over other businesses.

Many very affluent citizens try to avoid paying inheritance and other taxes through exploiting loopholes. They follow different social norms. When this tax avoidance exceeds legal action it is called tax evasion. Evasion can be made legal, and become avoidance, by changes to the law. The law on inheritance tax is being changed to allow a tiny number of people rich enough for their estates to be liable for inheritance tax to avoid paying a large part of their share of that tax. Currently, only about 7% of people have sufficient wealth to have inheritance tax levied on their estates after their death (Figure 17.1d shows how that rate varies across the country when expressed per 1000 deaths). Half of those people avoid the tax, at least in the short term. In the majority of cases the tax is delayed because a surviving spouse has inherited and the tax applies only upon that spouse's death, and then with a threshold of double the individual allowance.

In 2007/08 only 22,210 estates in Britain were found to be eligible for inheritance tax; some 557,499 people died in the calendar year 2007 (which ended a few months before that tax year), thus inheritance tax was payable on the estates of only around 3.98% of people who died in Britain in the latest year for which there is data. Very rich people

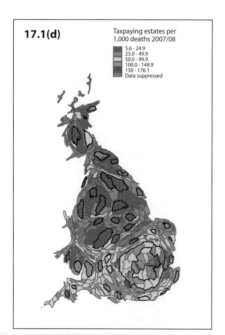

17.1(d)

Taxpaying estates per 1,000 deaths 2007/08

- 5.6 - 24.9
- 25.0 - 49.9
- 50.0 - 99.9
- 100.0 - 149.9
- 150 - 176.1
- Data suppressed

(d) 2007/08 inheritance tax-paying estates per 1,000 persons dying, local authorities, Britain.

Figure 17.2: 2007/08 inheritance tax-paying estates, numbers, regions and countries, Britain.

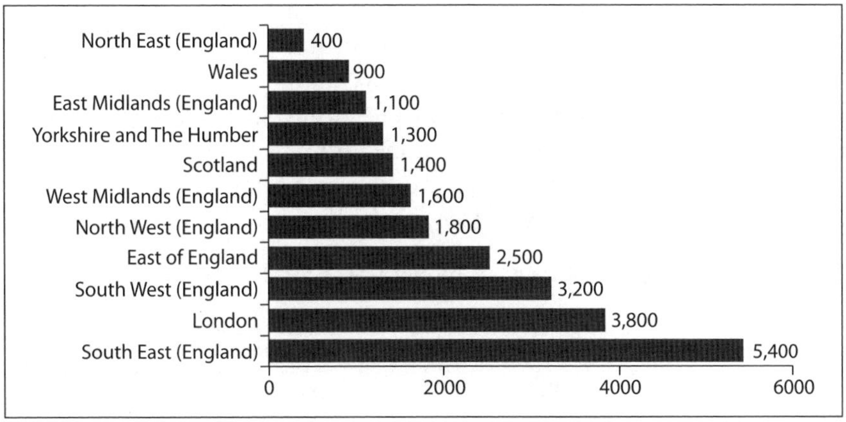

Source: Dorling and Thomas, 2011.

often spend a lot of money on legal advice and the setting up of trusts to enable them to avoid paying inheritance tax. Figure 17.2 shows on how many estates tax was paid by region in the latest year for which we have data.

More than 68,000 people died in the following 80 areas in one year, the highest number, over 2,500 a year, in Hull. Fewer than 20 of these people left estates large enough to be liable for inheritance tax in each of these places; in some probably no-one will have paid, because almost no-one is wealthy. We are almost all victims of tax evasion, but these are the places where the greatest victims of tax evasion, the poor, are most concentrated. These 80 places where there are least material riches left to inherit upon death are listed here, sorted from the most people dying a year whose estates are not liable for tax to the least:

Kingston upon Hull, Caerphilly, Falkirk, Neath Port Talbot, North Ayrshire (mainland), Knowsley, East Ayrshire, Middlesbrough, Redcar & Cleveland, Blackburn with Darwen, West Lothian, Barking & Dagenham, Telford & Wrekin, Halton, Ashfield, West Dunbartonshire, Nuneaton & Bedworth, Ipswich, Great Yarmouth, Tower Hamlets, Chesterfield, Easington, South Holland, Inverclyde, Torfaen, South Bedfordshire, Hartlepool, Derwentside, Burnley, Sedgefield, Gravesham, West Lindsey, Cannock Chase, Blyth Valley, Blaenau Gwent, Bolsover, Lincoln, Pendle, Hyndburn, Slough, Midlothian, Kettering, Wear Valley, Barrow-in-Furness, Copeland, Selby, East Northamptonshire, Boston, Blaby, Durham, Crawley, Wansbeck, Stevenage, Wellingborough, Rossendale, Merthyr Tydfil, Harlow, North Warwickshire, Redditch, Rushmoor, Tamworth, Ross & Cromarty, Caithness & Sutherland, Chester-le-Street, Forest Heath, Corby, Clackmannanshire, Melton, Oswestry, Eilean Siar, Alnwick, Berwick-upon-Tweed, Helensburgh & Lomond, Orkney Islands, Teesdale, West Moray, Shetland Islands, Lochaber, Skye & Lochalsh and Badenoch & Strathspey.

In contrast to the 80 areas above where, for all recorded purposes, practically no-one is rich enough to have inheritance tax levied upon death, Table 17.1 lists the 42 areas where the highest proportions of people had inheritance tax levied on their estates, some 5,390 estates in all. These areas account for just 8% of deaths in Britain, and yet some 24% of estates paying inheritance tax can be found in these areas, three times what would be expected were wealth equally spread around the country. The share of inheritance taxation requisitioned from these places will be far higher still because quite a few people in the wealthiest areas on this list are among the wealthiest people in the country and the world. Figure 17.3a shows these numbers

Table 17.1: 2007/08 inheritance tax, highest rates, local authorities, Britain.

Local Authority (in ascending order)	Number of tax-paying estates 2007/08	Number of people dying in 2007	Rate per 1,000 deaths
Lewes	100	1,056	94.7
Eden	50	527	94.9
Mid Sussex	120	1,258	95.4
Oxford	90	936	96.2
Hertsmere	90	927	97.1
Bromley	270	2,758	97.9
South Oxfordshire	110	1,123	98.0
Rother	130	1,327	98.0
Windsor & Maidenhead	110	1,120	98.2
New Forest	200	2,015	99.3
Wandsworth	170	1,707	99.6
Merton	130	1,285	101.2
East Dorset	100	988	101.2
Hart	60	592	101.4
Hammersmith & Fulham	100	968	103.3
Camden	130	1,252	103.8
Reigate & Banstead	130	1,233	105.4
Tandridge	80	752	106.4
East Hampshire	110	1,030	106.8
Sevenoaks	110	1,030	106.8
Horsham	130	1,209	107.5
Three Rivers	80	739	108.3
West Dorset	130	1,198	108.5
Winchester	120	1,089	110.2
Chiltern	80	723	110.7
Wokingham	110	965	114.0
Cotswold	100	857	116.7
South Hams	110	928	118.5
Chichester	170	1,429	119.0
Guildford	120	990	121.2
Harrow	180	1,464	123.0
Westminster	140	1,127	124.2
Mole Valley	110	840	131.0
Barnet	320	2,374	134.8
Kingston upon Thames	150	1,111	135.0
St Albans	140	1,006	139.2
Waverley	150	1,073	139.8
Richmond upon Thames	170	1,187	143.2
Epsom & Ewell	80	551	145.2
South Bucks	80	529	151.2
Elmbridge	180	1,123	160.3
Kensington & Chelsea	150	852	176.1

Source: Dorling and Thomas, 2011.

on the map, but the numbers are deceptive as death rates vary. In Edinburgh tax was found to be due on some 290 estates, for example, but over 4,300 people die each year in Edinburgh, so with 6.7% paying in the Scottish capital, there are many areas of England where far more are richer and even the wealthiest part of Scotland does not feature in this list.

Figure 17.3: **(a)** 2007/08 inheritance tax-paying estates, numbers, local authorities, Britain. **(b)** 2007 CO_2 emissions due to road transport (tonnes per person), local authorities, Britain. **(c)** Nations and regions. **(d)** Major towns and cities.

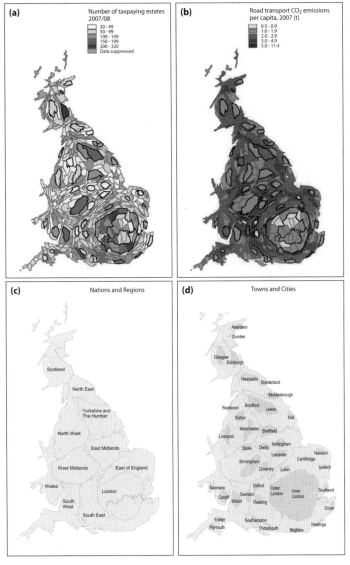

see colour version in plate section

Source: Dorling and Thomas, 2011.

Burning up the planet: CO$_2$

Recently estimates have been made of how much carbon dioxide (CO$_2$) pollution has been emitted from each region of Britain from domestic, industrial and transport activities, as well as how much is absorbed by local forestry and other carbon sinks. Industry and commerce produced slightly less CO$_2$ pollution than did all domestic and road use combined in Britain in recent years, but more than either of these two sources when each is measured alone. These official estimates of CO$_2$ emissions have been published for the years 2005, 2006 and 2007. Figure 17.3b shows just one of the many maps that can be produced from this data – the distribution of CO$_2$ emitted due to road transportation by area in 2007. Geographically road transportation emissions vary more than those for any other activity, with a twenty-fold difference between the most and least extreme local authority areas.

Environmental and political campaigners such as George Monbiot (2006) have explained repeatedly – and increasingly convincingly – the argument that we simply should not continue to pollute at the levels we do, especially in terms of how much additional CO$_2$ we cause to be emitted. This and emissions of other greenhouse gases are harming the environment and contributing to artificial global warming and the exhaustion of limited natural resources.

Just under a third of the emissions that have been measured and attributed to specific areas of the country are due to transportation pollution, mostly from petrol engine exhausts. Up to a further third of emissions are due to domestic pollution, mostly from the heating of homes. Finally, over a third of emissions in almost all areas are due to the activities of industry – again mostly caused by their consumption of energy either from the coal, oil and gas-fired electricity-generating power plants supplying that energy, or directly through the use of such fuels at the industrial plants themselves. These are – or should all be – well know facts about Britain, but people rarely get to see the maps of who pollutes the most and least and of what impact that has. If you want to know more about British society you can't avoid having to know a little bit more of its human geography (Dorling 2011).

References and further reading

DCLG (2010) *Local government contribution to efficiencies in 2010–11*, London: HMSO.

Dorling, D. (2011) *So you think you know about Britain*, London: Constable.

Dorling, D. and Thomas, B. (2011) *Bankrupt Britain: A post-recession atlas*, Bristol: The Policy Press.

Institute for Fiscal Studies (2010) *New IFS research challenges Chancellor's 'progressive Budget' claim*, IFS press release by James Browne and Peter Levell, August, www.ifs. org.uk/publications/5245.

Monbiot, G. (2006) *Heat: How to stop the planet burning*, London: Allen Lane.

Wilkinson, R and Pickett, K. (2009) *The spirit level: Why equality is better for everyone*, London: Penguin.

18

London's political landscapes[1]

Hennig, B.D. and Dorling, D. (2012) 'In focus: London's political landscapes', *Political Insight*, vol 3, no 1, p 38.

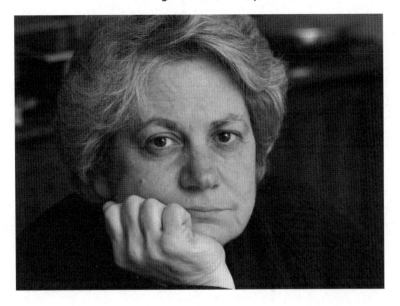

Ahead of London's 2012 mayoral vote we took a look at the geography of the 2008 London mayoral election (Figure 18.1).

2012 is not only the year of the London Olympics. In May, Londoners will decide on who they want to see leading their city for the next four years. The 2008 mayoral election in London was won by the Conservative candidate Boris Johnson, who secured 50 per cent of the votes after taking second preferences into account. But the political message from the last election goes beyond the usual fight between the Labour and Conservative parties over who has power in Britain's capital.

This map series shows the specific distribution of first preference votes for each of the candidates and their respective political party in the 2008 mayoral election mapped onto an equal population projection, where every Londoner is given exactly the same amount of space in the map. Instead of showing the total shares in comparison, the maps take the maximum share of votes into account. The range of

---

[1] Editorial Note: This very short article was written with Benjamin Hennig and he drew the maps. The maps shown here reveal how divided that city is through its voting, which shows patterns very similar to the geographies of good and poor health. Londoners were voting in 2012 whether to share more or less. They chose 'less'.

votes is shown in five graduated circles based on a natural breaks classification that highlights the variance of the particular support for a party's candidate across London.

Although the candidates of the smaller parties hardly stood a chance in taking over the job that currently pays an annual salary of £143,911, the electorate that voted for these candidates is just as concentrated in particular clusters across the city as are those supporters of the two main political camps. The geographical relevance of these patterns is a manifestation of the socioeconomic patchwork of a divided city.

Figure 18.1: Vote shares in the 2008 London mayoral election.

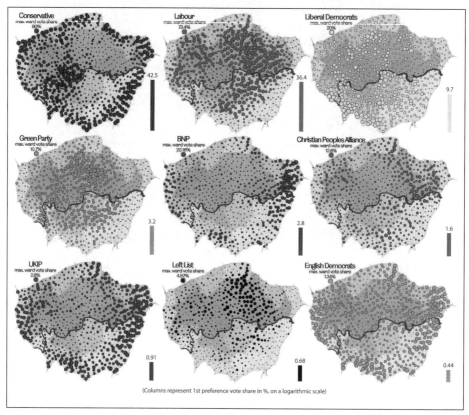

Source: Thanks to Michael Thrasher of the University of Plymouth for data used in these maps.

SECTION IV
Despair and joy

19

Preserving sanity when everything is related to everything else

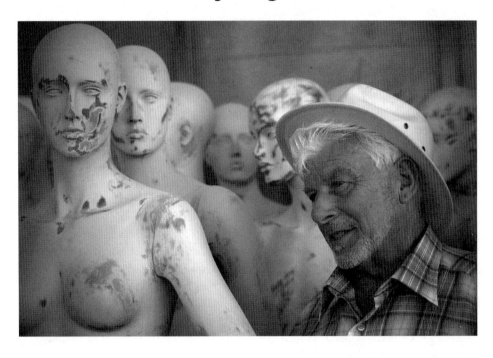

This section brings together issues of both despair and joy. It begins with the study of the depths of despair and an academic paper that has been edited down to a short commentary (see Chapter 20) concerning the predictability of the geography of suicide. It suggests that it is possible, with an accuracy of within a few dozen people, to estimate the numbers of those who will kill themselves within every parliamentary constituency of Britain each year. This is despite the fact that, for any single individual, such a prediction is almost impossible, and despite the fact that between these areas there are five-fold differences in their recorded annual suicide rates. Suicides are rarely reported in the press unless the victim is a celebrity, or more than one person dies at a time, or other people are killed (STV, 2012). They are rarely reported because they are so common. And in Britain in recent years the numbers of suicides have risen by at least 10 per cent.[1]

---

[1] Personal communication, June 2012, with David Gunnell, Professor of Epidemiology, University of Bristol. On the rarity of the reporting of suicide, note that between 2009 and 2011 just one police officer in England and Wales was recorded as having died as a result of homicide (*Hansard*, House of Commons Debate, 11 October 2011, col 331W), as compared with 55 suicides being recorded as the cause of death of police officers over the same period of time in the same two countries (*Hansard*, House of Commons Debate, 12 July 2012, col 294W).

Suicide and the long recession

> *Michael Marmot, a world expert in public health epidemiology, last week stated that we are in 'a public health emergency ... if you look across Europe at unemployment rates, a 1% rise in unemployment in a country is associated with a 0.8% rise in suicides'. According to the Campaign for a Fair Society, 25% of the cuts are falling disproportionately on 3% of the population, namely sick and/or disabled people in receipt of state support.* (Carty et al, 2012)

The number of suicides varies over time. It rises during bleak periods of increasing worklessness, and also during periods where greater selfishness is encouraged (see Chapter 21). However, at the same time as the suicide rate rises when political parties promoting *inequality* are elected, it is also one of the few causes of death that is more common in more *equitable* affluent countries.

Although poor mental health, the use of drink and drugs to self-medicate and the killing of others are all more common in more *inequitable* nations, people are *less* likely to turn the blame in on themselves and to quietly internalise despair in places where there are *greater* differences between income and wealth within a population. Within the most equitable of affluent nations, such as within the Scandinavian countries and Japan, suicide rates have tended to be higher than within the most affluent nations, such as Greece and Italy, with average rates of inequality (among OECD countries. However, recently, on the south-eastern edge of Europe:

> *In Greece, the suicide rate among men increased more than 24 percent from 2007 to 2009, government statistics show. In Ireland during the same period, suicides among men rose more than 16 percent. In Italy, suicides motivated by economic difficulties have increased 52 percent, to 187 [per million men] in 2010 — the most recent year for which statistics were available — from 123 in 2005.* (Povoledo and Carvajal, 2012)

By 2011 and into 2012 the situation in the north-west European periphery became worse:

> *... Irish suicide helpline 1life has revealed that it is struggling to cope with the near one hundred calls a day it is taking. The group has confirmed it received over 33,000 pleas for help in the past 12 months as the suicide rate rises dramatically. Experts fear that as many as 1,000 people will commit suicide in Ireland in 2012. The situation is so bad that police are watching known suicide spots like the quays in Dublin, Cork, Limerick and Waterford. The* Irish Independent *also reports that sea cliffs in Clare are under surveillance in a bid to thwart the growing numbers.* (Counihan, 2012)

Economic turmoil in the European periphery, from Greece through Italy, Spain, Portugal, Ireland, Britain and Iceland, was totally surpassed by the economic collapse that occurred in Eastern Europe after 1989, and which resulted in a far higher number of deaths from suicide as a result. When suicide rates are studied within one large highly unequal country, such as Russia, a series of unsurprising correlations between those rates and alcohol consumption are revealed (Pridemore, 2006). The more alcohol men drink, the more people (both men and women) kill themselves, but what causes more despair in one area compared to another? The following correlations reveal different trends for men and women's relative risks of suicide within 78 regions of Russia (the Chechen and Ingush Republics were not included because of the ongoing wars there):

- suicide and inequality have a negative correlation of –0.19;
- male suicide and inequality have a negative correlation of –0.22;
- female suicide and inequality have a negative correlation of –0.09.

The greater the inequality within a region in Russia the fewer men, in particular, are likely to commit suicide. For women there is hardly any statistical relationship between inequality and suicide. Inequality here is measured as the ratio between the top and bottom quintile incomes within each Russian region. The study also found an even stronger negative correlation of –0.37 between poverty (measured as the percentage living below a 1999 standard poverty line) and inequality – in Russia where there were more poor people there was more equality, presumably because the whole region was poorer. The highest suicide rates were found within the poorest areas, with a positive correlation between poverty and suicide of 0.33.

In Russia suicide is not most common within the most economically unequal of regions. So just as worldwide we find suicide rates are a little lower in more unequal countries, so within Russian regions we find the same relationship. Perhaps men have a little more hope in more unequal Russian regions of doing better? Or perhaps to survive in such regions it becomes more common to blame others rather than yourself for your misfortune? The differences between male and female rates should provide clues as to the mechanism operating.

A case could be made that because there are so many dissimilarities in the possible causes and circumstances (and most preferred methods) of male and female suicide, then suicide for men as compared to women could be considered as somewhat separate causes of death, particularly as they show such different trends over time (see Figure 19.1). Simply because the label 'suicide' is the same does not mean that causes need be that similar. This argument could also be used to suggest that causes are more likely to differ between those for young adults and those among older people. Notice that the repeated rises in suicide rates in Greece, Ireland and Italy referred to above were mostly, if not all, rising rates among men.

If further studies find that the negative correlation between suicide and inequality rates observed worldwide is male-dominated, that would suggest that it is possible that some men gain somewhat greater comfort (or hope of advancement) from being placed in more rigid rank ordering, even if for others the adverse consequences of such ranking is a key part of the underlying explanations of why some of them live shorter lives. Note how suicide rates fall faster for men during wartime (Figure 19.1).

Figure 19.1: Age-standardised suicide rates for ages ≥15 years in England and Wales (three-year moving averages), 1863–2007.

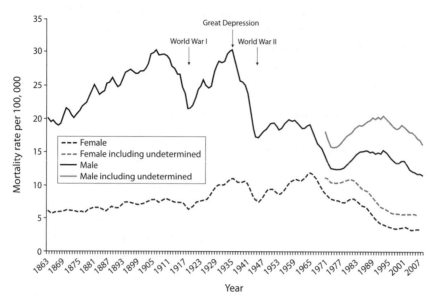

Source: Sebastian Kraemer, personal communication (2012)

Inequality and self-respect

There is a huge amount we do not know. When we ask people about their own health we find that, at the international scale, their responses tend to be inversely correlated with their actual life expectancy, but area rates of self-reported ill health and premature mortality are highly correlated within any country (see Chapter 22). Within any one country, especially within very small areas, where more people say they are sick, more people of their age group die. Between countries, those wealthy nations where people are more likely to report that they have worse health (when asked) tend to be home to citizens who, on average, live longer.

Everything is related to everything else, but near things are more related than distant things.[2]

The apparent contradiction above between what happens within a country and between countries frequently recurs. While in more *selfish times* suicide rates might rise within a more selfish country, such as Britain, in general the suicide rate is lower in more *selfish countries*. In less selfish countries with greater equality, people are allowed to compete on a more open playing field. It is suggested here that men may then be more likely to blame themselves for any failure, rather than claiming it is somebody else's, or society's, fault. That this is less the case for women requires

---

[2] Tobler's First Law of Geography: http://en.wikipedia.org/wiki/Tobler's_first_law_of_geography

further study, especially given that women are, in many countries, now allowed to compete and cooperate with men on more equitable terms than in earlier generations.

People living in harder circumstances tend to reassure themselves (and others) that all is fine more often; this matters for maintaining self-respect. The alternative, a little more truthfulness, is often simply too depressing. Alternative possibilities are that when a very bad situation is getting slightly better, people tend to be optimistic, but when a good situation starts to deteriorate, they tend to be pessimistic even if their personal situation is still much better than that found among most people in most other countries.

In more unequal countries people try to blame others more than themselves. It is worth thinking in this context about how, in an extremely affluent but unequal country such as Britain, 'immigration' can have risen to become the major political consideration in voters' minds during the 2001 and 2005 General Elections. Only the dire state of the economy pushed 'immigration' into second place as the 'most salient issue' during the 2010 General Election. More unequal countries make racial or ethnic differences both appear to be more real and to begin to matter more.

Immigration and slavery

Among rich countries rates of net immigration are greatest into the US, which has the highest number of poorly paid jobs available. Immigration is lowest into Japan, where the wages of the lowest paid fifth of people are proportionately the highest and where people are not segregated into rich and poor areas in most cities. It is not that citizens of the US are more open to immigration than those of Japan. Black American academics repeatedly report on how closed white American elite society is, but those elites create a demand for immigrant labour. Western academics often think of Japan as not particularly welcoming of immigrants, but it might be worth thinking just how welcoming Western countries are of people from places like Japan?

As economic inequalities increase, segregation by income, health and wealth also rises. Within the US, Britain and other countries that are becoming more unequal, poorer black and minority ethnic families become less free to choose their residential location. Racism becomes more acute. Private housing becomes more expensive, unemployment rises, and rents also rise where there are jobs; the freedom to choose where to live is then reduced further for all (see Chapter 23). The overall housing supply is increased but is shared out less and less well. Calls for more border controls to keep immigrants out become even shriller.

Everything is connected to everything else, but nearby issues in space become more closely linked in our imaginations than far away issues (for example, concern over our over-consumption of goods and the rubbish it creates tends to be greater than concern over the destruction of far-away rainforests or peoples). The ways in which we monitor, affirm and enforce citizenship and concern via border controls are closely linked to levels of inequality. In affluent unequal countries there is a tendency to despise immigrants more, while simultaneously creating more lowly paid jobs that often end up being carried out by immigrants (Chapter 24 gives one example of the behaviour that may then follow).

Immigration policies shape our ideas of who a country's citizens are, and who can be a citizen, even if border security is partly motivated by beliefs of improved security against terrorism. All this influences how anxious we are overall, how safe we tend to feel in general, both with others and with ourselves. When we start to treat those seen as both strangers and as economically at the bottom badly, it becomes easier to treat others who once were not strangers but who are now at the bottom with similar callousness (see Chapter 25).

Within a country, citizenship is important in so far as it can have an impact on how someone is treated under the law. When rights of entry into a country are restricted, 'immigrant workers' can become 'illegal workers' who have little or no legal recourse if they are being mistreated by employers. In the week in which I first put the chapters for this section together, the British government proposed that foreign domestic workers in Britain only be allowed to work for one family (the law had been changed in earlier years to prevent such absolute control). If the employing rich family was annoyed by its servants, its servants would have to leave not just their home, but also the country. The rich family could make their servants do whatever they wanted or face deportation: '... *tying domestic workers to one employer was in effect licensing slavery'* (Travis, 2012). This is a form of slavery that is currently most common in the most unequal of affluent countries (see Chapter 36) but is being resisted in Britain as activists try to prevent the country's current move towards becoming one of the most unjust of all the rich nations.

In Britain fighting against renewed slavery became the watchword of those concerned by growing inequality in the last week of February 2012 as companies started to refuse to accept the effectively unpaid slave labour of young people who back then were just starting to be forced to work for their food (the benefits they received were so low as to mainly only pay for food). The protests began after several hundred had all their welfare monies taken off them as 'workfare' replaced 'welfare'. Emma Harrison, the boss of one of the companies involved in the government's workfare scheme, A4e, was forced to resign. She had paid herself £8.6 million in the previous year alone, enough, it was written, to have created 4,000 *'real'* jobs as opposed to the slave labour of *'work for the dole'* schemes (Butler, 2012).

At the same time, the British government was also toying with reducing the 50 per cent tax rate for the richest 1 per cent (they then did this in the March 2012 Budget, memorably labelled the 'giveaway to millionaires'). Meanwhile, just across the channel in France, it was reported that there were proposals to raise the top rate of tax to 75 per cent (Chrisafis, 2012). A small strip of water can make two otherwise nearby places appear very far apart. In April 2012 the French voted overwhelmingly to give support to a Socialist candidate in the first round of their presidential election. That candidate won convincingly in the second round.

Meanwhile, in the UK, John Redwood, a far-right Conservative politician, had appeared on the BBC at the end of February, on *Question Time*. He advocated the call for further tax cuts for the richest 1 per cent. This 1 per cent was made up of people who had already paid themselves so much that they were now responsible, he said, for 30 per cent of all income tax payments (it may be a fraction lower – he did not seem very concerned with the accuracy of his statements). A few years ago their share of all income tax payments was 25 per cent, and, as the remaining 99 per cent of people in Britain became relatively poorer, the majority got to pay relatively less through direct taxes (but more of their income was taken through indirect taxes).

Profit and direct action

Within the UK, any sense that it would be better to share more (in England especially) appeared to be lost, but people were also searching for new ideas, so there was simultaneously renewed hope being expressed that another way was possible. Just as it appeared that those acting on the side of selfishness were going to take more and more for their small group of friends, many things began to go wrong within the British government in spring 2012. The word 'omni-mega-shambles' was coined toward the end of April that year (Bentham, 2012). Journalists and other pundits then began to try to search out what it could be that was making these politicians so incompetent, and there were many clues.

In the same week as John Redwood spoke on behalf of the very rich, Paul Ormerod, an economist, was reported explaining how our increasingly individualistic behaviour was becoming self-reinforcing because '… *we tend to cluster in self-reinforcing cliques'*. Paul also argued that the rich could be shamed into better behaviour (Hinsliff, 2012). The government began to claim that it was closing some tax loopholes for banks and for the rich. When publicly shamed, some bankers began not taking their bonuses.[3] Both were responses to successful shaming. However, at around the same time, a regular newspaper columnist, George Monbiot, reported how calls were being made to give companies actual votes (in proportion to their profits!) and that the government was suggesting that it was good that it was allowing large private corporations to appear to care about health or well-being while selling as many cigarettes, alcoholic drinks, weapons or environmentally destructive energy sources as they could:

> *British American Tobacco is promoting public health by educating and counselling its workers about HIV. The drinks giant Diageo is improving its waste water treatment process. Bombardier Aerospace is enhancing the environmental performance of its factories, in which it manufactures, er, private jets. RWE npower, which runs some of Britain's biggest coal and gas power stations, teaches children how 'to think about their responsibilities in reducing climate change'.* (Monbiot, 2012)

I did not have to work hard to search out these stories – many were taken from just one newspaper in the two or three days in which I wrote the first draft of this

---

[3] Some very prominent bankers were in effect sacked in July 2012, the most notable being Bob Diamond from Barclays.

chapter. The same newspaper in these same few days suggested that there might be an economic recovery because the Queen's Diamond Jubilee was due[4] (Inman, 2012), and that a major bank was paying even middle managers million pound salaries: *'One unidentified employee – described as "non-senior management" – got a signing-on fee of $3.5m'* (Treanor, 2012).

Within a few dozen metres of the offices of some of the bankers who were receiving million-pound-a-year salaries were the Occupy protestors, who were evicted from outside St Paul's Cathedral that same week in February. During early 2012 it felt like a great deal was happening all at once, but it takes a great deal happening all at once to ever so slightly change the most basic of opinions. Quoted in the same newspaper in the same week were the words of Conor Gearty, who explained that:

> *Minds are not changed by singular actions, however singular. They are changed when society comes to regard these singular actions as the rule rather than the exception, when common sense shifts on to the side of the erstwhile heretic.* (quoted in Colvin and Barda, 2012)

And then, just to keep up the oscillating story of people talking truth to power and power hitting back, the newspaper reported how the largest weapon-making companies of the world were getting richer and richer as the nations they sold to were becoming poorer and poorer during the global recession, the second largest of all the arms traders being the British (see Figure 19.2; Norton-Taylor, 2012).

There are now billions of people just struggling to get by, with a tiny few causing huge misery for countless others. That misery is misery whether it is caused by the making and selling of as many weapons as possible, or by trying to profit in other less immediately deadly ways: by selling alcohol or cigarettes, by polluting the air, by charging high rents or even by just charging great rates of interest on thousands of small loans so a middle manager can be given a £3.5 million a year salary. Human beings are not necessarily each other's best allies.

But what is there to turn to in place of continuously trying to 'rip each other off'? Many people are working for something much more than simply trying to profit from their neighbours (either near or far). These alternatives include: explaining that giving legal rights to corporations as if they were people is wrong, while not giving proper legal status to domestic workers creates slavery; exposing what is wrong within a supposedly good work programme; fighting for democratic change and a shift in understanding; learning how to shame bankers, journalists and politicians; exposing arms traders and corporate dictators; and effectively opposing changes that may mean any domestic worker who leaves a private household to escape abuse

---

[4] There was no economic recovery for the Jubilee. There probably would not have been even if it had not rained almost all of that weekend. Royal Jubilee's do not tend to result in great spending although the Silver Jubilee, in 1977, turn out in hindsight to have taken place at a point where we were most equal. They can be turning points.

will immediately face the prospect of being deported.[5] Journalists, much more often than academics, are best placed to chart out the possibilities of both despair and joy and reveal in which direction we are heading on any particular day or across any turbulent year. However, in quieter times, when it is not 'news', analysis is required, sometimes, academic analysis. Academic analysis also often underpins news stories (see the source of the newspaper graphic reproduced in Figure 19.2).

Figure 19.2: Top 10 arms producers in the world.

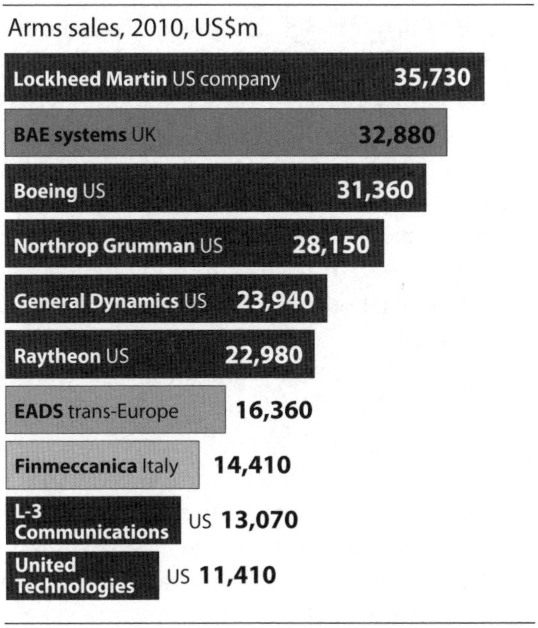

Arms sales, 2010, US$m

Lockheed Martin US company	**35,730**
BAE systems UK	**32,880**
Boeing US	**31,360**
Northrop Grumman US	**28,150**
General Dynamics US	**23,940**
Raytheon US	**22,980**
EADS trans-Europe	**16,360**
Finmeccanica Italy	**14,410**
L-3 Communications US	**13,070**
United Technologies US	**11,410**

Source: SIPRI (Stockholm International Peace Research Institute)

Every little action has a reaction

Every little action matters, from exposing great wrongs to just taking the time to write a letter, even a letter that is not published. Writing about the contents of the same newspaper a week before I read it to provide the examples shown here, a friend of mine wrote the following letter and sent it off. It shows how different people can have completely opposing views of the same world (Dorling, 2008). It wasn't published:

---

[5] Journalists lead the fight to try to extend human rights and maintain the ones we may soon lose; see Travis (2012).

Editor—Anne Milton's foggy statement about the cause of health inequalities – 'a complex web of factors' ('Cuts in children's services risk greater inequality, says expert', February 15) – is designed to obscure continuing abuses of power that maintain steep differences of wealth and privilege.

Wherever you look – senior civil servants' tax dodges supported by government, 'social cleansing' in London council housing, denationalisation of the greatest legacy of the 1945 government, covert selection in schools taken out of local authority control – you see an arrogant assumption of the rights of the powerful and a cynical rubbishing of disadvantage and disease, as if those in need had brought it upon themselves. Note Vince Cable's reminder (recollected by Suzanne Moore, 'Instead of being disgusted by poverty, we are disgusted by poor people themselves', February 16) that this is how fascism begins.

Since Margaret Thatcher dismantled the working class in the 1980s, Britain has been drifting towards a neo-Dickensian world of rich men and paupers. How can people stay healthy in such an insecure and offensive society? How can infants and schoolchildren flourish? The disgust that Suzanne Moore identifies as a 'growth industry' is an epidemic of gangster thinking, against which speaking up for equality, co-operation and social justice just sounds lame.

(Dr Sebastian Kraemer, Whittington Hospital, London)

When I first read this letter I had never met this friend; I just got emails from him occasionally and sent some back. I asked him if I could use his words here. Everything is related to everything else, near things tend to be more strongly related than far, but quite how you measure distance today is not how it used to be measured. Often being able to maintain a sense of sanity is realising that you have friends you have never met, realising that how you see the world is how many others see it too, and that you are not alone.

Losing sanity comes when you imagine your views to be supported by many others, but a multitude of admirers who do not exist or, more commonly, when you think you are alone in your thinking but are not.

References

Bentham, M. (2012) 'Minister told to get a grip over queue chaos at Heathrow', *London Evening Standard*, 27 April.

Butler, P. (2012) 'Why the work programme is a bad business', *The Guardian*, 28 February.

Carty, S., McArdle, J., Burnip, L., Jolly, D., Lisney, E., Scott, B., Preece, S., Martin, H., Rud, M. and McDougal, I. (2012) 'Abolish this harmful work capability test', Letter, *The Guardian*, 2 July (www.guardian.co.uk/society/2012/jul/02/abolish-harmful-work-credibility-test).

Chrisafis, A. (2012) 'François Hollande hits election trail in France's sixth biggest city: London', *The Guardian*, 29 February.

Colvin, N. and Barda, G. (2012) 'The fight for democratic change can't be left to Occupy', *The Guardian*, 28 February.

Counihan, P. (2012) 'Suicide rate rising rapidly in Ireland as recession grips', *Irish Central*, 6 February (www.irishcentral.com/news/Suicide-rate-rising-rapidly-in-Ireland-as-recession-grips-138771164.html).

Dorling, D. (2008) 'Looking from outside the goldfish bowl', *Significance Magazine*, vol 5, no 3, pp 122-5 (www.dannydorling.org/?page_id=589).

Hinsliff, G. (2012) 'Shame works on bankers, MPs and tabloids, however immune they seem', *The Guardian*, 28 February.

Inman, P. (2012) 'Is the worst finally over for the UK economy?', *The Guardian*, 27 February.

Monbiot, G. (2012) 'Britain is being rebuilt in aid of corporate power', *The Guardian*, 27 February.

Norton-Taylor, R. (2012) 'Arms sales rise during downturn to more than $400bn, report reveals', *The Guardian*, 29 February.

Povoledo, E. and Carvajal, D. (2012) 'Increasing in Europe: suicides "by economic crisis"', *New York Times*, 12 April (www.nytimes.com/2012/04/15/world/europe/increasingly-in-europe-suicides-by-economic-crisis.html).

Pridemore, W.A. (2006) 'Heavy drinking and suicide in Russia', *Social Forces*, vol 85, no 1, pp 413-30.

STV (2012) 'Mother killed son before taking own life', 29 February (http://local.stv.tv/edinburgh/news/299413-tributes-paid-to-woman-and-child-found-dead-in-house/).

Travis, A. (2012) 'New visa rules for domestic workers "will turn the clock back 15 years"', *The Guardian*, 29 February.

Treanor, J. (2012) 'HSBC paid 192 staff more than £1m', *The Guardian*, 27 February.

Suicide: the spatial and social components of despair in Britain, 1980–2000[1]

Dorling, D. and Gunnell, D. (2003) 'Suicide: the spatial and social components of despair in Britain 1980–2000', *Transactions of the Institute of British Geographers*, vol 28, no 4, pp 442-60.

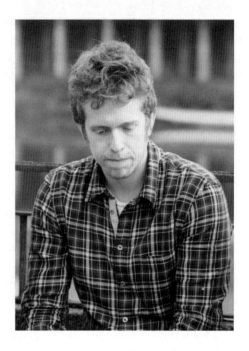

Summary

In this paper we show that, by accounting for the varying influence of just three area indicators of social isolation, it is possible to predict the number of deaths due to suicide and undetermined injuries (most of which are suicides) across a great many areas remarkably closely. The exceptions to this model suggest that in a few unique areas of the country other local, often historical and cultural or intrinsically geographical factors matter also.

These findings of the general predictability of suicide matter because suicide is such a common cause of death, particularly for the young. Between 1 January 1981

---

[1] Editorial Note: The introduction, a small section of results, two tables of modelling coefficients and the conclusion of the original paper are omitted from this version to save space.

and 31 December 2000, the underlying cause of the deaths of 130 000 people in Britain were recorded as being directly due to suicide, or in all probability being due to suicide. Collectively, these thousands of personal stories are brought together here to show how a pattern of despair in Britain over this period was spread across the country, affecting different places and different groups in society to differing extents over changing times.

The changing geography of despair can be shown to be largely the product of changing economic, social and demographic geographies. This chapter is concerned with determining the extent to which the stories of suicide in Britain were more than the sum of thousands of individual acts of misery and the extent to which they reflected the changing social structure of the country. Quantitative analysis is used to identify possible key trends with a more qualitative set of interpretations placed on the possible meanings of these findings. The chapter concludes by speculating on how current social trends may influence the future map of the extremes of despair in Britain.

...

Methods and data

The British censuses of 1981 and 1991 are used here to provide a series of measures of the extent to which places were socially integrated at the beginning of the 1980s and the 1990s.

To ensure that we are comparing the lives of roughly equal numbers of people, our spatial units of analysis are parliamentary constituencies as used to elect members of parliament in Britain in 1997 and 2001. These are not just sensible spatial units in terms of population size, they also allow for the differentiation of many inner city areas from suburbs, or remote rural areas from urban hinterlands and of towns from collections of villages. The small area census data from earlier years have been aggregated to these units so that the same areas can be compared over time (Mitchell *et al.*, 2002).

Analyses using administrative geographies (such as local authority districts) suffer from comparing areas of greatly varying populations. Comparing the tiny county of Rutland with the huge district of Birmingham is hardly comparing like with like. Furthermore, the densely populated large local authorities tend to contain the greatest variations in mortality rates and thus their use hides those spatial variations. We do not have access to comparable census or mortality data for Northern Ireland and so that province is excluded from this study.

For the mainland of Britain, in each constituency, we have divided the population by sex and into six age groups: 16–24, 25–34, 35–44, 45–54, 55–64, 65+. We have not considered suicide under the age of 16 (which is extremely rare). The choice of these age and sex groups is largely constrained by the variables that were disaggregated by age and sex in the two censuses we use. For each age/sex group we can measure three pertinent aspects of potential social isolation in society in each area at each point in time. These are: the proportion of people who are single; the proportion who have recently (in the last 12 months) migrated into the area; and the proportion who are not in work.

Figure 20.1 shows the national proportions of people in each age and sex group who were in each of the three categories of social isolation as measured by the 1981 and 1991 censuses in each area. It is important to remember that these measures are often combined in studies of the possible social influences on suicide not only with

Figure 20.1: Measures of social isolation in Britain by age and sex.

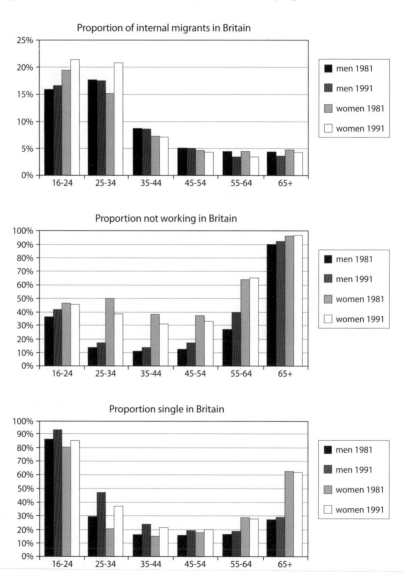

Source: 1981 and 1991 Census of Population for all of Britain.

each other, but also for all the different age and sex groups shown here (Whitley *et al.,* 1999; Congdon, 1996).

What Figure 20.1 illustrates is that at different points in people's lives, different social conditions are more or less unusual. We might therefore assume at different stages in people's lives, and varying for men and women, the possible influence of being in a particular group, or more indirectly of living in an area with a large proportion of other people being in a particular group, might not be particularly unusual and hence not particularly isolating for different people in different places at different times.

In the year before the census dates of 1981 and 1991, between 15 per cent and 22 per cent of people aged between 16 and 34 had migrated to their current place of residence in Britain. Migration is relatively common at these ages. Conversely, less than five per cent of people aged over 45 migrated each year in Britain. Being a migrant at older ages is a much more unusual situation to find yourself in. The extent to which migration is socially isolating might thus be assumed to be higher for older people in Britain. Migration can thus be assumed to be more isolating the fewer people of your age who migrate. Put another way, if you are a young migrant, you are likely to have more in common with a large proportion of other young people living in your area who have also migrated there in the last few years. It could be argued that if we had a measure of who was 'lonely' in each place in Britain this would be far more useful. We don't, but more important than that, loneliness can be the result of many things, just one of which is population mobility.

Figure 20.1 shows that there is an even wider variation by age and sex in a person's chances of not working in Britain. Not working is the norm for all people aged over 65 and for women aged over 55. However, between ages 25 and 44, only between 10 and 20 per cent of men do not work nationally. For women, not being in paid employment is much more common, as it is for everyone aged under 24. The extent to which being out of work is socially isolating is therefore clearly influenced by your age and sex. Being in work at older ages can put you in a small minority of your age group – and, as we see below, appears to correlate detrimentally with suicide rates.

Once you begin to decompose simple measures such as unemployment by age and sex, the importance of personal context becomes very clear and the problematic nature of interpreting a general all age/sex group 'unemployment rate' becomes apparent. Again, it could be argued that long-term unemployment might be a more appropriate measure. Unfortunately, various governments made over 30 changes to the official definition of unemployment over this period and so any consistent measure of the changing geography of long-term unemployment is almost impossible to derive. The measure we use is whether people self-defined themselves to be not employed at the census dates, a measure largely independent of official manipulation.

Finally, in discussing Figure 20.1, it is normal to be single beneath the age of 25, and over the age of 64 for women. However, being single between ages 35 and 64 puts you in a small minority of the population of your age and sex group and is presumably more socially isolating (although the extent to which this very broad generalization may hold should be expected to reduce over time as increasing numbers of people cohabit). The statistics shown in Figure 20.1 are national averages and therefore mask the large amount of geographical diversity in the extent to which people may find themselves to fall into different categories. Nevertheless, they demonstrate the very great influence of age and sex on all these potential measures of social isolation. How old you are and whether you are male or female is usually more influential than where you live in determining your chances of being in a particular social group. Of all our measures, the proportion of people who are either single or married initially appears to be the most tangential measure of whether they are likely to be in a happy relationship. We would agree with this, but there is no census box to tick 'are you happy', and despite the bad press that marriage often gets, analysis of the British Household Panel Study has found marriage to be the single most effective contributor to personal happiness (apparently worth the same as an annual £72,000 rise in income(!) according to the Strategy Unit, 2003). Finally, marriage rates will, to a small extent, reflect religious beliefs, which have been known since Durkheim's work to influence suicide rates.

In total, we are considering 641 areas, two time periods, six age groups and both sexes for three variables of potential influence. We did model the groups together too, but found that the differences between the coefficients by age and sex were great enough to suggest that separate models were more appropriate (see below). Thus, in any particular area at any one period, we have just three measures to model the suicide rate for each group in the population. As these are the same three measures for all groups, we can then compare their relative predictive powers between age/sex groups and time periods to gauge the extent to which these models suggest that different factors matter more or less for these different groups of the population, as expressed through the complex 'response' of suicide to social isolation.

The mortality data used for this study were obtained from the Office of National Statistics and the General Registrar's Office for Scotland. All deaths recorded to have occurred between 1981 and the end of 2000 were included where they had a valid postcode (well over 99% of cases). The postcode of usual residence was used to assign the death to a parliamentary constituency. Causes of death were recorded using the International Classification of Deaths version 9 (ICD9) in all cases except for Scotland in 2000, where causes of death were recorded by ICD10. These causes were converted back to ICD9. All causes recorded as ICD9 E950–E959 ('Intentional self harm') and E980–E989 ('Injury undetermined whether accidentally or purposely inflicted') were included under the definition of suicide used here. The resident 1981 population and the 1991 population corrected for the under-enumeration of that census were used as denominators for the calculation of suicide rates.

From here on, for simplicity, we use the terms 'suicide' to refer to all these deaths, whether 'undetermined' or not. We chose to include undetermined deaths (those given open verdicts by coroners) because previous analyses of national suicide data for England and Wales have shown that such deaths tend to follow a very similar pattern to suicides – other than there being slightly more doubt involved over the level of intent (Charlton et al., 1992; Kelly and Bunting, 1998). All violent or unnatural deaths are investigated by coroners in England and Wales, and Scotland;

based on their inquiries, a verdict of homicide, suicide, accidental death or an open verdict is given. Where there is uncertainty about whether the deceased intended to kill themselves, an open or accidental verdict may be given. Research indicates that most deaths given an open verdict are in fact suicides (Linsley *et al.*, 2001).

Changes in the lethality of commonly used methods of suicide can have important impacts on secular trends in suicide and more recent trends may have had an impact upon the spatial distributions that we are studying here. Trends in Britain in the last four decades have been influenced by changes in the toxicity of the domestic gas supply (Kreitman, 1976), fitting cars with catalytic converters (Amos *et al.*, 2001) and the toxicity of drugs commonly taken in overdose (Gunnell *et al.*, 1999a).

Figure 20.2: Suicide rates in Britain by age and sex, 1981–90, 1991–2000.

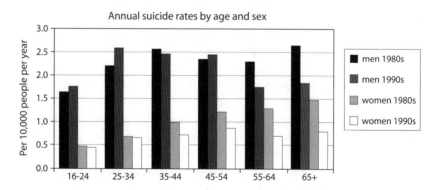

Source: Individual mortality records for Britain 1981–2000 and population estimates.

Figure 20.2 shows the suicide rates for the 12 age/sex groups during the 1980s and 1990s. The rates are higher for men and rose for men aged under 35, but fell for men aged 55 and over. The lower rates for women fell even further for women aged 35 and over in the 1990s. These changes are most likely due to the changing lethality of methods used at different ages at different times, as just discussed (in particular, the reduced toxicity of certain prescribed drugs), but they may also be partly due to the rising social status of women in society.

The rates of suicide have changed markedly in some groups of the population in differing directions, while the underlying measures of social integration (in Figure 20.1) suggest that changes in these factors between the 1980s and 1990s have generally been less striking. However, for men aged 25–34, their rising rates of not being in work and of being single coincide with a rising suicide rate (Gunnell *et al.*, 1999b; but see Crawford and Prince, 1999). For this reason, we should not in general expect changes in social isolation to be an explanatory factor for the changes in suicide rates in Britain during the period 1981–2000. However, as we show below, the geographical pattern of social isolation is strongly coincident with the geographical distribution of suicide rates in Britain, and so we are interested in for whom that relationship is strongest and how the possible geographical relationships between suicide rates and social isolation have been changing over time for different groups of the population.

...[2]

Results

...

The following graphs (Figure 20.3) allow easier interpretation of the data presented in Tables I and II [tables shown only in original paper], and encourage comparison of the changing relative spatial importance of different factors for different groups. They highlight interesting trends in the magnitude of the influence of different factors on suicide rates as age increases and between the two sexes. Curves have been fitted to the coefficients in the graphs as we hypothesize that these relationships are changing fairly smoothly with age.

Associations with migration were stronger than were those with the other factors examined. The first graph charts the coefficients for migration from the 24 separate models. High migration into an area has its lowest effects on the population aged under 35 for whom migration is a more common activity (see Figure 20.1). The ecological influence of migration peaks for men aged 55–64 in both the 1980s and 1990s. At these ages the proportion of the population dying due to suicide over ten years increases roughly three-fold for every additional ten per cent migrating into an area in a year at the start of those ten years. The greatest influence in any one constituency of this factor is in (what is now) the Cities of London and Westminster constituency where, in the 1980s, 40 per cent of this age-group migrated in between 1980 and 1981. The suicide rate in the 1980s in this constituency for this age and sex group was 9.6 per 10,000 per year, over four times the national rate.

The second graph in Figure 20.3 shows how the influence of living in an area where many people are not working is strongest for men between the ages of 25 and 44 and that the importance of this factor rose over time for these groups. For the most extreme constituency in the 1990s, Liverpool Riverside, where 44 per cent of men aged 25–34 were not working in 1991, the suicide rate in this area in the 1990s for this group was 3.0 per 10 000 per year. The model over-predicts suicide rates here, but as we see later Liverpool is a special case and Liverpool Riverside[3] is one of a group of constituencies where the models in aggregate tend to over-predict the expected number of suicides there, given prevailing social conditions.

The proportion of people not working in an area has almost no effect on suicide rates for people aged between 45 and 64. Interestingly, over the age of 64 the higher

---

[2] Editorial Note: A short section on methods and two tables of results have been removed at this point from this condensed version of the original paper.

[3] Editorial Note: The better-known, unsanitised, older name of this constituency is Liverpool Toxteth.

Figure 20.3: Influences on suicide by age and sex, 1981–1990, 1991–2000.

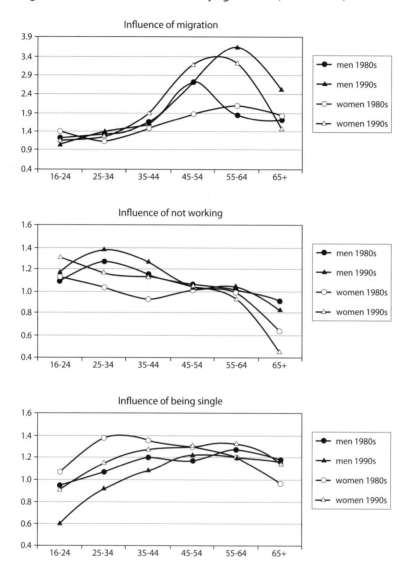

Source: Likelihood ratio coefficients from Tables I and II [shown in the original full version of this paper].

the proportion of people not working at these ages, the lower the local suicide rate, this effect being strongest for women in the 1990s. Because all four coefficients (for men and women for both the 1980s and 1990s) are lower than one, it would appear that this detrimental impact of elderly people working on the suicide rates of the elderly is unlikely to occur by chance. All four coefficients were significant at the five per cent level, as Tables I and II demonstrated. Put another way, for people of retirement age, those living in areas where more than average numbers of people are actually retired are at significantly lower risk of suicide in their old age.

The third graph in Figure 20.3 also shows how a factor thought to influence suicide rates can have opposing effects at different ranges of the age scale. Living in areas where a high proportion of your age and sex group are single was associated with reduced suicide rates for the youngest age group of men in the 1990s and a small detrimental effect for older groups. A similar effect is seen for men aged 25–34 by the 1990s. For women, the negative influence of living in an area with a high proportion of single people rose to a peak around ages 25–34 in the 1980s and then fell; however, the peak shifted to 55–64 in the 1990s. For men, the peak occurred in later years at both decades. Looking in particular at men aged 45–54 in the 1990s; the area with the highest proportion being single was Holborn and St Pancras, 46 per cent being single at these ages. The rate there over the ten years of the 1990s was 4.6 per 10,000 per year, 2.2 per 10,000 per year higher than the national average rate of 2.4 per 10,000.

In general, the 24 models cope reasonably well, with areas of unusually high or low suicide rates. The overall fits of the models are weaker where there appears to be a higher degree of apparently random variability in suicide rate in what otherwise appear to be areas of quite average social conditions (see Figure 20.4 and below). When we consider areas which are not modelled well (listed below), a variety of possible factors are found rather than evidence that one or two key variables were missing from these models.

Finally, we can consider where there appears to have been a significant large change in the influence of a particular factor on suicide. We do this by noting which coefficients have 95 per cent confidence intervals that do not overlap between the two decades. Four significant changes have occurred:

- For men aged under 35, the beneficial effect of living in an area where being single is more common has increased.
- For people aged 35–44, the harmful effect of living in an area where many men of these ages do not work has increased.
- For men aged 55–64, the harmful effect of living in an area of high migration has increased.
- For women aged 25–34, the harmful effect of living in an area where many are single has fallen, for younger women the beneficial effect has risen, while for women aged 65+ harmful effects have risen.

Reliability of the model

A conventional multiple regression model only 'explains' a minority of the geographical variation in suicide rates for any particular age and sex group of the population in any one ten-year period. Proportions of variance accounted for through negative binomial regression are less simply described. However, when all 24 separate models are put together to predict the total number of suicides in any one place over 20 years the fit of the model appears to be very good (see Figure 20.4), with the correlation between the number of observed and expected deaths due to suicide being 0.856 (the same correlation to three decimal points being achieved through either method of modelling). This suggests that it is mainly random variation (which is cancelled out when we aggregate) which is responsible for any apparent weakness in the individual models. In looking at where the overall fit of the models is worse, we can perhaps begin to see other geographical factors that might be influencing the rates of suicide in particular areas.

Figure 20.4: Aggregate fit of the 24 separate models for all areas.

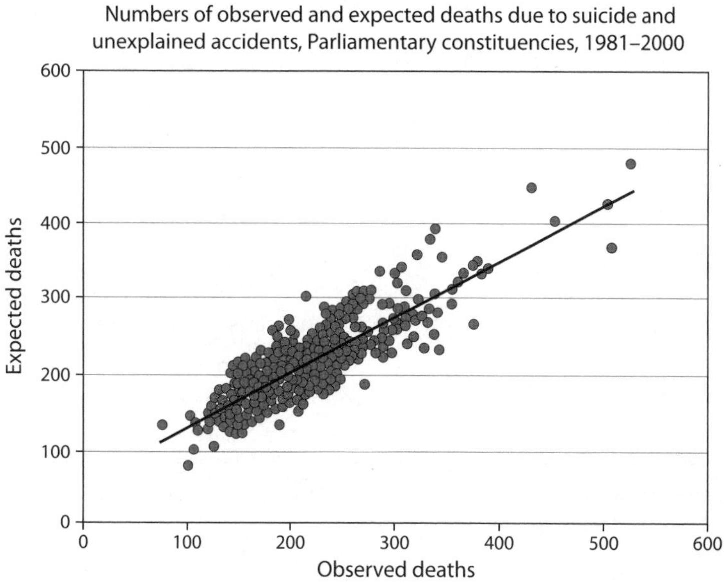

Numbers of observed and expected deaths due to suicide and unexplained accidents, Parliamentary constituencies, 1981–2000

Note: The observed numbers of deaths are the totals of all those which took place within each constituency over 20 years. The expected numbers are the sum of the 24 seperate linear models, multiplying for each constituency for each age and sex group and at each time period the numbers of people living in a particular social situation by the coefficient from the model for the estimated effect of living in that situation on the group suicide rate.

Table 20.1 lists the 20 parliamentary constituencies where the number of suicides is over-predicted the most and Table 20.2 lists the 20 where the rate is under-predicted the most. These places are unusual because their rates of suicide are unusually high or low, not because of an artefact of the particular model used to predict their suicide rates. Of the top 20 areas where we would have expected there to have been more deaths due to suicide than there were, five are in Merseyside (marked by an ★ in the table) in an area where traditionally there have been a high number of practising

Table 20.1: Areas where the models over-predict suicides in total, 1981–2000.

Observed	Expected (from model)	Difference (%)	Parliamentary Constituency
77	134.0	-74	Islwyn
104	151.7	-46	Aldridge-Brownhills
146	206.4	-41	Walsall North
215	302.6	-41	Hackney North and Stoke Newington
145	201.9	-39	North Durham
183	254.7	-39	Liverpool, West Derby*
151	209.7	-39	Sheffield, Brightside
150	208.1	-39	Walsall South
156	214.0	-37	Bootle*
145	198.9	-37	Mole Valley
132	180.1	-36	Sheffield, Attercliffe
199	267.1	-34	Liverpool, Walton*
188	252.1	-34	Hendon
154	204.4	-33	Enfield, Southgate
171	226.0	-32	Knowsley South*
153	202.1	-32	Louth and Horncastle
155	202.1	-30	West Bromwich West
135	175.9	-30	Blaenau Gwent
174	225.3	-30	Knowsley North and Sefton East*
162	209.4	-29	North West Durham

Source: Mortality data and the results of applying all 24 models. The difference is the percentage fewer deaths observed compared to model predictions.
* in Merseyside.

or believing Catholics. However, until 2001 census results are released we will not be able to confirm any religious influence (and even then different Christian denominations in England and Wales will not be differentiated). It is intriguing that a factor such as religion which was identified at the very beginning of the social study of suicide may still be important today (Durkheim, 1897). For more recent studies of the potential importance of religion, see Neeleman and Lewis (1999) and Neeleman *et al.* (1997).

Of the remaining 15 areas in Table 20.1, several others are also places which attracted a high level of Irish immigration in the past (such as those in County Durham) and hence which may still have unusually strong Catholic communities. Others have distinctive and larger than average ethnic minority populations as identified by the 1991 census (e.g. Hackney), again with possible high concentrations of people adhering to religions that proffer strong views on suicide (or which help build strong communities that this form of modelling clearly misses).

Table 20.2 lists those places where there have been more suicides than our models would predict. Again the discrepancies are small – between 26 and 131 more deaths

Table 20.2: Areas where the models under-predict suicides in total, 1981–2000.

Observed	Expected (from model)	Difference	Parliamentary Constituency
272	183.6	33	Inverness East, Nairn and Lochaber
271	186.9	31	Ross, Skye and Inverness West
189	131.6	30	Caithness, Sunderland and East Ross
327	231.4	29	Halifax
341	243.1	29	Glasgow Shettleston
208	150.5	28	Aberavon
374	270.9	28	Glasgow Springburn
507	375.5	26	Vauxhall
102	76.1	25	Western Isles
232	173.7	25	Banff and Buchan
313	236.1	25	Brighton, Kemptown
240	181.6	24	Argyll and Bute
295	225.6	24	Truro and St Austell
211	162.3	23	Central Fife
290	223.4	23	Glasgow Anniesland
318	245.1	23	Blackpool North and Fleetwood
336	259.1	23	Glasgow Maryhill
289	226.1	22	Rochford and Southend East
283	221.5	22	Slough
246	192.7	22	Pendle

Source: Mortality data and the results of applying all 24 models. The difference is the percentage excess of deaths predicted over and above those which occurred.

in each place over 20 years than we would predict from their social circumstances (1–7 more deaths per year). Many of the top 20 areas where there were more suicides than the model predicted are some of the poorest places in Britain. Parts of Glasgow and Manchester stand out here (but, interestingly, not Liverpool – areas of which appear in Table 20.1 above). Some very remote rural areas also have higher numbers of suicides than the models in aggregate can account for: remote parts of Scotland and Cornwall, for instance.

The ecological effects of poverty and/or extreme rural isolation (Middleton *et al.*, 2003a, 2003b) may thus be missing from the model, but there are an equal number of places in the top 20 under-predicted constituencies where neither of these factors are in place. Why, for instance, should suicide rates be higher than expected in Slough unless John Betjeman's observations on that area were particularly apposite? In general, when looking at these unusual places the degree to which they diverge from the general model is small and explicable in a number of cases as being probably due to factors not well correlated to the three we have used to model local suicide rates nationally.

The above two tables concentrate on the 40 areas out of all 641 British parliamentary constituencies for which the models work least well. Figure 20.4 (above) which showed the relationship between the observed and expected number of deaths for all constituencies illustrated how a series of individual models, none of which account for a majority of the variation between areas in suicides for their particular age and sex groups, can produce an aggregate model in which the large majority of the variation between areas is accounted for. As we suggested above, the most likely explanation for this is that the errors from the various individual models tend to cancel each other out at the aggregate level. This suggests that those errors were largely random. Thus, by accounting for the varying influence of just three social indicators of isolation for the different age groups, sexes and at different time periods, it is possible to predict the number of deaths due to suicide and undetermined accidents across a great many areas quite closely. That does not, however, mean that what we have measured explains the rates, simply that it either does, or alternatively, that our measures simply correlate well with whatever actually does explain them.

Discussion: one person's meat is another's poison?

Using social statistics to model the number of deaths by suicide for relatively small geographical areas and for particular age and sex groups would not normally be expected to produce results that generate an extremely close fit between the observed and expected numbers of cases. Even looking at deaths over 20 years, there are still areas where for particular age and sex groups no deaths from this cause are recorded and the deaths rates being modelled are still very small with a high degree of randomness to their distribution. Furthermore, expecting three crude ecological factors to account for the majority of the spatial variation in suicide rates assumes a world in which the major influences on people's lives are three measures made of the average state of the lives of the nearest (at most) 5000 people to any one individual at two points in time (1981 and 1991). The fact, therefore, that a very large amount of the spatial variations in suicide rates between areas can be modelled by just three social factors is thus remarkable and requires careful interpretation.

The three factors that we have measured may well be proxies for other things that influence suicide rates. Below we take each factor in turn and suggest what proxies might be at play. What is equally surprising about how well these models fit in aggregate is that they only look at the circumstances of people of the same age and sex as the 'at risk' group. The models take no account of the social circumstances of people of the opposite sex or of all other ages. One would expect that if a woman lived in an area where a great many men were out of work then her life might be somewhat blighted by this, but we do not try to take account of these influences (we have looked at some of these statistical relationships and found them not to be at all strong – i.e. we tried to model the rates of suicide of men of a particular age using the social circumstances of women of that age as well as men's and *vice versa*).

What is also surprising is that two snap-shot measures taken in the first year of a ten-year period should have a strong predictive effect for the subsequent ten years.

Rates of unemployment change quickly. Local unemployment rates in 1981 and 1991 are hardly a good guide to worklessness in 1989 and 1999. Furthermore, the rate of recent in-migration was found to be a significant predictor of local suicide rates for all groups other than men aged 16–24 in the 1990s and women aged 25–34 in the 1980s. Recent in-migrants might themselves be at greater risk of suicide, presumably, on average, having fewer local social contacts in the area they have migrated into than those that they had left behind. More importantly, a high rate of in-migration in one year in an area suggests that many more of the population living there will have been migrants in the less recent past. Additionally, for those people living in the area for longer, their neighbours and potential local friends are more likely to have changed recently and thus local social ties in general are likely to be more fluid. Why though would this have its most detrimental effects upon men and between the ages of 35 and 64?

Men are traditionally seen as less adept at maintaining social ties and so perhaps migration can increase the chances of them losing the ties they do have as physical distance increases. Below the age of 35 migration is more common, almost becoming expected for people aged 18–21. Over the age of 64, you progressively begin to lose more local friends and neighbours of your age from death than from them moving physically away. Also in old age, living in an area of relatively high in-migration for your age group may simply imply that you have moved to a 'retirement area', which by definition should expect a high rate of in-migration (but not necessarily of out-migration as, again, people leave through death rather than migration). The fact that the relative influences of migration (under age 55) appear to have remained stable between the 1980s and 1990s suggests that these are long-term influences.

Explanations for the largest change there has been – the influence of migration rising for men aged over 55 and women aged over 45 – are unclear and require further research.[4] Secondly, the rate of people not working appears to only have had a strong detrimental effect for men aged between 25 and 44 and women aged 15–24, but that effect increased in intensity between the 1980s and 1990s. Unemployment is known to be associated with an increased risk of suicide at both the individual and population level (Lewis and Sloggett, 1998; Gunnell *et al.*,1999b). A relatively high local rate of unemployment also tends to imply that jobs in general are less secure in a particular area and that those jobs that are there may be less well-rewarded financially. Thus the impact of unemployment may also be wider than simply affecting the unemployed themselves.

The consistent categories of economic activity used in this study also included students as 'not working' and thus the small significance of not working below age 25 is not unexpected. What was surprising was to find all the ecological effects of the local proportion of people not working to collapse to near unity for people between the ages of 44 and 65. Perhaps the group of men of these ages who could choose to

---

[4] Editorial Note: It is almost entirely internal migration within Britain that accounts for particular areas having a high in-migrant rate. Migration from overseas was far rarer during these years than was the case after the year 2000 and, following both the early 1980s and early 1990s recessions, there were brief periods of net emigration from England and Wales. See Figure 24.1, Chapter 24, p 242, this volume.

retire early saw beneficial effects from this which balanced out the negative effects of being forced not to work for those men of these ages that did want (or had) to work? Over age 64 the picture is clear again. Living in a place where people over retirement age tend to work increases the chances of someone over this age of dying due to suicide. Perhaps where you cannot choose to enjoy your retirement without working (and/or if your neighbours cannot), this appears to indicate that there is slightly less to live for – particularly for women aged over 64.

Lastly, the influence of living in areas with a high proportion of people who are single in your age group appears most detrimental for people aged over 34. For women in the 1980s aged under 35, this was one of the few influences which had a greater negative effect on them than on men. However, the influence of being single has fallen for women in the 1990s in general (except above age 55). Our consistent measure of being single is actually of not being married and so as cohabitation increases (an increase which is measured as more people being single here) it is not surprising to see the influence of marriage on younger people fall. It is thus somewhat surprising that the influence has not fallen for men aged 45–54.

Just as migration and not working can be proxies for other things, so too can being single. Most obviously, people are less likely to have (or be living with) children if they are single and having responsibilities for children reduces an individual's chance of dying from suicide (a decreased risk of suicide has been found for mothers of babies in their first year of life; Appleby, 1991). Conversely, as being single becomes the norm for younger age groups, then it is interesting to see the local rate becoming an apparently protective factor for men as a group aged under 35 by the 1990s. Put another way, there are more suicides than average in areas where men tend to marry younger nowadays. However, these areas also tend to be poorer areas and so it would be misleading to assume a direct influence of young marriage on raising suicide rates.

...

References

Amos, T., Appleby, L. and Kiernan, K. (2001) Changes in rates of suicide by car exhaust asphyxiation in England and Wales, *Psychological Medicine*, 31, 935–9.

Appleby, L. (1991) Suicide during pregnancy and in the first postnatal year, *British Medical Journal*, 302, 137–40.

Charlton, J., Kelly, S., Dunnell, K., Evans, B., Jenkins, R. and Wallis, R. (1992) Trends in suicide deaths in England and Wales, *Population Trends*, 69, 10–16.

Congdon, P. (1996) Suicide and parasuicide in London, *Urban Studies*, 33, 1137–58.

Crawford, M.J. and Prince, M. (1999) Increasing rates of suicide in young men in England during the 1980s: the importance of social context, *Social Science and Medicine*, 49, 1419–23.

Durkheim, E. (1897, 1952) *Suicide*, London: Routledge and Kegan Paul.

Gunnell, D., Wehner, H. and Frankel, S. (1999a) Sex differences in suicide trends in England and Wales, *Lancet*, 353, 556–7.

Gunnell, D., Lopatatzidis, A., Dorling, D., Wehner, H., Southall, H. and Frankel, S. (1999b) Suicide and unemployment in young people. Analysis of trends in England and Wales, 1921–1995, *British Journal of Psychiatry*, 175, 263–70.

Kelly, S. and Bunting, J. (1998) Trends in suicide in England and Wales, 1982–1996, *Population Trends*, 92, 29–41.

Kreitman, N. (1976) The coal gas story: United Kingdom suicide rates, 1960–71, *British Journal of Preventive and Social Medicine*, 30, 86–93.

Lewis, G. and Sloggett, A. (1998) Suicide, deprivation, and unemployment: record linkage study, *British Medical Journal*, 317, 1283–6.

Linsley, K. R., Schapira, K. and Kelly, T.P. (2001) Open verdict v. suicide – importance to research, *British Journal of Psychiatry*, 178, 465–8.

Middleton, N., Gunnell, D., Whitley, E., Frankel, S. and Dorling, D. (2003a) Urban–rural differences in suicide trends in young adults: England and Wales, 1981–1998, *Social Science and Medicine*, 57, 1183–94.

Middleton, N., Whitley, E., Frankel, S., Dorling, D. and Gunnell, D. (2003b) Suicide risk in small areas of England and Wales 1991–1993, *Social Psychiatry and Psychiatric Epidemiology*, 39, 45-52.

Mitchell, R., Martin, D., Dorling, D. and Simpson, S. (2002) Bringing the missing million home: correcting the 1991 SAS [Small Area Statistics] for undercount, *Environment and Planning A*, 34, 1021–35.

Neeleman, J. and Lewis, G. (1999) Suicide, religion, and socioeconomic conditions. An ecological study in 26 countries, 1990, *Journal of Epidemiology and Community Health*, 53, 204–10.

Neeleman, J., Halpern, D., Leon, D. and Lewis, G. (1997) Tolerance of suicide, religion and suicide rates: an ecological and individual study in 19 Western countries, *Psychological Medicine*, 27, 1165–71.

Strategy Unit (2003) Life satisfaction: the state of knowledge and implications for Government Cabinet Office, London (http://www.cabinet-office.gov.uk/ innovation/2001/futures/ attachments/ls/paper.pdf). Accessed 10 October 2003.

Whitley, E., Gunnell, D., Dorling, D. and Davey Smith, G. (1999) Ecological study of social fragmentation, poverty and suicide, *British Medical Journal*, 319, 1034–7.

21

How suicide rates have risen during periods of Conservative government, 1901–2000

Shaw, M., Dorling, D. and Davey Smith, G. (2002) 'Editorial: Mortality and political climate: how suicide rates have risen during periods of Conservative government, 1901–2000', *Journal of Epidemiology and Community Health*, vol 56, no 10, pp 722-7.

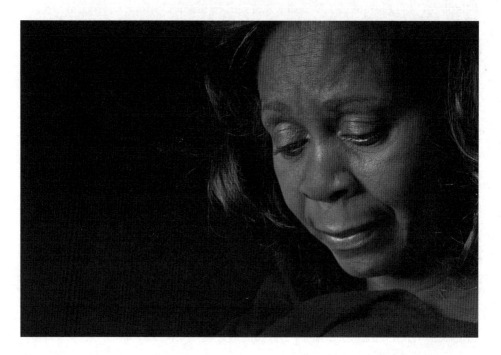

Mortality and political climate

The paper by Page and colleagues[1] adds to a growing literature that considers the effect of the political environment (whether from the point of view of which political regime holds power or considering in more detail the proportion of population voting for particular parties) and mortality.[2] In this case the specific cause of death

---

[1] Editorial Note: This paper was original written in response to: Page, S.A., Morrell, S. and Taylor, S. (2002) *Suicide and political regime in New South Wales and Australia during the 20th century*, 56, 766-772.
[2] Davey Smith, G. and Dorling, D. (1996) "I'm alright, John": voting patterns and mortality in England and Wales, 1981–92, *BMJ*, 313:1573–7. 2 (see Figure 41.2, p 378, this volume); and Kelleher, C., Timoney, A., Friel, S., *et al.* (2002) Indicators of deprivation, voting patterns, and health status at area level in the Republic of Ireland, *Journal of Epidemiology and Community Health*, 56:36–44.

in question is suicide, and the paper thus adds to a long tradition of research in sociology and epidemiology on factors beyond the individual that influence societal rates of suicide.[3]

The findings by Page *et al.* suggest a dose-response or perhaps 'true' effect such that during the 20th century the presence of Conservative governments at both State and Federal level in Australia were associated with higher suicide rates. Crucially, the effect is strongest when both levels of government are Conservative, with adjusted relative risks of suicide of 1.17 for men and 1.40 for women compared with years of administration by both State and Federal Labor governments.

What can we infer from the findings of this study? The best societal conditions to minimise suicide rates are as follows: have both a State and Federal Labor regime, economic stability, be at war, control the availability of sedatives, and avoid drought. However, the implications of these results for reducing population suicide are unclear. The controlling of sedatives is perhaps the easiest to implement, but what about war? The authors' results suggest that not all wars have the same effect on suicide rates; considering all-cause mortality might change the perception of war as a positive factor in population health. While Wilkinson[4] argues that the increased sense of social cohesion brought about by facing a common enemy resulted in an improvement in overall life expectancy in Britain during the Second World War, it is not always the case that national wars are based on national unity, as American opinion regarding the Vietnam war testifies. Moreover, it would obviously be morally indefensible to suggest pursing war as a strategy in order to reduce suicide rates.

The interpretation of the effects of economic conditions (indexed by changes in GDP) is also problematic, seeing as periods of economic depression are associated with higher suicides rates among men, but times of economic depression and expansion are associated with higher suicide rates among women. For women, economic stability, or incremental rather than rapid economic change, seems to be most beneficial. The study period for these analyses covers almost the entire 20th century—during which time the role of women, and their economic participation, has changed dramatically. Women may suffer in times that are economically tight as they are often in the position of serving as a reserve army of labour and, in the private sphere, have the responsibility for managing family budgets and somehow making ends meets. In times of economic boom, they may not enjoy as rapid access to better work opportunities and other aspects of social success as do their male counterparts. Taking into account the proportion of women in the labour force,

---

[3] Durkheim, E. (1897, 1952) *Suicide*, London: Routledge and Kegan Paul; Ashford, J.R. and Lawrence, P.A. (1976) Aspects of the epidemiology of suicide in England and Wales, *International Journal of Epidemiology*, 5:133–44; and Charlton, J., Kelly, S., Dunnell, K., *et al.* (1993) Suicide deaths in England and Wales: trends in factors associated with suicide deaths, *Population Trends*, 71:34–42.

[4] Wilkinson, R.G. (1996) *Unhealthy societies: the afflictions of inequality*, London: Routledge.

and perhaps the proportion of women in public life (see Lynch *et al.*[5]), may help to explain this finding.

Page and colleagues seem to favour a psychosocial over a materialist interpretation[6] of their results—suggesting that a greater proportion of the population are living in conditions of hope under Labor governments. Suicide is clearly a psychosocial outcome, but even in this case the fundamental determinants may lie outside of the psychosocial domain.[7] The variable 'political regime' could be substituted by an indicator of the egalitarian and redistributive qualities of tax and welfare policies— the direction of the results would almost certainly be similar (Labor governments historically having being more redistributive than Conservative ones), but the interpretation would be very different. The authors reasonably argue that people think that life is less worth living when there is less worth living for. Thus the fundamental determinant is the degree to which fiscal policies compensate for the general tendency of some people to have increasingly more than others, policies which lead to greater fairness.

Governments are changeable within democratic societies, and at least in Britain health care is an issue of considerable electoral importance. Health itself, as compared with the National Health Service, has not been a high profile issue around elections, however. But demonstrations of mortality outcomes of selection of a particular political party illustrates what must—potentially—be modifiable influences on population health. To test the generality of Page and colleagues' findings we have crudely examined the same issue in British data.

To what extent are the results for Australia reflected in Britain?

Suicide rates in Australia tended to rise during Conservative periods of rule over the course of the past century. Similar results—with respect to attempted suicide—have previously been reported for Britain.[8] In this short response, given problems of data availability, it is not possible to replicate the Australian results exactly. However, it is relatively simple for anyone with access to the World Wide Web to conduct a very crude analysis that produces uncannily similar statistics within England and Wales— albeit for men and women combined.

The fact that suicide rates are affected by the political, economic, and cultural environment in which people in England and Wales live has been demonstrated many

---

[5] Lynch, J.W., Davey Smith, G., Hillemeier, M. *et al.* (2001) Income inequality, the psychosocial environment, and health: comparisons of wealthy nations, *Lancet*, 358, 200.

[6] Lynch J.W., Davey Smith, G., Kaplan, G.A. *et al.* (2000) Income inequality and mortality: importance to health of individual income, psychosocial environment, or material conditions. *BMJ*, 320:1200–4; and Marmot, M. and Wilkinson, R.G. (2001) Psychosocial and material pathways in the relation between income and health: a response to Lynch *et al., BMJ*, 322, 1233–6.

[7] Editorial Note: The rapid and almost immediate reduction in suicides that followed the Labour government victory in Britain in 1997 coupled with very little material gain at the bottom of society would suggest that a psychosocial interpretation, in hindsight at least, in the case of Britain is more plausible.

[8] Masterton, G. and Platt, S. (1989) Parasuicide and general elections, *BMJ*, 298, 803–4.

times. Even very short-term effects have been noted, such as suicide rates rising by 17% in the four weeks after the death of Diana, Princess of Wales.[9] Suicide rates in Britain have tended to follow economic trends such as the unemployment rate, but that in turn is partly a product of political decisions and it is clearly not by chance that the unemployment rate in Britain peaked during long periods of largely Conservative administration during the 1930s and 1980s. Thus, treating unemployment as the cause may not get to the underlying modifiable factor, which may be the package of economic and fiscal policies introduced by a particular regime. How then does the century's trend in suicide compare to the trend in political control?

Table 21.1: Suicide rates per million, England and Wales, 1901–98, by prime minister.

Period	Suicide rate	Main prime minister in power in each five years
1901-1905	101	Balfour (Conservative 1902-1905)
1905-1910	102	Campbell-Bonnerman (Liberal 1905-1908)
1911-1915	96	Asquith (Liberal 1908-1916)
1916-1920	85	Lloyd George (Liberal 1916-1922 & WW1)
1921-1925	101	Baldwin (Tory 1923-24, 1924-1929)
1926-1930	123	Baldwin (Tory 1923-24, 1924-1929)
1931-1935	135	MacDonald (Lib/Tory coalition 1931-1935)
1936-1940	124	Chamberlain (Conservative 1937-1940)
1941-1945	92	Churchill (Conservative 1940-1945 & WW2)
1946-1950	106	Attlee (Labour 1945-1951)
1951-1955	107	Churchill (Conservative 1951-1955)
1956-1960	116	Eden (Conservative 1955-1957)
1961-1965	137	Macmillan (Conservative 1957-1963)
1966-1970	118	Wilson (Labour 1964-1970)
1971-1975	101	Heath (Conservative 1970-1974)
1976-1980	112	Callaghan (Labour 1976-1979)
1981-1985	121	Thatcher (Conservative 1979-1990)
1986-1990	118	Thatcher (Conservative 1979-1990)
1991-1995	110	Major (Conservative 1990-1997)
1996-1998	103	Blair (Labour 1997-present)

Source: http://www.statistics.gov.uk/statbase dataset 'Deaths (per million population) from injury and poisoning: external cause and year of registration or occurrence, 1901–1998'.

---

[9] Hawton, K., Harriss, L., Appleby, L., *et al.* (2000) Effect of death of Diana, Princess of Wales on suicide and deliberate self-harm, *British Journal of Psychiatry*, 177, 463–6.

Table 21.1 shows the crude suicide rate in England and Wales for 1901–1998 per million people per year. Suicides are defined on a consistent basis by the Office for National Statistics as being equivalent to E950-E959 between 1901 and 1960 and including deaths from external causes in which intent was undetermined thereafter (E980-E989). Equivalent data for Scotland are not available (data on all or the part of Ireland under the rule of Britain during this period are also not available). The data are provided by ONS for every five years of the century and are the only consistent data on suicide over the century easily available on the web. Here we have simply added the name of the longest serving prime minister during each five year period to this list of rates along with their political affiliation for the majority of that period (Table 21.1).

The century began with a Conservative government and a suicide rate of just over 0.01% of the population per year. The Liberal government first elected in 1906 enacted policies that were increasingly socially progressive under the leadership of David Lloyd George. As the table shows overall suicide rates fell during this period of Liberal government—to an all-time low that coincided with the First World War. After the First World War rates rose with a succession of barely interrupted Conservative administrations. Rates reached an all time high coincident with the coalition government of 1931–1935. This government was lead by Ramsay MacDonald who left the Labour party in 1931 to lead the largely Conservative and Liberal coalition of that time. A cynic might suggest that if there's anything worse than a Conservative government for suicide rates, it is one led by an ex-Labour party leader. However, unemployment also peaked to its maximum for the century in these years. Rates of suicide (and unemployment) remained high under Chamberlain's leadership and only fell substantially with the outbreak of the Second World War; but suicide rates under a Conservative wartime administration were higher than under a Liberal one.

Postwar suicide rates under the 1945–1951 Labour administration were lower than at any time since 1925. However, after the political fall of that famously progressive government they rose steady over the next 15 years—under Churchill, then Eden, and then Macmillan (the later rise is only partly attributable to the change in classification noted above). They fell quickly under the next Labour administration of Harold Wilson and then, for the first and only time, fell under a Conservative government—the administration led by Edward Heath between 1970 and 1974. The large majority of this fall can, however, be attributed to the switch from coal gas to natural gas in the period leading up to Heath's term of office[10] (that is similar to the effect of sedative legislation found in Australia). It is probable that if the substantial fall attributable to this method of suicide being withdrawn were accounted for we would actually find a rise in the real rate under that government's tenure—but this is only a very crude analysis.

---

[10] Kreitman, N. (1976) The coal gas story: United Kingdom suicide rates, 1960–71, *British Journal of Preventive and Social Medicine*, 30, 86–93; and Kendell, R.E. (1998) Catalytic converters and prevention of suicides, *Lancet*, 352:1525.

Ignoring the 'blip' of the Heath years, rates were lower under Callaghan than Wilson but jumped up dramatically with the election of the final Conservative administration of the century, initially lead by Margaret Thatcher. They fell with the election of the more moderate John Major and fell again under Tony Blair. If recent annual figures are studied then the fall can be seen to have actually occurred between 1995 and 1996 (see Table 21.2). Nevertheless, yet again the election of a supposedly more progressive government coincides with a longer term reduction in suicide rates. After a slight rise in suicide rates during their first few years in office (when the fiscal plans of the previous Conservative government were adhered to and before new policy initiatives were in place) suicide rates have fallen.

To compare these trends to the Australian case we need to see how the rate of suicides in Conservative periods of government compares with that generally experienced under Labour (and Liberal) prime ministers. The average crude suicide mortality rate in the 20th century in Britain under Labour and Liberal administrations was 103 deaths per million per year. During the 20 years from 1921 to 1940, almost all under Conservative administrations, the rate was 1.17 times that. During the 15 years of almost all Conservative rule from 1950 to 1965 it was again 1.17 times, and during the 10 years 1981–1990 encompassed by Mrs Thatcher's rule it was 1.16 times, the rate under Labour and Liberal governments. The overall effect on suicide rates in Britain is similar to that which is seen for Australian men; Australian women are more responsive (in terms of suicide rate changes) to Conservative elections than are Australian men or the overall British population.

Table 21.2: Suicide rates per million, England and Wales, 1991–2000.

Year	Suicide rate
1991	118
1992	115
1993	105
1994	106
1995	107
1996	101
1997	103
1998	106
1999	106
2000	101

Source: http://www.statistics.gov.uk/ statbase dataset, 'Deaths (per million population) from injury and poisoning: external cause and year of registration or occurrence, 1901–1998', for 1991–1998, and for 1998, 1999 and 2000, ONS Mortality Statistics: Cause, Series DH2, Nos 25, 26 and 27, London: The Stationery Office.

Who commits suicide under Conservative regimes?

Finding a rise in national suicide rates during periods of Conservative administration does not indicate which groups in society might be most adversely effected by such administrations. However, cross sectional data for geographical areas can be used to show that suicide rates tend to be higher in areas where fewer people vote Conservative. Building on earlier work[11] we have correlated suicide rates within parliamentary constituencies with voting behaviour during parliamentary elections. Taking directly age-sex standardised suicide rates for the four periods 1981–85, 1986–1990, 1991–95, 1996–2000 and relating them to the proportion of the electorate who voted Conservative in each parliamentary constituency at the general elections of 1983, 1987, 1992, and 1997 produces correlation coefficients of −0.23, −0.34, −0.48, and −0.47 respectively (all p<0.05). Thus throughout the 1980s and 1990s suicide rates were progressively higher where fewer people voted for the party that won all but the last of those elections. Put bluntly, this suggests that while a Conservative government is associated with a higher suicide rate, living in an area with a high proportion of Conservative voters is associated with a lower risk of suicide (and by extension—putting aside concerns regarding the ecological fallacy—Labour voters suffer as a result of the higher suicide rates engendered by Conservative governments).

Conclusion

During the 45 (Tory) years of excess suicide mortality identified above some 238,431 people died as a result of suicide. If the excess is 17%, then the conclusion is that roughly 35 000 of these people would not have died had these Conservative governments not been in government. This is one suicide for every day of the century, or more appropriately, two for every day that the Conservatives ruled.

---

[11] Davey Smith, G. and Dorling, D. (1996) "I'm alright, John", voting patterns and mortality in England and Wales, 1981–92, *British Medical Journal*, 313, 1573–7.

22

The inequality hypothesis: thesis, antithesis, and a synthesis[1]

Dorling, D. and Barford, A. (2009) 'The inequality hypothesis: thesis, antithesis, and a synthesis', *Health & Place*, vol 15, no 4, pp 1166-9.

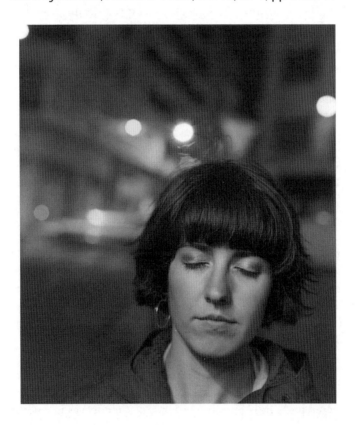

In the pages of [*Health and Place*] Min Hua Jen, Kelvyn Jones and Ron Johnston recently presented a paper claiming to have evaluated Richard Wilkinson's hypothesis that social inequality damages the health of populations (Jen *et al.*, 2008). It was an interesting paper with findings not originally recognized in Wilkinson's hypothesis, but it suffers from one major flaw: the findings are not a direct evaluation of Richard Wilkinson's hypothesis. We show why below. It is important to point this out as the balance of much very new evidence now points towards inequality having damaging effects on society in all kinds of ways (Wilkinson and Pickett, 2009), not

[1] Written in response to Jen *et al.*, 2008.

just in terms of health (but for a review of that see Ram, 2006) and it would be unfortunate if the value of these new findings were cast into doubt by studies that did not evaluate the actual hypothesis, but something else, which in turn turns out to be quite interesting.

In hindsight it is easy to see how Jen *et al.* could have thought that they were evaluating the inequality hypothesis. Part of the argument of their paper is that quite complex methods of synthetic data creation and multilevel modelling are needed to evaluate the inequality hypothesis. This might be the case, although others find the existing evidence in support of Wilkinson's hypothesis to be near overwhelming (Dorling *et al.*, 2007). However, it is possible that it was dealing with that complexity of synthetic data and multiplicity of hypothesized levels which led to the very simple oversight we highlight below. We should note that our response is far from being a simple critique, as we find Jen *et al.*'s analysis and findings very interesting, just in a way that they didn't. ...

Jen *et al.* show that it is possible to generate synthetic data to suggest that the patterns observed by Wilkinson could have occurred without the mechanisms he suggests. Wilkinson is the best known advocate of the theory that among affluent nations, life expectancy is lower in more unequal nations because inequality of itself has a detrimental effect on the health of people who live in more unequal societies. A large amount of his life's work has been spent collecting evidence to support this hypothesis. An alternative hypothesis is that more unequal societies simply contain more poor people who are disproportionately likely to die young producing the outcome without any so-called contextual effect, but simply as the result of the composition of all those individual life chances. It is possible to produce synthetic data that supports the compositional story but, of course, it is equally possible to produce synthetic data that would support the contextual story. So we look no further at that part of the story here.

There is a paucity of good quality comparable health data available at the individual level to exhaustively test the inequality hypothesis and the idea that inequality hurts all members of an unequal society, not just the poor (although for a good collection of work that does support the hypothesis see Marmot, 2004). If it were the case that the rich benefited in terms of their health from living in an unequal society, but the poor suffered just a little bit more, as Jen *et al.* (in effect) suggest, then there may be little incentive for the rich to support redistribution other than for purposes of charity, altruism or a commitment to social justice. Alternatively, if on aggregate all social groups living in an unequal society suffer from the effects of such inequality, albeit to different extents, and all would benefit from redistribution from rich to poor in terms of health and life expectancy, albeit far more for the poor than the rich, but still a benefit for all, then the argument for redistribution is very hard for those in power to evade. Thus the political stakes could not be higher as to whether it is composition or context that causes life expectancy to be lower in more unequal countries.

Would it benefit almost everyone in more affluent countries to live in more equitable societies, or would the rich lose out substantially in terms of their health status were they to sacrifice some of their wealth to make the poor in their countries less poor? The truth may lie somewhere in between these two extremes, but if the analysis that Jen *et al.* have carried out is true, then the truth lies only at one extreme of the range of possibilities. Redistribution would harm the rich. Fortunately for the rich, even more fortunately for the poor, there is a 'killer' flaw in this argument. The killer flaw is that Wilkinson's hypothesis is about actual experienced health, and most vitally, premature death, whereas Jen *et al.* use what they think is a proxy for that: self-rated health.

Jen *et al.* quote only one source (Idler and Benyamini, 1997) to suggest that self-rated health 'is closely related to mortality at an aggregate level' (Idler and Benyamini, 1997, p 201). Unfortunately Idler and Benyamini's study was of community level research, not of international comparisons. At the community level, when comparing neighbourhoods within a town, or even towns within a country, what people say about their health is a good proxy for their actual health as measured by mortality rates. However, as the geographical scale is increased the closeness of that relationship reduces, and at the international level it appears to invert for rich countries—as we show below. Those rich countries in which people rate their health the best tend to be those countries in which people live shorter lives. People in more unequal countries, it turns out, appear a little more confused about the status of their health, or those in more equal countries are more prone to express pessimism. Either way, experiments with international survey data on self-rated health cannot be used to discredit the inequality hypothesis.

Between the community and the international level, studies that involve more than one nation have pointed towards there being an ambiguity that grows with spatial scale between what people say about their health and their actual health outcomes. Within the British Isles it is now well known that people in Wales tend to report worse health status than they experience in terms of premature mortality, while people living in Scotland are more likely to be optimistic about their health status when asked (in comparisons to actual life expectancy). England sits in between the other two countries both geographically and in terms of the slopes of relationship between self-rated health and life expectancy. Within each of these three countries the relationship looks like a good proxy. It is only when all three are compared that it becomes clear that there are cultural differences between how different geographical groups describe what are most probably similar actual states of health (Shaw *et al.*, 2008).

In their claim to have discredited the Wilkinson hypothesis Jen *et al.* use survey data for 15,292 individuals taken from the World Values Survey (WVS) sampled in Wave 3 of that study (1995–1996) across 12 OECD countries (Australia, Finland, Germany, Japan, Mexico, New Zealand, Norway, Spain, Sweden, Switzerland, Turkey, USA). For their study to actually discredit Wilkinson, measures of self-rated health according to that survey undertaken in those countries have to be related to health as measured by Wilkinson, in other words have to be related to life expectancy. In Table 22.1, we show the proportions of people in a later wave of the same survey, in those same countries, describing their self-rated health as good or better in 2005, and the national levels of life expectancy as reported to the nearest whole year, for men and women combined, by the World Health Report 2005 (WHO, 2005).

Table 22.1: Self-rated health and life expectancy for OECD countries.

Health is good (%)	Life exp. (years)	Country
54	82	Japan
76	81	Australia
74	81	Italy
78	81	Sweden
83	81	Switzerland
72	80	France
80	80	Spain
73	79	Britain
66	79	Finland
67	79	Germany
71	79	Netherlands
82	79	New Zealand
80	77	USA
64	74	Mexico
68	70	Turkey

Sources: World Values Survey (2005) and WHO (2005).

Norway is no longer included in the survey, but Britain, France, Italy and the Netherlands are now included, so these are all included in the table. Excluding them has little effect on what follows. The correlation coefficient between the two columns of figures shown in Table 22.1 is +0.19; hardly a 'close relationship'. If the two poorest OECD countries are removed, the two to which Wilkinson would not claim his theory to apply (Mexico and Turkey), then the correlation becomes –0.24. The relationship is inverted.

There is thus a tendency for people in the affluent OECD countries to report their health as good or very good more often in countries with lower expectations of life. A small part of this tendency is that because people in more equal countries live longer on average they will tend to be a little older on average, but that will only be a very slight effect. It is not the explanation as to why only 58% of people in Japan say their health is good or very good as compared to 80% of folk in the United States. Furthermore in their study Jen et al. do not standardize by age so they are reporting on the same phenomena that we are showing here. It may well be there appears to be no contextual effect that increases people's chances of telling someone taking a survey that their health is good for people living in more equitable affluent countries. That clearly does not mean that there is no contextual effect on actual experienced health.

Wilkinson does not claim his arguments apply to countries that have not reached a particular income threshold. In Mexico and Turkey enough people still suffer from abject poverty such that simple lack of money kills enough; people experience obviously worse health, and die many years less on average than in other OECD countries. That is why the two lower dots look so out of place in Figure 22.1. Once those dots are excluded it is possible to begin to see that, if anything, there is an inverse relationship between life expectancy and self-rated health. In affluent OECD countries where people on average live longer, they are less likely to rate their health as 'good' or very good'.

Figure 22.1: Self-rated health (%) and life expectancy (years).

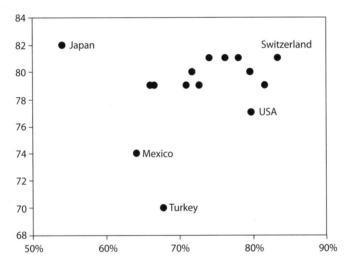

Source: Table 22.1 (*OECD countries in 2005*).

It has been hypothesized that one way to cope with living in an extremely unequal affluent society is to feign optimism, to be strong, have high self-belief, convince yourself that you are special, more able than others: you are strong, you will survive, prosper, get to the top of the pile, achieve the dream, even though you realize that most around you will not. The experience of living in Harlem in New York with its very high murder rate and very low suicide rate is often discussed in this context.

You do not last long in an environment like Harlem if you internalize your concerns. Better to let your anger out, and when asked how you are, say you are doing '*just great*' (Wilkinson and Pickett, 2009). In contrast in more equitable nations, such as France, it is oft quoted that the French will reply when asked whether they are happy: '*only an idiot would answer yes*' (obviously not answering in English). Similarly, of people in OECD countries the Japanese are the most likely to be realistic (if not pessimistic) about their personal state of health, while living the longest of people in all these countries. There is less need to fool yourself that all is well in more equitable countries.

So what have Jen *et al.* discovered if not that Wilkinson (and all his supporters) are incorrect? Well, they may have discovered the beginnings of a stream of evidence to help explain one of the greatest conundrums facing researchers interested in the worldwide effects of inequality on people in rich countries today. Most things are worse in more unequal rich countries. People die younger on average, their education is worse at school, they are more likely to resort to drugs, have sex when very young (and usually when also very drunk), become pregnant as a young teenager, end up in prison as a young adult, become depressed in mid-life, suffer from debt in later life, are much more likely to be murdered even.

Life is more grim in more unequal rich nations. However, despite all this, including worse rates of measured mental health, people in more unequal rich countries are not more likely to kill themselves than are people in more equitable affluent nations. In fact, if anything, suicide rates are highest in the more equitable of rich countries.

It has been hypothesized that it is harder to blame others, or 'the system', for your woes in countries where people are more equal. People are more likely to internalize their concerns, not to lash out, they blame themselves more, and do not talk themselves up. At the extreme more kill themselves. Before that extreme it would appear that more admit their own health to be poor; poorer than it actually is in relation to others living in more unequal countries, but perhaps poor as far as they are really concerned.

Have Jen *et al.* found the beginnings of evidence to help understand the long hypothesized link between equality and suicide? They do not mention it in their paper, but Wilkinson's hypothesis has never been successfully applied to suicide rates, in fact almost the opposite occurs. An hypothesis that stretched back to Emile Durkheim observing that countries in which suicide was more common over a century ago tended to have lower murder rates.

The link between equality and suicide is perhaps most well known in the stories of severe melancholy and the suicides of early socialists (see Dixon, 2008; Livesey, 2007). Equality can be hard to deal with, not as hard on society as a whole as inequality and its consequences, but hard on otherwise affluent individuals to both accept and live with that acceptance. If you come to believe that people are equal, you have to believe that there is nothing that special about your abilities. Academics are typical in disliking this understanding, working in a system which constantly requires them to be clambering for attention. Who wants to say that their collection of university degrees is more a result of their head-start in life, than their claim to either innate intelligence or great toil? If equality is good, then academic elitism and one-upmanship is not that useful, so it helps to try to be constructive rather than just find criticism.

Grand theories such as the inequality thesis are currently out of vogue in an academia where the fashion of the day is to say that everything is all very complicated and contingent. Grand theories are, by their nature, unlikely to be true. That is because they tend to contradict each other so only a few can hold water and most have to be wrong. However, a Grand theory may be proposed that turns out largely to appear to hold water.

The most extensive review of the literature undertaken so far, albeit from a partisan source (Wilkinson and Pickett, 2006), clearly shows the balance of academic evidence currently to be in favour of the hypothesis that inequality is bad for societies. Jen *et al.*'s contribution describes itself with a remarkable lack of contrition as '… *a significant addition to the substantive literature*' (Jen *et al.*, 2008, p 203). In the cold light of equality it is simply another paper in the smaller camp opposing the hypothesis; this paper that you are currently reading is simply yet another paper in the camp supporting Richard Wilkinson.

Is it really as tit-for-tat as that? Jen *et al.* claim to have found the hypothesis to have been '… *based on a statistical artefact*' (p 204). We use the simple statistical artifice of the graph, table and correlation coefficient reported above to refute this. But surely something better is possible than one academic paper merely cancelling out another, a bit of sly innuendo that the other side have not quite been smart enough (that really is not our aim at all), a little sad showing-off (on our part)[2] to a potential journal audience of, at the very most, just a few hundred readers interested in this debate? That would all be a bit of a tragic waste of time!

One great product of the inequality hypothesis is that if you do come to believe that greater equality is good for all, and all are essentially capable of making contributions, are all of remarkably equal ability, all deserve a pretty equal share and equal say, then you look more closely for what good can come out of discoveries such as that of Jen *et al.* rather than simply dismissing that study as suffering itself from the authors not have noticed the statistical artefact that international self-rated health is not a good measure of the actual direction of health inequalities between affluent countries. The good that can come out of Jen *et al.*'s study is not that it shows any problem with Wilkinson's work, but that it does reveal remarkable variations in how people in different affluent countries describe their own state of health in ways that clearly are not well reflected by how long they tend to live.

For people in more inequitable countries, such as the United States, clearly more will be suffering ill health for mortality rates to be so high there. The fact that they do not report that, the fact that they even report the opposite, raises the possibility— the potential synthesis—that inequality leads to people being more likely to think

---

[2] Editorial Note: It is possible that often academic debate is as simple as *tit for tat*. This footnote is an example of *tit*. Where debate becomes confrontational that can be useful in illustrating how academics, just like any other group, can take offence easily. This is especially the case in more unequal settings such as in the very competitive and machismo world of US and UK health inequalities research. For the *tat* to which this note is *tit*, see: Johnston, R.J., Jen, M. and Jones, K. (2009) On inequality, health, scientific progress and political argument: A response to Dorling and Barford, *Health & Place*, 15, 4, pp 1163–65, ISSN: 1353-8292 10.1016/j.healthplace.2009.06.004, which opens with: '*To accuse us of "sly innuendo" suggesting that "the other side have not been quite smart enough" through "a little sad showing-off" involving "a bit of a tragic waste of time" is just a parody of science.*' You'll notice that we said '*on our part*' implying that we were '*showing off*', in (failed) self-depreciation. In debate under strained circumstances others quickly look for insults, always concerned over whether they are receiving enough respect. This is a normal human response to living under unusually high inequality. It has traditionally been identified amongst men living in prisons, so it is interesting to see it in universities too.

positively in more unequal countries. We know from the famous 'Lake Wobegone effect' and the numerous examples given of it that are mostly taken from the United States, that people in the United States are remarkably more likely than in other countries to say that they think they are particularly able individuals.

The Lake Wobegon effect is for people's optimism to overcome their abilities to estimate. It is named after the fictional lake town where '*all the women are strong, all the men are good looking, and all the children are above average*'. The large size of the majority of Americans who say they are individually in the upper reaches of intelligence distributions, income distributions, and that good things are more likely to happen to them, they are better drivers than most (and so on and on) has until now largely been anecdotal testament to this (Gilbert, 2006). Similarly, anecdotal stories of people in Japan being less likely to attempt to take personal credit for their social position and standing, of people in France laughing off the idea of using American-style terms when asked how they are doing today, of Scandinavians being dour and unassertive, and so on, have also been largely anecdotal.

There are grains of truth in many stereotypes, they point towards something. The something they seem to be pointing to here is that in more equitable countries such as Japan, France, and the states of Scandinavia, you are less likely to pretend to others that all is ok and you are better than most, and you are less likely to pretend to yourself that you are well when you are not. You may be a better judge of your own situation in a more equitable country, and that is not always a boon.

It is possible that suicide levels are higher in countries where people have not had to be brought up always looking for the bright side of life to get through life. After all, in more equal countries if you are poor and ill you have decent health services to fall back on; and you may be less likely to feel you have to convince the World Values Survey research team, and yourself, among others, that you are fit, healthy, or 'the best'. In the United States the best you can do if you are poor and ill, is often to try to tell yourself that you are neither really ill, nor that poor, and that things will get better soon.[3] It is either that, or accept the truth, and the truth is far more frequent premature death than in any other rich nation.

References

Dixon, T. (2008) *The Invention of Altruism: Making Moral Meanings in Victorian Britain*. Oxford: Oxford University Press.

Dorling, D., Mitchell, R. and Pearce, J. (2007) The global impact of income inequality on health by age: an observational study, *British Medical Journal*, 335, 873-875 [reproduced as Chapter 32 of this volume].

Gilbert, D. (2006) *Stumbling on Happiness*, London: Harper Collins.

Idler, E.L. and Benyamini, Y. (1997) Self-rated health and mortality: a review of twenty-seven community studies, *Journal of Health Social Behavior*, 38, 21–37.

---

[3] See Chapter 34, this volume, for an elaboration of this argument.

Jen, M.H., Jones, K. and Johnston, R. (2008) Compositional and contextual approaches to the study of health behaviour and outcomes: using multi-level modelling to evaluate Wilkinson's income inequality hypothesis, *Health & Place* 15, 1, 198–203.

Livesey, R. (2007) *Socialism, Sex, and the Culture of Aestheticism in Britain, 1880–1914.* Oxford: Oxford University Press.

Marmot, M. (2004) *The Status Syndrome: How Social Standing Affects Our Health and Longevity*, London: Bloomsbury.

Ram, R. (2006) Further examination of the cross-country association between income inequality and population health, *Social Science and Medicine*, 62, 779–791.

Shaw, M., Davey Smith, G., Thomas, B. and Dorling, D. (2008) *The Grim Reaper's Road Map: An Atlas of Mortality in Britain*, Bristol: The Policy Press.

Wilkinson, R.G. and Pickett, K.E. (2006) Income inequality and population health: a review and explanation of the evidence, *Social Science Medicine* 62, 1768–1784.

Wilkinson, R. and Pickett, K. (2009) *The Spirit Level: Why More Equal Societies Almost Always Do Better*, London: Allen Lane.

World Health Organisation (2005) *World Health Report*. Geneva: WHO.

World Values Survey, 2008. Official Data File v.20081015, 2005 World Values Survey Association, http://www.worldvaluessurvey.org, Aggregate File Producer: ASEP/JDS, Madrid.

23

Housing and identity: how place makes race

Dorling, D. (2011) *Housing and identity: How place makes race*, Better Housing Briefing 17, London: Race Equality Foundation.

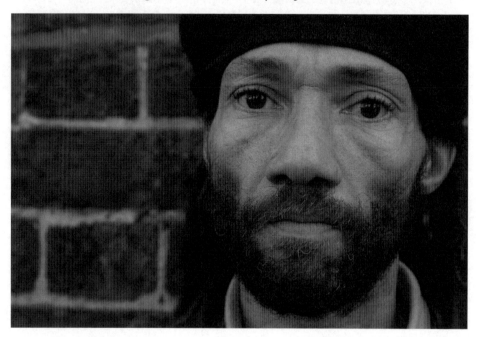

Suffering no serious invasion or revolution for almost a millennium, the social geographical arrangement of Britain is unusually rigid. Whereas in the USA, inner cities, declining suburbs and poorer outlying settlements are often allowed to decline further into ghost towns, in Britain, over the last century, areas that might have been abandoned as slums have generally been rebuilt as new social housing or mixed tenure, and former housing stock has been replaced with homes deemed to fit the social make-up of the area. This policy has had the effect of preserving differences between neighbourhoods, allowing places such as south-central Manchester to be rebuilt regularly, and preserving the social geography of Inner London for over a century, despite successive waves of immigration (Orford *et al.*, 2002).

Indeed, many of what were the poorest parts of Britain a century and a half ago are still the poorest parts today. In England, life expectancy was lowest in Salford and Oldham in 1851 and 140 years later it remained lowest in those same towns (Dorling, 1995). This is despite a complete turnover of population due to death and high out- and in-migration rates, which replaced a partly Irish-origin population with people of South-Asian origin.

In Whitechapel in London, similar stories are told of Huguenot, then Jewish, then Muslim populations each replacing one another. In every case, the housing system into which new arrivals have had to fit – ghetto housing in Whitechapel; cheap, less stereotyped private renting later; social housing later still – has helped define a group as a particular minority, until another group takes its place. It is the place that carries the stigma over time, far longer than differing groups of people or differing races do.

Housing inequalities in Britain

In other European countries, people tend to rent more and buy later. In Britain we are drawn to home ownership which leads to divisions in housing quality based on wealth. In turn, racial divisions in wealth mean that housing quality is often also very unfairly distributed by race, and a number of housing issues disproportionately affect black and minority ethnic families:

- There is now eleven times less public green space in areas where 40 per cent of the population are from black and minority ethnic groups compared to areas where just 2 per cent are from such groups (CABE, 2010).
- The percentage of school children aged over ten who share a bedroom with an adult or a sibling of the opposite sex rose from 8 per cent in 1999 to 15 per cent by 2005 (this is known as the bedroom standard; HMSO, 2003). These children are disproportionately from black and minority ethnic groups and such overcrowding is most common in London, an area with one of the highest proportions of black and minority ethnic groups in the UK (Dorling, 2010, p 117).
- The majority of children living above the fourth floor in England are from black and minority ethnic groups (2001 Census national statistics table).
- Homelessness rates rose by 14.5 per cent for black and minority ethnic households between 1998 and 2006, despite falling by 8 per cent overall; for African and Caribbean households, these homelessness rates increased by 25 per cent and 42 per cent respectively (Roberts and McMahon, 2008, pp 17–18; Dorling, 2009).
- Some 33 per cent of Pakistani and Bangladeshi households live in unfit dwellings, compared to 6 per cent of white people (Roberts and McMahon, 2008, pp 17–18).

This [chapter is drawn from an] opinion piece [which] introduces some recent advances in the social sciences concerning race and place. In particular, it draws on work from the USA on wealth and race, work from Britain on the current crisis in housing, and observations made in the best-selling popular social science book, *The Spirit Level* (Wilkinson and Pickett, 2009, p 178).

Wilkinson and Pickett observe that in more equitable societies, race is a much less salient issue, and where inequalities in income and wealth are high, race matters more: in effect, different places and times make race matter more or less. This [chapter] concentrates on how the operations of the housing market help that to occur, and raises the possibility of a 'right-to-sell' policy to alleviate the harmful effects of the not-really-free market.

How place makes race

The argument that social inequalities maintain and, in some cases, create racial divisions is not new, but it has been built on greatly in recent years (Dorling, 2010, pp 159–70 and p 346, footnote 33). Racial inequality can be established and controlled only when there are strong spatial residential divisions and when certain racial groups are confined to living in certain streets or housing blocks. [The argument in this chapter] extends the adage that '*The soil grows castes; the machine makes classes*' (Young, 1958, p 21) by also arguing that '*housing separates races, the home creates gender*'.

Social divisions are pertinent to a particular geography and time in history and may grow and diminish in importance. The following four examples, given in the chronological order in which they have come to the fore, are relevant to people in Britain. Each scenario has not necessarily been subsumed by the next and sometimes old divisions are reintroduced from abroad.

1 Caste divisions became established in feudal farming societies where relationships were ordered primarily around the connection between people and the soil. They become untenable outside of rural village settings. People do not fit naturally into castes and castes are not a natural division of humanity. Farming in the North China plain was carried out successfully for millennia without caste systems (Frank and Gills, 2006).

2 Class divisions became established in newly industrialised societies where relationships were ordered primarily around the connection between people and the machine. They become untenable outside of factory-town settings. People do not fit naturally into classes and classes are not natural divisions of humanity. Markets operated successfully for millennia before the invention of free-market capitalism (Lohmann, 2009).

3 Gender divisions are peculiar to particular times and places and are rapidly changing. The home is the most palpable location in which gender categorisations are made and maintained: '*Women do two-thirds of the world's work, earn one-tenth of the world's income, and own less than one-hundredth of the world's property*' (MacKinnon, 2006, p 21). Established gender divisions become untenable as the nature of homes changes, as we have fewer children, live on our own more often and for longer. Gender divisions in Britain are wide, but were far greater a century ago and are far greater in other continents today.

4 Racial categorisation is most acute in the city and its quarters. It was in the city where ghettos were first formed. Only since the 1960s has the word 'racism' appeared in dictionaries and the word 'racist' is even more recent (Leech, 2005, pp 1–5). Jewish people, persecuted for years on religious grounds, are now seen as racially persecuted. Like poverty, racism has not always been with us and, also like poverty, only recently have very large numbers of people become committed to its eradication (Goldberg, 2009, p 370).

Race and housing

Britain is one of the most unequal of the world's richest twenty-five countries. Only three countries have higher income inequalities, and even Israel, the country with the greatest religious divides, has lower inequalities in income than Britain (Dorling, 2010, p 327). One result is that when people without many financial assets enter Britain from abroad, they are placed at the bottom of a very long housing ladder.

Income and wealth inequalities in Britain are now as wide as they were a century ago, when Jews fleeing pogroms in the East faced overcrowding in the Whitechapel ghetto (Vaughan and Geddes, 2009). The history of British fascism dates from that time, with similarities in the myths spread about Jews then, to those spread about Muslims today.

We no longer have ghettos in Britain, but we do have very poor quality housing for those at the bottom. This has the effect of linking the racial identity of new immigrants to particular residential locations and to particularly obvious points in a widely and tightly stretched social hierarchy. If our housing system were less polarised, it would be harder for racial divisions to be maintained. New minority groups would not be so easily identified if our 'skid rows' were not so obviously on the slide downwards.

Britain has some of the smallest housing units in Europe when floor space per person is measured. At the same time, and not unconnected, Britain also has some of the most inefficient policies when it comes to the use of our housing stock. More people own two or more homes in Britain than in other countries of similar population density (such as the Netherlands), which limits the availability of housing for the rest of the population.

Furthermore, the inefficient private rented sector has been allowed to grow rapidly while the efficient social housing sector has been deliberately shrunk. In contrast to the private sector, there are usually fewer under-occupied or empty social housing properties at any one time (Dorling, 2010, p 248). Recent changes in tenure and inequality have been the result partly of a rising political geography of fear, which is not unrelated to racial prejudice.

The political geography of wealth in the USA

People do not happily polarise, but they will vote and act to polarise out of fear. When no alternative to abandoning poorer areas and poorer people seems apparent, otherwise well-meaning people may act selfishly, exercising choice over where they live in order to attempt to keep their living standards stable. In the 1970s, in contrast to today, white families in both the USA and Britain had greater freedom to choose residential locations, because of greater consistency in housing costs across different places (Frank, 2007).

Black and minority ethnic families have been less free to choose residential location in recent history even if financially secure. They could face acute racism if they moved into the wrong block or street. As private housing became more expensive, the freedom to choose where to live reduced further, even though the supply of housing increased. This is partly because increased supply allowed a small group to buy several homes each, but also because location matters more in a country which is more economically segregated.

Assets in the USA were and remain an embarrassing topic for discussion. During the run-up to the election of Barack Obama, following a great deal of controversy, it was revealed that American Senator and later Republican presidential nominee, John McCain, owned at least eleven homes for his personal use (Halbfinger, 2008).

Recently, Massachusetts' Brandeis University's Institute on Assets and Social Policy produced a widely covered report which showed that, from 1984 to 2007, the wealth gap between white and African-American families had, on average, grown by $75,000 between single pairs of families. Even excluding equity in housing, the average white family in the USA saw its median holding of wealth grow from $22,000 to $100,000 over these twenty-three years. For African-American families, median wealth levels had remained at about $2000 when measured in constant dollars (Shapiro *et al.*, 2010).

While it might be expected that wealth gaps between racial groups were related to differences in employment, the Brandeis University report argues that job achievement does not '*adequately predict family wealth holdings*' (Shapiro *et al.*, 2010, p 2). Instead, it is differential rates of inheritance of wealth, especially of property, which is the main cause of rapidly rising wealth inequality between white and African Americans.

Those with assets can, through institutions like banks, gain interest by lending to those with less. The Brandeis report found that deregulation of the lending market saw increased debt among poorer African-American families and that '*the segmentation of the mortgage lending market highlights a general trend in lending in which low-income people and consumers of colour pay more for accessing credit*' (Shapiro *et al.*, 2010, p 3).

The political geography of wealth in Britain

Although economic and racial divides are not as acute in Britain, they are moving in the US direction. It is possible to compare John McCain's eleven homes with an estimate for the Conservative leader (and now Prime Minister), David Cameron, who does not think he owns a fourth home ('*I don't think so – not that I can think of*'; Dougary, 2009, p 8). In polite British society, talking about the distribution and ownership of housing can cause a little squirming, but it is vital if we are to understand 'how place can make race'.

Few admit to buying a home in the suburbs to get away from the poor. Instead, they blame schools, or the attractive décor, or the air, but the evidence of higher and higher prices being paid for otherwise identical homes betrays beliefs, rising prejudices and fears. The mantra that began in the 1970s and became a loud chant by the 1990s was: 'location, location, location'. This was not always down to 'white flight', but instead to the flight of the modestly supported from the poor, the average away from those of modest means, of the affluent from the average, or the very rich from the affluent.

Geographical segregation by ethnicity has fallen in Britain, but between 1968 and 2008 rose for Britain's richest people, who now live in a more tightly defined set of areas than before (Dorling, 2010, pp 124–6). Once economic polarisation begins, it is hard to reverse: attitudes harden, fear grows on fear, people know less and less about each other and imagine more and more. As the very richest gain second homes, in Chelsea and the Cotswolds, in Manhattan and Maine, they complain of limited community cohesion, when they themselves have so many homes that they cannot even know their neighbours, let alone 'muck in' with them.

Offering solutions

That how we live is how we must live, isn't necessarily so. In Britain we have a nationalised state-run health system which caters for the vast majority of citizens. The USA did not make that choice and suffers the lowest life expectancy in the rich world partly as a result (Wilkinson and Pickett, 2009). Neither Britain nor the USA has chosen nationalisation in housing, but the current housing and liquidity crisis could be the impetus needed for some new initiatives.

Our current over-reliance on the housing market ensures that more people are badly housed than need be, that we take too little care of our housing stock, that we maximise short-term profit to sell poorly maintained properties to gullible first-time buyers, and that we rack up enormous debts that benefit only the few rich individuals who earn huge quantities through 'interest'.

In Sheffield as of 2010, 100,000 families were waiting for council homes after the implementation of market mechanisms into social housing through the 'choice-based lettings' scheme. Private landlords rarely have the wellbeing of their tenants as their paramount interest and would be unlikely to survive for long in the private market making enough profit from their investments if they did. Social divisions and racial divides are exacerbated by reliance on private provision when there could be much more public good.

Just as most people choose not to be solely responsible for educating their children or providing their families with health care, a mixed state–market housing system would see the state take control of housing when people would prefer not to take responsibility for a building. When you are young and mobile, or old and immobile, it makes least sense to own your own home – while it helps the young to be footloose, older people may find their housing needs change quickly as their physical abilities change.

The right-to-sell

A better mixed state–market system could be achieved by introducing a 'right-to-sell' to accompany the 'right-to-buy', or, in other terms, a 'National Health Service for housing'. Right-to-sell could both stabilise the housing market and reduce social polarisation. Pilot versions have already been introduced in all four countries of the UK for the most vulnerable households, and in England the extended right could improve considerably opportunities for poorer black and minority ethnic groups.

At its most simple, the right-to-sell is just the opposite of the right-to-buy and it can co-exist with that right. It gives mortgagees the right to become tenants, and private tenants the right to become social housing tenants, without moving home. It has the short-term benefit of reducing repossessions in a market crash and the long-term benefit of preventing segregation based on high rental prices, since high rent could no longer force poorer families from newly expensive neighbourhoods.

If a household were to exercise the right-to-sell, the title of their home, and any capital and debts associated with it, would be transferred to a social landlord and they would become tenants within those same four walls. People losing their jobs [see Figure 23.1[1]] need not also lose their home. Children need not lose their school and school-friends. Private landlords could not simply evict families if they wanted to increase the rent. Families could choose to sell their landlord's property to a social landlord (or another better private landlord). The private landlord would receive some recompense, just as the state receives recompense when the right-to-buy is evoked.

Right-to-sell in practice: MRS and MTR

The last British (New Labour) government did institute a partial right-to-sell. It was called the 'Mortgage Rescue Scheme' (MRS). A recent evaluation found that, between January 2009 and March 2010, 629 applications to the scheme were made, resulting in 613 mortgagee families staying in their homes as housing association tenants (as reported in July 2010). The report also stated that: '*MRS provided former borrowers with a profound sense of relief from the anxieties associated with potential homelessness, offering them a "lifesaver", "hope" and a "light at the end of the tunnel"*' (CLG, 2010, p 5).

The evaluation of the MRS also found that there was much less demand for the government's other scheme, the 'shared equity' option, with only sixteen households being accepted across all of England for that more complicated solution (CLG, 2010). It would appear that it is preferable to know either that you are responsible for the upkeep of a property or that someone else is, and not to share that responsibility in some way. Right-to-sell schemes allow households to move between times when

---

[1] Editorial Note: Figure 23.1 has been added to the original article to illustrate how unemployment was rising at the time of writing. The unemployed were reported, in 2012, to include over half of all young black men aged under 25 in the workforce. Note that over half of young black women in Britain were unemployed and searching for work in 2009 but no comment was made at that time. Part of the reason was that banks in London quickly cut back on contracting the firms that cleaned their offices and made them so shiny. Unemployment rose for these women because of that. It then fell again as so many had to take any job going. There is a wide error range around these figures because the authorities do not consider youth unemployment a serious enough issue to warrant the collection of better quality data. Instead we have to rely on a sample survey. See also how rates for young white people are climbing but are not yet as high as those suffered by both young black men and young black women in 2006. Rates for older groups are generally lower, normally higher for men than women, black than white, poor than affluent, north than south, disabled than able-bodied, less-qualified than more-qualified, and almost all these social gaps are widening as we are less and less in it together.

Figure 23.1: Unemployment rates of men and women, black and white, aged 16–24, 2006–11, Q4, United Kingdom.

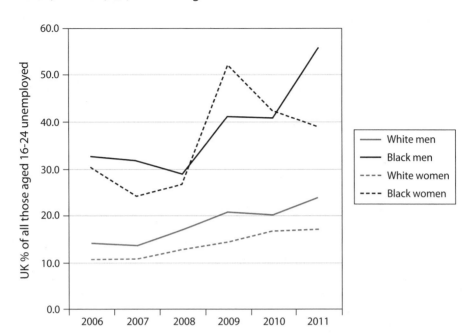

Source: Drawn from data at: http://www.guardian.co.uk/news/datablog/2012/mar/09/black-unemployed-young-men. Sourced in turn from the Labour Force Survey, 2012.

they are best able simply to be tenants, or best able to look after the long-term repair of the property as well, which is what ownership should mean.

The present government's MRS scheme is more generically known as a 'Mortgage to Rent' (MTR) scheme. There are now many of these to be found in fledgling states around the world, all designed to help households who own their homes, but now have little chance of sustaining a mortgage. In England, the registered social landlord (RSL) purchases the property and the applicant pays rent to their landlord (instead of their old mortgage) at a level that it is calculated they can afford, given a full assessment of household finances.

These schemes are generally initially available only to the most vulnerable households, usually those with children, who are likely to require homelessness assistance if left unaided. The new coalition government has expressed a preference for people who fall on hard times to move or be moved away from prosperous areas – the opposite of the direction of these schemes (Dorling, 2011). As part of the Comprehensive Spending Review of 20 October 2010, the government also announced a series of cuts to housing benefits in England to accelerate the process of clearing some areas of poorer people.

In Wales, there is a Mortgage Rescue Scheme similar to that available in England until recently, but it has a greater chance of survival, as the Welsh Assembly Government appears to have a very different agenda from that of Westminster (Welsh

Assembly Government, 2010). Any family falling behind with mortgage payments is advised to contact their local council, where a housing options team, homelessness team or housing strategy officer will advise on the appropriate course of action. It can be argued that this kind of assistance and caring for neighbours is part of what makes Wales a *Big Society*.

The Scottish Mortgage to Rent scheme has been very successful and, following its introduction in 2003, is much more advanced than in England (Bramley *et al.*, 2008). The scheme differs slightly in the detail from the English and Welsh models, but in general is very similar: '*offering households the opportunity to change the tenure of their home from owner occupation to a tenancy in the social rented sector*' (Bramley *et al.*, 2008, para 3.5). However, with a stronger culture of social housing, it can be argued that the Scottish system also represents a *Bigger than English Big Society* model, where people look out for each other and eviction is frowned upon. With housing as a devolved responsibility for the Scottish Parliament, it looks as though the Scottish scheme will, at least in part, survive the coming cuts.

In Northern Ireland, repossessions doubled between 2007 and 2009. In response, Margaret Richie, the new Housing Minister (appointed in February 2010) suggested the 'need for a full mortgage rescue scheme' (Richie, 2010). However, she continued by reporting that although a pilot scheme had assisted 373 people and prevented twenty-nine home repossessions, at that time she was unable to secure funding to extend the scheme. The finance minister was a member of the Democratic Unionist Party and Ms Richie a member of the Social Democratic and Labour Party, two parties which have traditionally been associated with Protestant and Catholic divisions in Ireland.

Conclusion

Where people live in the world largely determines the groups they are born into, whether that group might be race, religion, caste or creed. At the micro-level, your postcode determines a great deal of your future. Where your mother and father lived in Britain from the point of your gestation is enough to largely predict many life outcomes far better than knowing if you are to be born male or female, or even black or white, especially with regard to education. In the recent past, especially in the 1970s, it mattered far more if either your mother or father (or both) were not white. Now class, as mediated through place, can often be just as important, if not more so.

The right-to-sell would mean that children would not have to move school when their parents fell on hard times. It would mean that new property would become available in the long term in the social housing sector, scattered across cities and breaking the relationship between concentrations of ethnicity and concentrations of poverty.

Introducing the right-to-sell would make a child's race less of an acute predictor of their outcomes in life, because the strong connections between race, wealth, housing and, hence, location and education would be slightly, but surely, weakened. The right-to-sell would reduce the advantages of those who currently have most advantages in life – so we should expect that those who own the most property might oppose it. It would be helpful if it could be explained to large property owners how their lives would benefit from not living in a society where so many others felt so often to be on the edge of destitution, unsure of whether they will be able to afford to stay in their home.

In mainstream policy circles, the right-to-sell was unthinkable before the current crisis. However, a housing market in danger of failure and the threat of mass repossessions may force governments to seriously consider how it could work more widely. This is even true with a Westminster government hostile to ideas such as this: the market might just demand it, as housing demand falls, along with rising government spending cuts.

The right-to-sell differs from allowing housing associations to take vacant properties off the open market in that possession under the right-to-sell is achieved without eviction. The idea could be introduced by making it available to the most obviously needy cases – not just the most vulnerable households, but all people with dependent children, for instance, especially those not within the bedroom standard. The natural extension of the right-to-sell would allow tenants to swap private landlord, to shop around for a better landlord, without having to move home.

In England, the government is currently withdrawing even further from having an interest in providing adequate housing. In summer 2010, it suggested that it would withdraw any oversight for how much housing should be built in a year. Regional plans had varied from the South East Region (excluding London) allowing up to 39 000 dwellings a year to be built up to 2026, while only some 7660 a year would be built in the North East. None of these targets is likely to even remain as a target, let alone be achieved. However, Britain has enough housing for all already. What we need much more of is repair rather than rebuilding. Above all, we need to better share our resources in a country that is becoming relatively poorer. The strongest reasons not to share are racist reasons.

References

Bramley, G., Kofi Karley, N., Morgan, J., Lederle, N., Sosenko, F., Stephens, M., Wallace, A. and Littlewood, M. (2008) *Research to Evaluate the Operation and Impact of the National Mortgage to Rent Scheme*, Edinburgh: The Scottish Government (web report), www.scotland.gov.uk/Publications/2008/12/11115931/0 (last accessed January 2011).

Commission for Architecture and the Built Environment (CABE) (2010) *Green Space and Race: The connections between health, ethnicity and inequality*, London: Commission for Architecture and the Built Environment.

Communities and Local Government (CLG) (2010) *Evaluation of the Mortgage Rescue Scheme and Homeowners Mortgage Support: Executive summary for interim report* (edited by S. Wilcox, A. Wallace, G. Bramley, J. Morgan, F. Sosenko and J. Ford), London: Communities and Local Government, www.communities.gov.uk/ documents/ housing/pdf/1648144.pdf (last accessed January 2011).

Dorling, D. (1995) *A New Social Atlas of Britain*, Chichester: Wiley.

Dorling, D. (2009) *How Much Evidence Do You Need?*, www.sasi.group.shef.ac.uk/publications/2009/EHC_Dorling_response.pdf (last accessed February 2011).

Dorling, D. (2010) *Injustice: Why social inequality persists*, Bristol: The Policy Press.

Dorling, D. (2011) 'Clearing the poor away' in Yeates, N., Haux, T., Jawad, R. and Kilkey, M. (eds) *In Defence of Welfare: The impacts of the Comprehensive Spending Review*, London: Social Policy Association.

Dougary, G. (2009) 'Who is David Cameron?', *The Times*, 16 May [the key quote on homes is on p 8], www.timesonline.co.uk/tol/news/politics/article6267193.ece?token=null&offset=0&p ge=1 (last accessed January 2011).

Frank, A.G. and Gills, B.K. (2006) *The World System: Five hundred years or five thousand?* (2nd ed.), Abingdon: Routledge.

Frank, R.H. (2007) *Falling Behind: How rising inequality harms the middle class*, University of California at Berkeley: University of California Press.

Goldberg, D.T. (2009) *The Threat of Race: Reflections on racial neoliberalism*, Oxford: Blackwell.

Halbfinger, D.M. (2008) 'The McCain properties', *New York Times*, 23 August, www.nytimes.com/ref/us/politics/mccain-properties.html (last accessed January 2011).

HMSO (2003) *Housing (Overcrowding) Bill*, as introduced in the House of Commons on 22 January 2003 [Bill 46], www.publications.parliament.uk/pa/cm200203/cmbills/046/en/03046x--.htm (last accessed January 2011).

Leech, K. (2005) *Race*, London: SPCK.

Lohmann, L. (2009) *When Markets Are Poison: Learning about climate policy from the financial crisis, Briefing 40*, The Corner House, www.thecornerhouse.org.uk (last accessed January 2011).

MacKinnon, C.A. (2006) *Are Women Human? And other international dialogues*, Boston, MA: Harvard University Press.

Orford, S., Dorling, D., Mitchell, R., Shaw, M. and Smith, G.D. (2002) 'Life and death of the people of London: a historical GIS of Charles Booth's inquiry', *Health & Place*, 8, 1, pp 25–35.

Richie, M. (2010) *Speaking in the Mortgage Rescue Scheme Social Development Northern Ireland Assembly debate*, 9 February 2010, 3:15 pm, as reported at www.theyworkforyou.com/ni/?id=2010-02-09.5.32 (last accessed January 2011).

Roberts, R. and McMahon, W. (2008) *Debating Race, Ethnicity, Harm and Crime*, London: Centre for Crime and Justice Studies.

Shapiro, T.M., Meschede, T. and Sullivan, L. (2010) *The Racial Wealth Gap Increases Fourfold, Research and Policy Brief*, Massachusetts: IASP, The Heller School for Social Policy and Management, Brandeis University, http://iasp.brandeis.edu/pdfs/Racial-Wealth-Gap-Brief.pdf (last accessed January 2011).

Vaughan, L. and Geddes, I. (2009) 'Urban form and deprivation: a contemporary proxy for Charles Booth's analysis of poverty', *Radical Statistics*, 99, pp 46–73.

Welsh Assembly Government (2010) *Mortgage Rescue Scheme* [advice web pages], wales.gov.uk/topics/housingandcommunity/housing/private/buyingandselling/mortgagerescue/?lang=en (last accessed February 2011).

Wilkinson, R.G. and Pickett, K. (2009) *The Spirit Level: Why More Equal Societies Almost Always Do Better*, London: Allen Lane.

Young, M. (1958) *The Rise of the Meritocracy 1870–2033: An essay on education and equality*, London: Thames and Hudson.

Figure 23.2: Ernest Burgess's scheme of 'urban areas', 1929 (The University of Chicago Press)

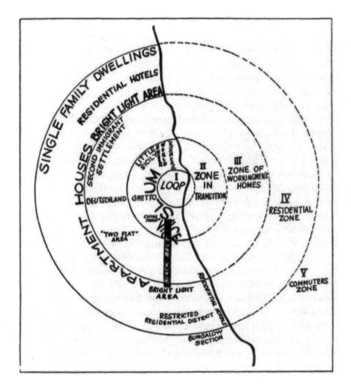

Note the area labelled 'Black Belt' in South Chicago.

Source: http://publishing.cdlib.org/ucpressebooks

24

Border controls? Here's a long line of reasons to relax

Dorling, D. (2011) 'Border controls? Here's a long line of reasons to relax', *The Guardian*, 8 November.

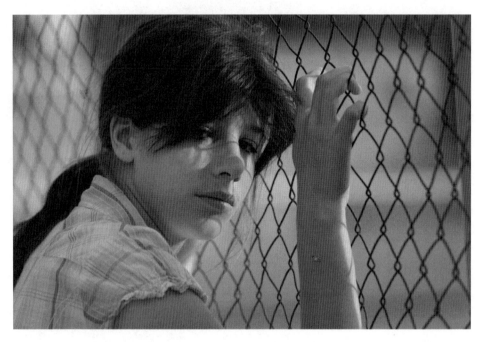

Queuing at border controls serves little purpose – the queues are as much about image as impact, and the image is not welcoming

I landed in Heathrow last Friday on a direct flight from Athens. I walked off the flight, and then through what appeared to be mile upon mile of corridors, until eventually getting to passport control. There I queued very briefly, watching three or four people with biometric passports trying to use the automatic channel. Eventually, when the camera didn't recognise their faces, they were waved through to a human officer. "Put your feet on the footprints", the immigration officer kept on telling the confused and mostly elderly travellers, who were struggling to work out what to do. "I only speak English", she kept on repeating. If I had to spend all day saying "Put your feet on the footprints", I thought to myself, I might try to learn how to say it in Greek or French or German.

I was only at passport control for less than a minute. Maybe I was benefiting from being at the very tail end of the '*"reduced security and passport regime" that is thought to have lasted until last week*'.[1] If so, I was very grateful. You catch a train through a city in economic meltdown. You queue your way out of one airport. You sit in a cramped tube of metal and hurtle over Europe. You arrive in Heathrow, still have the train, tube and train to go before you are home. The last thing you want is someone making you queue within what is supposed to be a free movement of labour zone because they want to give the impression that they are being 'tough on immigration', or that this queuing will somehow make us all safer.

Politicians say one thing when they want to sound tough in public, but – as Theresa May herself admitted – instruct their officials to relax checks on EU passport holders in private. Then, they have to be tough again when someone leaks the relaxation. …Tired middle-aged professors of human geography like me might moan about queuing for longer. But people travelling with children, or the truly elderly, or simply those who find standing for long hard have far more to moan about. Others could face hours of questioning because they don't appear to be European enough.

The amount of hassle experienced in aggregate will be directly proportional to the number of people employed to hassle. Just as crime rises when more police officers are employed. What would actually reduce illegal immigration or reduce terrorism is only tangentially related to border controls.

If heavily policed border controls had a great effect on illegal immigration, the US would not be home to so many undocumented migrants. It is a high demand for cheap labour in countries with wide income inequalities that pulls in migrants. It is wide international inequalities in income that push them. People move to where there is demand for them and away from where there isn't [see Figure 24.1].[2] Over the medium term, border controls do little but encourage some to stay for fear that they might not be able to return if they left.

If border controls reduced terrorism, the UK could have contained the violence of '*the troubles*' within Northern Ireland. Instead, border controls are a short-term palliative: something that can reduce the anxiety and alleviate slightly the concern, but not an option that even pretends to begin to address what underlies any motives for trying to stoke up terror in the first place. Border controls have effects, but they are almost all short-term effects, which can be worked around by people with a little

---

[1] Travis, A. (2011) 'Theresa May admits authorising reduced passport checks', *The Guardian*, 7 November.
[2] Editorial Note: Figure 24.1 has been added to the original article to illustrate how immigration rates were changing at the time it was written and to compare those changes to the same period after every other UK recession of the last century. In the recessions of the 1970s, 1980s and 1990s there was net annual emigration from Britain for at least the first three years. However, in the much more severe worldwide depressions of 1930–34 and 2008–12 there was net immigration to the UK, partly as prospects were often even worse abroad, perhaps also because leaving the UK was more difficult in such straitened times. Note that in all cases over time the lines slope down as the situation returns to normal. Normal, in 2012, means net annual in-migration of roughly a quarter of a million people. This is only if the official figures are to be believed. As I write, the 2011 census results have not yet been released and so the latest migration figures cannot be verified. Those statistics shown here prior to 2008 are most reliable as they have all been adjusted to match census data.

power, as smugglers always have. Border controls today are as much about image as impact, and the image is not very welcoming.

To be honest, having spent a week in Athens puts having to queue (or not) in Britain into a different perspective. At least when you queue you have an idea that there is something worth queuing for. You might say that it is good that we have more stringent border controls in Britain and Ireland than elsewhere in the EU. But how would you feel if one day it was Britain facing economic meltdown, and when you tried to fly to Spain for the weekend you got taken aside into a little room at Madrid-Barajas airport and grilled about why you were trying to leave the UK?

You might like being an alien in your own continent. Personally I feel safer being a citizen of something a little larger than one small country.

Figure 24.1: Net annual emigration from England and Wales after the onset of recession – first six years, numbers of people per year.

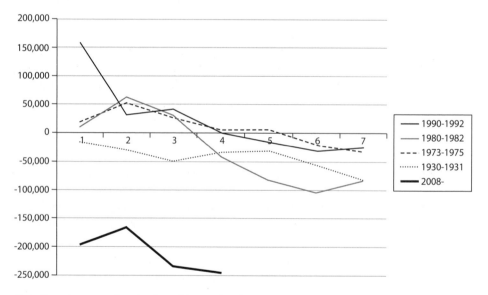

Note: Negative net emigration is positive net immigration.

Source: Office for National Statistics, Migration Statistics Quarterly Report, November 2011 (figures for year ending June, except for final figure - year ending March), and 'Migration: A long-run perspective', http://www.ippr.org/ publications/55/1688/migration-a-long-run-perspective.

Figure 1.3: An example of airbrushing and what non-misleading advertising would look like (see page 14).

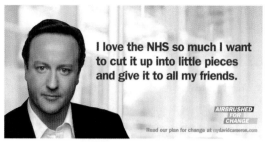

Source: www.mydavidcameron.com/posters/cam-nhs1

Figure 2.1: The localities of cholera, Manchester, 1832 (see page 18).

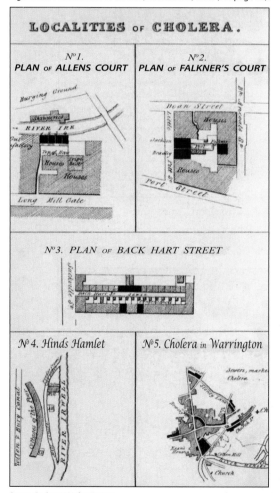

Source: Gaulter, 1833, frontispiece.
www.archive.org/stream/originandprogre00gaulgoog#page/n10/mode/2up

Figure 2.4: Cholera in Leeds in 1832 (section of map) (see page 26).

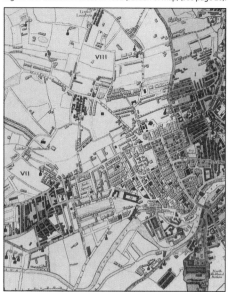

Source: http://www.bl.uk/learning/images/makeanimpact/publichealth/ large 12727.html

Figure 2.5: If pounds were pixels – one of many hundreds of images of dissent in 2012 (see page 29).

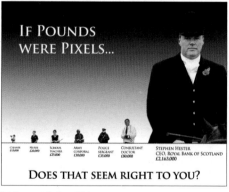

Note: Image created by Duncan Rickelton
Source: http://zoom.it/yE58

Figure 2.7: Picture drawn in chalk by Joe Hill, Manchester Piccadilly (see page 32).

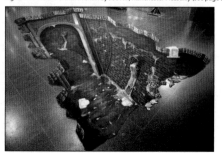

Source: BBC (2010): Temporary drawing made on the concourse floor. 'United Utilities say that Mancunians flush away thousands of incorrect items, such as make up wipes and ear buds, a year, causing sewers to block and toilets and drains to flood.'
http://news.bbc.co.uk/local/manchester/hi/people_and_places/newsid_9135000/9135707.stm

Figure 2.8: Two pages from Gaulter's work on the 1832 Manchester cholera outbreak (see page 35).

118

because its sewers were in a worse condition. The truth is that in the greater part of Manchester there are no sewers at all, and that where they do exist they are so small and badly constructed that instead of contributing to the purification of the town, they become themselves nuisances of the worst description. Recently two or three have been formed or enlarged on a scale of dimensions somewhat more adequate to the functions which they have to fulfil, but to make the *subterranean* of this vast town what it ought to be, and to excavate under its whole surface a complete order of primary and secondary drains, would require an expenditure of not less than three hundred thousand pounds. The labours of the night-man and scavenger do something towards the abatement of this evil; but it is necessary that those of the latter should be placed under better regulations, while in the formation of new streets it ought to be imperatively required that the *subterranean* and pavement of the street be constructed and rendered complete before the houses are built.

Two more remarks are suggested by the consideration of the generating causes of cholera. First, it is to his complete protection from their influence that the rich man is indebted for his immunity from cholera quite as much if not far more, than to any remarkable freedom from the agency of the predisposing causes, which his wealth confers. The contrast between the localities which the rich and poor

119

inhabit, exhibits perhaps the most striking example of the substantial advantages, as far as health is concerned, which affluence can bestow, by enabling its possessor so to construct and fix his residence as to place himself and his family beyond the reach of every ordinary source of malaria. In ancient times the importance of such a choice was not understood, and in towns accordingly the better classes who inhabited dwellings almost as small, ill ventilated, and badly placed, as the poor of our own days, fell victims in far more equal numbers to the epidemics that then preyed upon the land. Even during the progress of cholera in some cities where the local partition between the two great classes of society has been less marked, the disease has attacked both rich and poor in their promiscuous habitations with almost indiscriminate severity, as in Moscow, where one hundred and twenty-four nobles died of the disease.

2.—It may be thought visionary perhaps, but I am disposed to ascribe a large share of the exemption from cholera, which the working classes of this town enjoyed during the epidemic, (an exemption which has been happily extended to the manufacturing districts generally) to the cotton factories in which they work. It was impossible, at least in this town, not to be struck with the fact, that of the whole number of the Manchester cases very few indeed were employed in factories at all, and that of these a pretty large proportion were at the

Source: www.archive.org/stream/originandprogre00gaulgoog#page/n128/mode/2up

Figure 3.1: Detail of *Charles Booth's descriptive map of London poverty 1889* (see page 38).

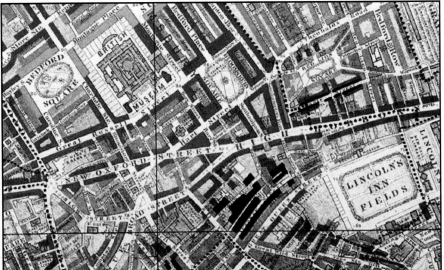

Note: Yellow indicates the highest social class, black the lowest.

Source: *Charles Booth's descriptive map of London poverty 1889*, with introduction by D.A. Reeder, Publication No 130, London; London Topographical Society, 1984.

Figure 3.3: London poverty (1896 and 1991) and mortality (1990s) (see page 43).

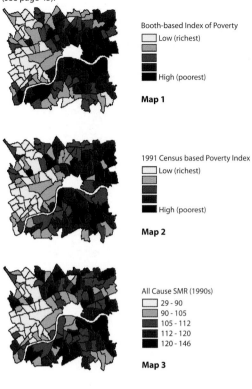

Booth-based Index of Poverty
☐ Low (richest)
☐
☐
☐
■ High (poorest)

Map 1

1991 Census based Poverty Index
☐ Low (richest)
☐
☐
☐
■ High (poorest)

Map 2

All Cause SMR (1990s)
☐ 29 - 90
☐ 90 - 105
☐ 105 - 112
☐ 112 - 120
■ 120 - 146

Map 3

Figure 17.1: **(a)** 2010–11 reduction in main revenue grant allocations (%), local authorities, England. **(b)** 2009 proportion of employees in the public sector (%), local authories, Britain. **(c)** Projection of unemployment rates given a 25% cut in public sector employment, local authorities, Britain. **(d)** 2007/08 inheritance tax-paying estates per 1,000 persons dying, local authorities, Britain (see page 175).

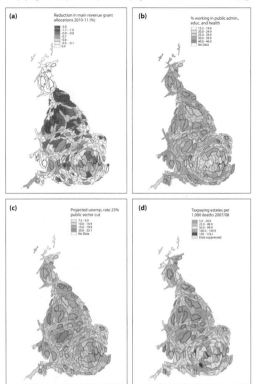

Source: Dorling and Thomas, 2011.

Figure 6.2: David Cameron and his Health Secretary, Andrew Lansley, meet nurses during a visit to the Royal Salford Hospital in Manchester on 6 January 2012 (see page 38).

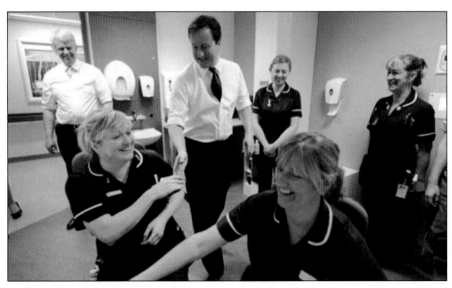

Source: Photograph: John Giles/Press Association (2012)

Figure 17.3: **(a)** 2007/08 inheritance tax-paying estates, numbers, local authorities, Britain. **(b)** 2007 CO_2 emissions due to road transport (tonnes per person), local authorities, Britain. **(c)** Nations and regions. **(d)** Major towns and cities (see page 179).

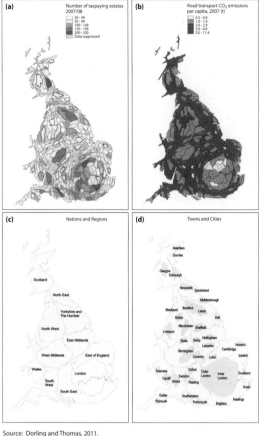

Source: Dorling and Thomas, 2011.

Figure 28.1: Global life expectancy slope index of inequality (in years) (see page 268).

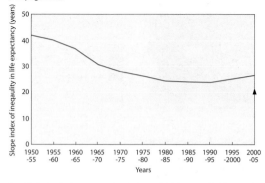

Note: Black triangle shows estimated index in 2000-05 with impact of AIDS removed.

Source: Calculated for this paper from World Health Organization routine data, and the United Nations population and HIV/AIDS wall chart 2005, www.un.org/esa/population/publications/POP_HIVAIDS2005/HIV_AIDSchart_2005.pdf (accessed July 2005).

Figure 28.2: Life expectancy (in years) by continent 1950–2005, world (see page 269).

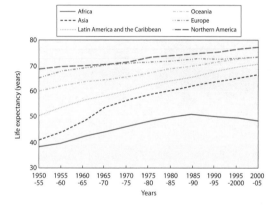

Source: Calculated for this paper from World Health Organization routine data.

Figure 18.1: Vote shares in the 2008 London mayoral election (see page 182).

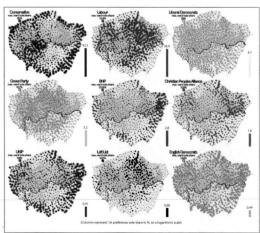

Source: Thanks to Michael Thrasher of the University of Plymouth for data used in these maps.

Figure 28.3: Average wealth per capita in dollars corrected for purchasing power parity ($PPP) (see page 270).

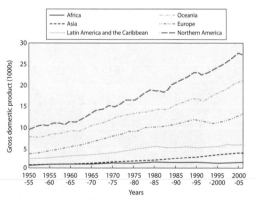

Note: Then: $1 = £0.6, €0.8

Source: UNDP data accessed via www.worldmapper.org.

Figure 28.4: Slope index of inequality for global wealth in dollars corrected for purchasing power parity ($PPP) (see page 271).

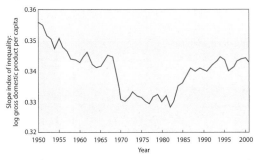

Note: Then: $1 = £0.6, €0.8.

Source: UNDP data accessed via www.worldmapper.org.

Figure 29.1: Mortality rate by age, men and women in 1850, 1900, 1950 and 2000, all affluent countries of the world at each point in time (see page 274).

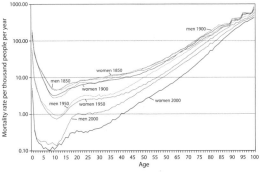

Source: The Human Mortality Database and calculations by the author, see: www.mortality.org/

Figure 30.1: Sex ratio of mortality (male/female rate) for the richer countries of the world, 1850–2000 (see page 280).

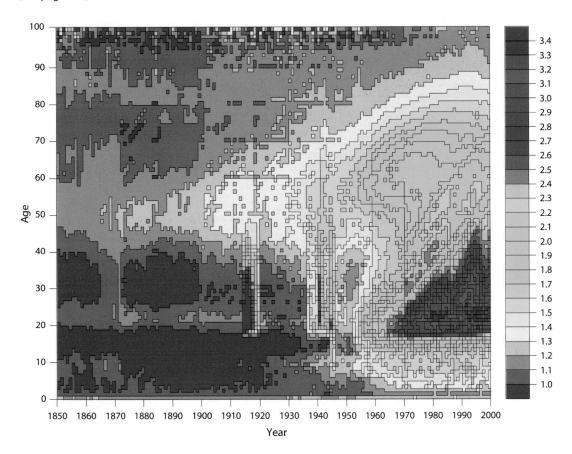

Source: The Human Mortality Database and calculations by the authors, see www.mortality.org/

Figure 30.2: First derivative of sex ratio of mortality, showing change in the ratio for the richer countries of the world, 1850–2000 (see page 281).

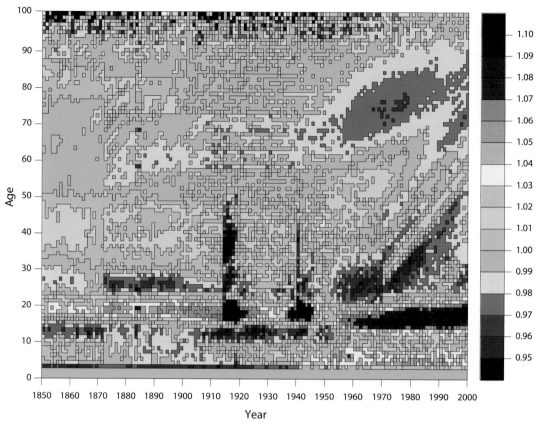

Source: The Human Mortality Database and calculations by the authors, see www.mortality.org/

Figure 30.3: Male : female mortality ratio by age in the rich world by 10-year cohort, 1850–1990 (see page 285).

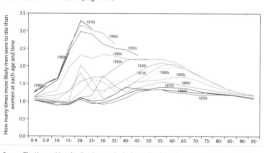

Source: The Human Mortality Database and calculations by the author, see: www.mortality.org/

Figure 30.4: Mortality rates in the 'affluent world', selected single years for ages 10 and 30, male and female, 1841–2000 (see page 287).

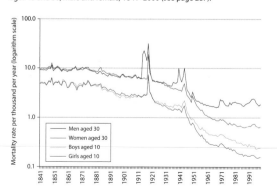

Source: The Human Mortality Database and calculations by the authors, see: www.mortality.org/

Figure 31.1: Physicians per head and child mortality (aged 1 to 4), countries of the world, 2002 (see page 290).

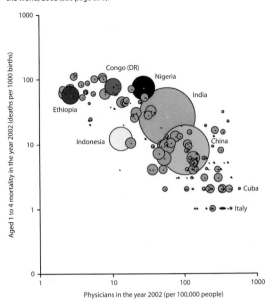

Note: Territories of the world drawn as circles with area in proportion to births. Both axes are drawn with a log scale here.

Source: www.worldmapper.org

Figure 31.2: Territories of the world drawn with area in proportion to deaths at ages 1–4, 2002 (see page 291).

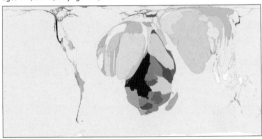

Note: This image is of the world as shaped when drawn in proportion to the more than 3 million children who die each year aged between 1 and 4 (inclusive) almost all from superficially easily preventable causes. In most cases their death is not simply due to the lack of intervention of a trained physician. However: 'There are more nurses from Malawi in Manchester than in Malawi and more Ethiopian doctors in Chicago than Ethiopia', G. Kinnock, 4 April 2006, Strasbourg: http://www.welshlabourmeps. org.uk/gk/gk_press/healthbudget04.04.06.htm.

Source: www.worldmapper.org

Figure 31.3: Territories of the world drawn with area in proportion to physicians, 2002 (see page 291).

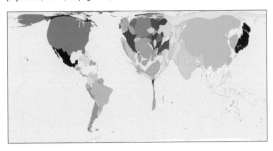

Note: There are more than two working physicians for every child that dies aged 1 to 4 worldwide each year. A traditional map in which territories are shaded according to the ratio of the population to physicians gives the reader little real impression of just how geographically concentrated physicians are: most into just a few territories worldwide.

The proof that a map of this kind could be drawn was made in 1975 when A.K. Sen published 'A theorem related to cartograms' (in American Mathematics Monthly, 82, 382-385). The first fully working practical realisation of that proof did not emerge until 30 years later and the latest version at time of writing is: Newman, M. (2006) Cart: Computer software for making cartograms [online]. University of Michigan. Available from: http://www-personal.umich.edu/%7Emejn/cart/ [accessed 5 July 2006].

Source: www.worldmapper.org

Figure 31.4: Territories of the world drawn with area in proportion to population, 2002 (see page 292).

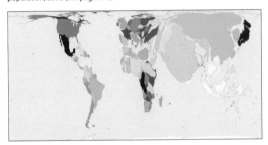

Note: Some 200 territories of the world are ranked according to their populations' weighted average score on the United Nations Development Programme's Human Development Index for 2002. That ranking is then used to determine the original colours used in these maps, from the poorest in red, through the rainbow shades, to the country with the highest index, Japan, in violet. 2002 is also the year from which the world population is drawn that is used to scale each territory according to its area.

Source: www.worldmapper.org

Figure 31.5: Territories of the world drawn with area in proportion to land area (see page 292).

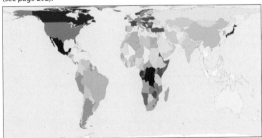

Note: This equal area projection appears very similar to that reproduced by Arno Peters and adopted by many parts of the United Nations as a more equitable projection than traditional world maps. However, this and Peter's projection, give most prominence to where there is most land – not most people. 'Africa's population density of 249 people per 1,000 hectares is well below the world average of 442 However, a great deal of the total destruction of the natural environment is occurring in the region. Poverty is a major cause and consequence. The area of Africa on the population cartogram is roughly half what the continent is on the equal land area map as a result of population density across Africa being almost half the world average.' (United Nations Population Fund, The State of the World Population 2001; Chapter 2: Environmental Trends: http://www.unfpa.org/swp/2001/english/ch02.html).

Figure 31.6: Territories of the world drawn with area in proportion to physicians, 2002 (see page 293).

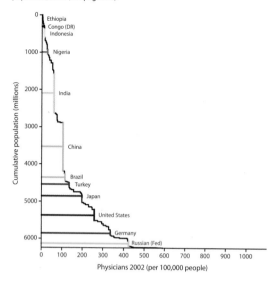

Note: On this graph the area of each territory is proportional to the number of physicians who work there, as also in Figure 31.3 above, but here information on geographical location is lost so that territories can be ordered by rates. The area to the left of the line is thus proportional to absolute numbers. This image is another example of an anamorphis where area is drawn in proportion to a count, in this case numbers of physicians.

Source: www.worldmapper.org

Figure 31.8: Anamorphosis in medicine and politics, from anatomy to subterfuge (see page 295).

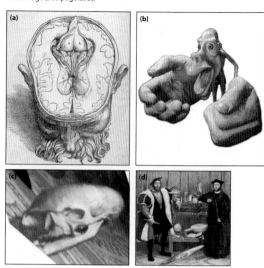

Note: Ambassadors engage in diplomacy in the interest of their country but, not necessarily, in the interest of others.

Sources: (a) Dissecting the cortex: taken from Vesalius' De humani corporis fabrica, 1543 [On the Fabric of the Human Body] now published online: http://vesalius.northwestern.edu/. This image sourced from: http://pages.slc.edu/~ebj/iminds01/notes/L1-Descartes-bats/s8-vesalius.html (b) Homunculus; taken from http://wwwppeda.free.fr/progressions/3/homunc_sens_grand.jpg (c) Detail of skull, transformed with photo software and derived from Holbein's 'The Ambassadors' (d) From http://www.dodedans.com/Eholbein.htm (accessed 26 October 2006)

Figure 31.7: Territories of the world drawn with rectangular area on this graph in proportion to deaths at ages 1–4, 2002 (see page 294).

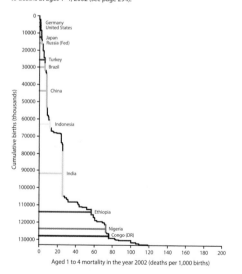

Note: All territories of the world are shown in this image and thus there is a minute space to the left of the line to represent the death of each child aged 1 to 4 that occurred in this one year. Worldwide 3,200,000 are estimated to have died, give or take well over 100,000 as recording is so poor. Some dozen territories that are home to over half the world's population have been labelled as, unlike on a map, it is far from obvious where places are on a graph.

Source: www.worldmapper.org

Figure 31.9: Physicians per head and child mortality (aged 1 to 4), countries of the world, 2002 (see page 296).

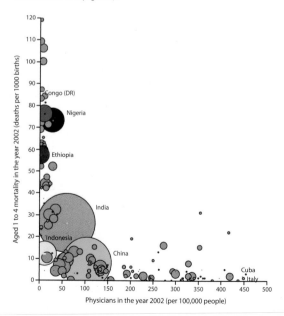

Note: Cuba is the most easterly circle, Sierra Leone the most northerly, and the most prominent circle to the south west extreme of the distribution is Malaysia. Here the territories of the world drawn as circles with area in proportion to births. Both axes are draw with a linear scale.

Source: www.worldmapper.org.

Figure 32.1: Association of income inequality and affluence with mortality in the 30 countries of the OECD, around the year 2000 (see page 304).

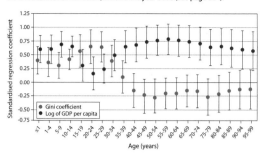

Note: Income inequality measured as the Gini coefficient, and affluence as the log of gross domestic product (GDP) per capita adjusted to ensure purchasing power parity. A higher regression coefficient indicates a closer correlation with mortality rates of either log GDP or Gini at those particular ages. Only data for 30 affluent countries are used here and GDP alone only comes to have a significantly greater effect than inequality after age 40. A higher correlation implies that the possible link is stronger, and that the influence of the factor is greater at those ages.

Source: Calculated by the authors from data provided by: Lopez, A., Ahmad, O., Guillot, M., Inoue, M., Ferguson, B. (2001) *Life tables for 191 countries for 2000: data, methods, results.* Geneva: World Health Organization (GPE discussion paper No 40) and United Nations Development Programme. Table 14 (Gini index of income inequality) in: *Human development report 2004.* Geneva: UNDP, 2004.

Figure 32.2: Association of income inequality and affluence with mortality in all countries worldwide, around the year 2000 (see page 305).

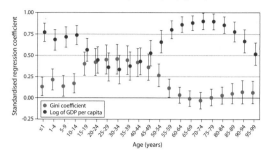

Note: Income inequality measured as the Gini coefficient, and affluence as the log of gross domestic product (GDP) per capita adjusted to ensure purchasing power parity. A higher regression coefficient indicates a closer correlation with mortality rates of either log GDP or Gini at those particular ages. Data for almost 200 countries are used here and GDP is seen to matter more at younger and older ages, but even with so many poor countries included inequality has a clear influence between ages 15 and 50.

Source: Calculated by authors from data provided by: Lopez, A., Ahmad, O., Guillot, M., Inoue, M., Ferguson, B. (2001) *Life tables for 191 countries for 2000: data, methods, results.* Geneva: World Health Organization (GPE discussion paper No 40) and United Nations Development Programme. Table 14 (Gini index of income inequality). In: *Human development report 2004.* Geneva: UNDP, 2004.

Figure 32.3: The world's countries drawn with area in proportion to the number of people living on ≤$10 a day, 2002 (see page 305).

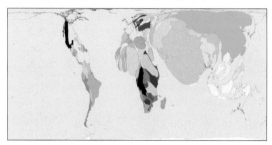

Note: In 2002, some 3.5 billion people, then more than half the world population, survived on the equivalent, or less, of what $10 in the United States of America would buy a day.

Source: From Worldmapper, www.worldmapper.org/display.php?selected=153

Figure 32.5: The world's countries drawn with area in proportion to the deaths of adults aged 25-29 years inclusive, 2001 (see page 307).

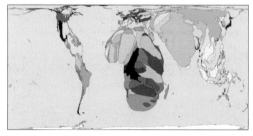

[Editorial Note: Some 1.5 million adults of these ages die every year. The original version of this figure had shown the map for children aged 1 to 4, but 4, but that map was shown earlier in this book as Figure 31.2 on p 291 of Chapter 31, so an older age group is shown here.]

Source: Worldmapper, http://www.worldmapper.org/display_extra.php?selected=535

Figure 32.4: The world's countries drawn with area in proportion to the gross domestic product per capita of people adjusted for purchasing power parity, 2002 (see page 306).

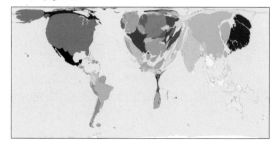

Note: In 2002 roughly $50 trillion was 'earned' a year worldwide, $7800 per person, or $21 on average a day, as measured in dollars, given what a dollar then bought in the United States of America.

Source: Worldmapper, www.worldmapper.org/display.php?selected=170.

Figure 35.1: Map of the world with countries resized according to the total amount of US treasury securities that were held in each place, July 2011 (see page 319).

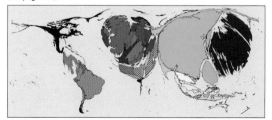

Source: Figures published by the US Treasury. Map created by Ben Hennig. See text for why some parts are dotted and some shaded with a criss-cross pattern.

UNEQUAL HEALTH

Figure 37.1: Public Health Spending: Worldmapper Poster 213 (see page 334).

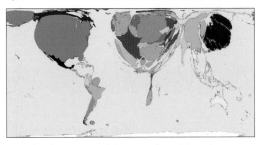

Note: The figure shows a cartogram in which territories are drawn with their area in proportion to the values being mapped. Territories are shaded identically on all cartograms here to aid comparison with the world cartograms shown in Figures 32.2 to 32.6 which employ identical shading. For detail on shading see http://www.worldmapper.org.

Source of data used to create map: United Nations Development Programme, Human Development Report 2004.

Figure 37.2: Private Health Spending: Worldmapper Poster 214 (see page 334).

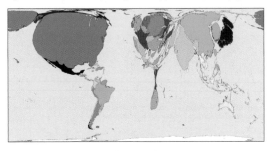

Source of data used to create map: United Nations Development Programme, Human Development Report 2004.

Figure 37.3: People dying over age 100: Worldmapper Map (see page 336).

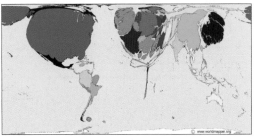

Note: The map shows the number of all 100-year-olds who died in 2001. The estimates come from the World Health Organization's Burden of Disease Estimates, published in 2006.
For further information on these mortality estimates (first made for 1999), see http://whqlibdoc.who.int/hq/2001/a78629.pdf

Source of data used to create map: Lopez, A., Ahmad, O., Guillot, M., Inoue, M. and Ferguson, B. (2000) *Life tables for 191 countries for 2000: data, methods, results.* Geneva: World Health Organization (GPE discussion paper No 40).

Figure 37.4: Early Neonatal Mortality: Worldmapper Poster 260 (see page 336).

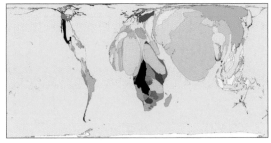

Source of data used to create map: World Health Organization, 2005, World Health Report, Basic data.

Figure 37.5: HIV/AIDS Prevalence: Worldmapper Poster 227 (see page 338).

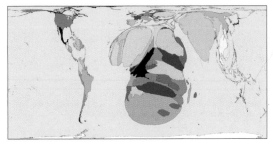

Source of data used to create map: United Nations Development Programme, Human Development Report 2004.

Figure 37.6: Malaria Cases: Worldmapper Poster 229 (see page 339).

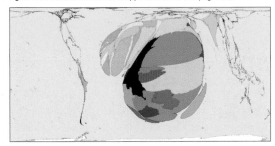

Source of data used to create map: World Health Organization and UNICEF, World Malaria Report 2005.

Figure 41.1: The survivors and deceased lists by social class, RMS Titanic, 1912, viewed in Singapore in 2012 (see page 377).

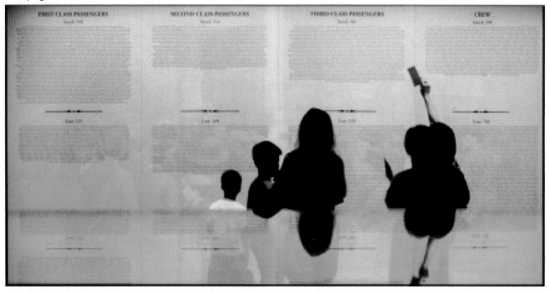

Source: Image included in *The Guardian* newspaper, 11 April 2012, of people at an exhibition in Singapore (the world's most unequal rich country) looking at the RMS Titanic survivor lists

Figure 42.1: Major life themes by age in Britain (aged 15–97), frequency of reporting events in the last year concerning subject (see page 393).

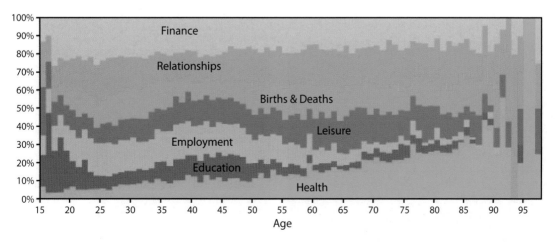

Source: British Household Panel Study questions asked between September 1992 and December 1992 on what happened of significance to all study members or to a a a member of their family.

Figure 43.2: Childhood cases of diarrhoea in the world today (see page 406).

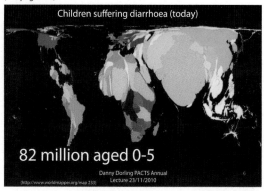

Note: Area of each country proportional to numbers suffering (total area is equal to 82 million children aged under six).

Source: World Bank's 2005 World Development Indicators, from the series named Diarrhoea prevalence (% of children under 5) (SH.STA.DIRH.ZS). The underlying source that the World Bank cites is the United Nations Fund for Children's (UNICEF) publication, *The State of the World's Children*.

Figure 43.4: The life expectancy gap between the extreme districts of Britain (see page 408).

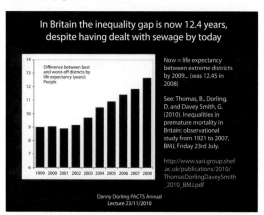

Source: Office for National Statistics and General Registrar Office (Scotland) estimates of life expectancy by local authority, three-year moving averages.
By 2008-10 the gap had grown to 12.65 years: http://www.guardian.co.uk/news/datablog/interactive/2011/oct/20/life-expectancy-map-local-authority-uk.

Figure 43.6: Deaths in the world today due to road traffic collisions (see page 410).

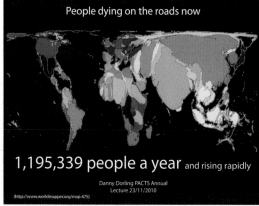

Source: World Health Organization's (WHO) Global Burden of Disease (GBD) statistics on death and disability worldwide in 2002. In 2002 road traffic accidents (now more commonly labelled 'crashes') caused 2.1% of all deaths worldwide in 2002, an average of 191 deaths per million people per year. This number is rising rapidly.

Figure 43.3: Deaths due to diarrhoea in the world today (see page 407).

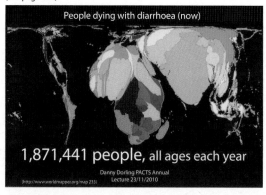

Note: Area proportional to number of deaths.

Source: The data used here are from the World Health Organization's (WHO) Global Burden of Disease (GBD) statistics on death and disability worldwide as measured in 2002. Diarrhoeal diseases, ICD U010, (causing 17% of deaths worldwide included in the category: Infectious and parasitic diseases).

Figure 43.5: Deaths in the world today with polio as underlying cause (see page 409).

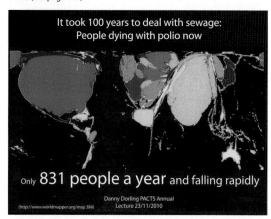

Source: World Health Organization's (WHO) statistics for 2002, as reported in Worldmapper. Most of the polio deaths that year were of people who had been severely disabled by polio years before who eventually died because of polio's long-term effects. Poliomyelitis caused 0.0015% of all deaths worldwide in 2002

Figure 43.8: Some early maps of social divisions which influenced public health (see page 412).

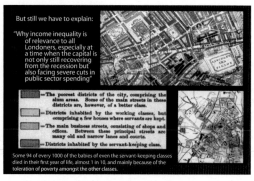

Source: Dorling, D. (2012) *Fair play: A Daniel Dorling reader on social justice*, Bristol: The Policy Press, reproducing figures in turn produced under the direction of Charles Booth and Benjamin Seebohm Rowntree, but drafted by others with data collected by yet others that they employed.

Figure 43.9: Two world wars, the smoking cloud, emancipation and repeated recessions (see page 413).

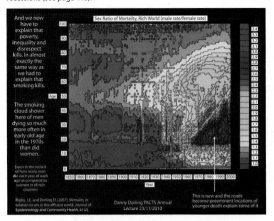

Source: The data used here were drawn from the Human Mortality Database collated by John R. Wilmoth (Director, University of California, Berkeley) and Vladimir Shkolnikov (Co-Director Max Planck Institute for Demographic Research). Access is free and may be found here: http://www.mortality.org/

Figure 43.10: Deaths of children aged 5 to 10 in Britain not attributed to disease (2006–07) (see page 415).

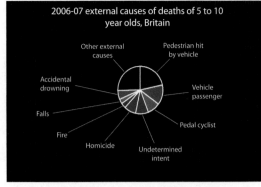

Source: Shaw, M., Davey Smith, G., Thomas, B., and Dorling, D. (2008) *The Grim Reaper's road map: an atlas of mortality in Britain*, Bristol: The Policy Press, relying in turn on data supplied by the Office for National Statistics and General Registrar Office (Scotland).

Figure 43.11: Underlying cause of deaths of children aged 11 to 16 in Britain (2006–07) (see page 417).

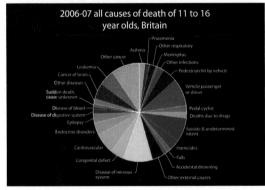

Source: Shaw, M., Davey Smith, G., Thomas, B., and Dorling, D. (2008) *The Grim Reaper's road map: an atlas of mortality in Britain*, Bristol: The Policy Press, relying in turn on data supplied by the Office for National Statistics and General Registrar Office (Scotland).

Figure 43.12: Deaths of children aged 11 to 16 in Britain not attributed to disease (2006–07) (see page 418).

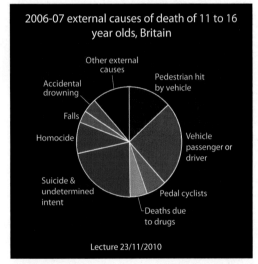

Source: Shaw, M., Davey Smith, G., Thomas, B., and Dorling, D. (2008) *The Grim Reaper's road map: an atlas of mortality in Britain*, Bristol: The Policy Press, relying in turn on data supplied by the Office for National Statistics and General Registrar Office (Scotland).

Figure 43.13: Underlying cause of all deaths of people aged 17 to 19 in Britain (2006–07) (see page 419).

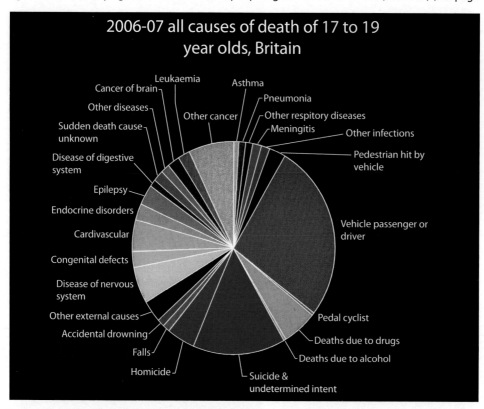

Source: Shaw, M., Davey Smith, G., Thomas, B. and Dorling, D. (2008) *The Grim Reaper's road map: An atlas of mortality in Britain*, Bristol: The Policy Press. relying in turn on data supplied by the Office for National Statistics and General Register Office (Scotland).

Figure 43.14: Deaths of people aged 17 to 19 in Britain not attributed to disease (2006–07) (see page 420).

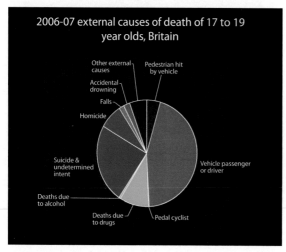

Source: Shaw, M., Davey Smith, G., Thomas, B., and Dorling, D. (2008) *The Grim Reaper's road map: an atlas of mortality in Britain*, Bristol: The Policy Press, relying in turn on data supplied by the Office for National Statistics and General Registrar Office (Scotland).

Figure 43.15: Underlying cause of all deaths of people aged 20 to 24 in Britain (2006–07) (see page 423).

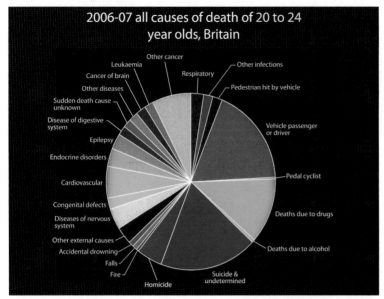

Source: Shaw, M., Davey Smith, G., Thomas, B., and Dorling, D. (2008) *The Grim Reaper's road map: an atlas of mortality in Britain*, Bristol: The Policy Press, relying in turn on data supplied by the Office for National Statistics and General Registrar Office (Scotland).

Figure 47.1: Population growth 1990–2015 – total change projected on a gridded cartogram (see page 446).

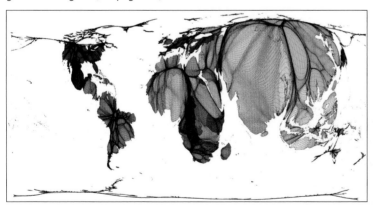

Source: Map drawn by Ben Hennig, using SEDAC data, the GPWv3 gridded population of the world, from Columbia University.

Figure 47.2: Population decline 1990–2015 – total change projected on a gridded cartogram (see page 446).

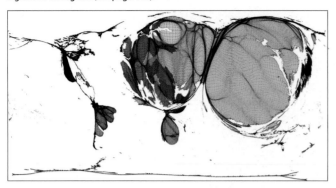

Source: Map drawn by Ben Hennig, using SEDAC data, the GPWv3 gridded population of the world, from Columbia University.

Figure 47.3: Population growth and decline 1990–2015 – areas of population increase or decrease shaded on an equal population gridded cartogram (see page 447).

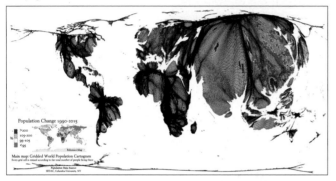

Note: Red areas are experiencing most population growth, blue areas most decline.

Source: Map drawn by Ben Hennig, using SEDAC data, the GPWv3 gridded population of the world,

Figure 48.1: Upper-class individuals are more likely to engage in unethical behaviour (see page 450).

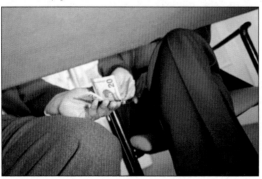

Source: Thinkstock, http://www.nsf.gov/news/news_summ.jsp?cntn_id=123301

Figure 48.2: Impact of the taxation and benefit changes, 2010 to 2014 (see page 452).

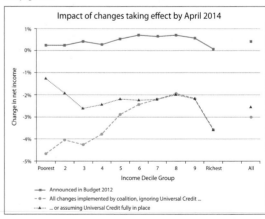

Note: The original graph was produced by the IFS and ignores measures affecting mainly the very rich. These budget measures included changes to taxation law proposed in the budget to prevent very rich people pretending they are giving money to charity, but giving it to something they have set up to look like a charity, to avoid paying tax. That proposal was not implemented, the reason given being that it would apparently affect genuine large charitable donations.

Source: Joyce (2012, slide 12)

25

'Poor kids', interview with Kerry O'Brien[1]

Dorling, D. (2011) 'Poor kids', Interview with Kerry O'Brien, Four Corners, Australian Broadcasting Corporation, 3 October, online transcript.

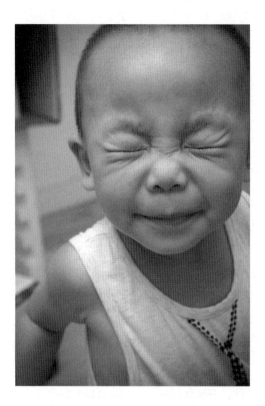

KERRY O'BRIEN, PRESENTER: Poverty from the mouths of little children; children who represent something like 25 per cent of Britain's next generation. And even as they speak their numbers are likely to be growing.

There is no faster route to poverty than unemployment, and Britain, Europe and the US are all teetering on the brink of a second recession since the global financial crisis. Governments in both regions are facing harsh austerity measures as they try to turn their massive sovereign debt around. Some European cities already have more than 20 per cent of their workers unemployed.

Danny Dorling is an academic author whose book, *Injustice: Why social inequality persists*, argues that the rise in Britain's wealth disparity through the period from

---

[1] The interview was part of Four Corners' screening of the True Vision documentary 'Poor kids'.

Thatcherism and Blair's New Labour through to the present day is unsustainable. He says the story in America is similar.

I recorded this interview with Danny Dorling from our London studio.

KERRY O'BRIEN: Danny, how did the documentary on the poor children of Britain impact on you? How did their stories gel with your statistics?

PROFESSOR DANNY DORLING, UNIVERSITY OF SHEFFIELD: The stories they tell and the story of the documentary gels very closely to what the statistics say. But when you hear the stories coming out of the mouths of children it's very different from when somebody like me says this is going on.

KERRY O'BRIEN: You've said that Britain's inequality today is as bad as it was in Dickensian times. How do you justify such a big call?

DANNY DORLING: You measure it. So there are several ways in which we measure it. One is the life expectancy gap between areas. Now, people live a lot longer than in Dickensian times, but in Dickensian times there were gaps of 10, 11, 12 years between poor cities and richer suburbs. Those gaps narrowed since the Victorian times. They narrowed particularly by the 1960s and 70s but they've widened again so that between different parts of Britain now, some people in entire cities can expect to live, men, 12, 13, 14 years less than men in some affluent parts of London.

KERRY O'BRIEN: But surely on other measures like health, education and housing the standards would have to be better than they were in Dickensian times, Victorian times?

DANNY DORLING: The average standard is better but the gaps between people have widened again. Another example to give you – if you're looking at inequality in income, one per cent of people in Britain round about 1920 were taking almost a fifth of all income, the richest one per cent. That declined but it's gone back up to the richest one per cent taking nearer a fifth of all income again now, and that leaves far less income for everybody else.

KERRY O'BRIEN: So why, in your view, has the gap between rich and poor grown so dramatically in the past 40 odd years through both Conservative and Labour rule?

DANNY DORLING: It's not Party Politics; it's not a particular set of politicians who have gone one way or the other. The gap was narrowing all the way from the late 1920s through to the 1970s with different politicians in power at different times.

It was under, in America, the Reagan years, in Britain under the Thatcher years, when the tide was changed, but the increase in inequality has happened in many parts of the globe, it's just been allowed to happen more ferociously if you like in Britain and in the United States than say in mainland Europe.

KERRY O'BRIEN: This is the trickle-down theory you're referring to, that if you create more wealth at the top it trickles down to all levels.

DANNY DORLING: There was more faith in trickle-down in the United States than in Britain, and more faith in it in Britain than in much of the rest of the rich world. For us in Britain, it became patently obvious, by the end of the 1980s, by the start of the 90s, that the trickle-down wasn't trickling down.

So having faith in something that doesn't work is certainly a problem.

KERRY O'BRIEN: The impacts of the global financial crisis are clearly still being felt. One recent study has suggested that the impacts of recent recession in Britain, on measures like household income, have only really started to show up this year. Would you expect recession to widen or narrow the inequality gap?

DANNY DORLING: What normally happens when there are recessions, particularly that following the great crash in 1929, is that the gaps narrow because the rich lose more, say of their share income. This hasn't happened since 2008.

In Britain, house prices have carried on going up in the middle of London where the very richest people live, so their wealth has gone up and up. But in the rest of the country housing prices are dropping, incomes are dropping, average living standards for average people are dropping and they're dropping fastest for people at the bottom because of benefit cuts.

So this is an unusual recession and, with the cuts so far, what's happening in Britain is that the rich are actually getting richer, the average is getting slightly poorer and the people who are poor are doing much, much worse than they were two or three years ago because a whole set of things are being taken away from them.

KERRY O'BRIEN: Where do the working poor feature in this equation of inequality?

DANNY DORLING: Half the people who are officially classified poor, half the families officially classified as poor in Britain, contain at least one person who's working, who's being paid a wage. We have a minimum wage but that minimum wage is not enough to get that family out of poverty. And what this shows you is that jobs alone are simply not enough.

What you need, to have a much lower rate of poverty, is a much more narrow income distribution, so fewer people are being paid enormous salaries and fewer people are being paid tiny salaries. That's how you get rid of, or reduce, child poverty to some of the lowest levels in the rich nations of the world; it is by not having a really wide distribution of incomes [see Figure 25.1[2]].

---

[2] Editorial Note: Figure 25.1 has been added to the original transcript as it was a still from the film being discussed, which had just been shown in Australia. It illustrates the faces of those children the viewers had just been listening to immediately before this interview.

Figure 25.1: Sam and Kayleigh from the BBC's 'Poor Kids', June 2011.

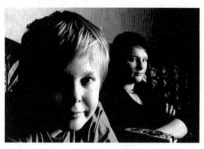

Source: http://www.bbc.co.uk/blogs/tv/2011/06/poor-kids.shtml

KERRY O'BRIEN: What would you regard as an acceptable wealth gap?

DANNY DORLING: When you ask people what kind of gaps are acceptable they tend to say fairly narrow gaps, or what somebody like me thinks is fairly narrow, so somebody earning 10 times more than somebody else.

Now chief executives of the biggest companies in Britain are earning at least 300 times more, 300 times more than the average worker. Recently government in Britain looked at imposing a 20 to 1 ratio in the public sector: the idea that nobody paid by government should earn 20 times more than somebody else paid by government in that same organisation. But the government here rejected implementing it.

So people want gaps which are much smaller, which are say a 10 to 1 or even 6 to 1, but we currently have 20 to 1 and even higher in the public sector, or 300 to 1-plus in the private sector.

KERRY O'BRIEN: You've said the British are now the Americans of Europe. What do you mean by that?

DANNY DORLING: It's not a great compliment about modern America. For instance, the British (per head) lock up more people in their prisons than anywhere else in Western Europe. We have well over 80,000 people locked up and it's rising rapidly since the riots this summer. America has 2 million people locked up.

America is one of the few big, rich countries in the world where you have people going hungry and having to be given food stamps in large numbers. But Britain is the country most similar for that and it's moving towards the American degree of inequality and normality and from my point of view this is a tragedy, because there is no need in these incredibly rich countries for children to be born into and be growing up in the kind of poverty that the documentary has just shown.

But the reason for it isn't a lack of money, the reason for it is a lack of imagination and people thinking you have to have a cut-throat, dog-eat-dog society, otherwise your whole country won't do okay and these children will have to grow up in poverty because it's somehow necessary for economic competitiveness. It's just stupid and it's wrong, and we learnt before it was stupid and it's wrong, the question is how long it will take us to learn again.

KERRY O'BRIEN: When you see someone like Warren Buffett calling for the rich to be taxed more, where do you think he's coming from[3]?

DANNY DORLING: There are lots of people right at the very top, within the top one per cent of the richest one per cent, who want the gaps to narrow, who've seen that the trickle-down fantasy doesn't work, who don't want to live in countries where they have to have bodyguards. There really are. If you want to see what extreme inequality is like, then you need to look at Brazil or South Africa.

KERRY O'BRIEN: Do you have any doubt that there is a connection between the recent riots in Britain and the inequality that you've measured?

DANNY DORLING: Recently two economists have done a brilliant job of showing (when they've used data for the last 100 years – from disorder in Germany in the 1930s right through to Greece in 2010) a statistical relationship that's very strong between government cutbacks, between inequalities rising and social disorder.[4]

So when people think that things are getting worse and a government doesn't have their general interest at heart and is willing for the rich to get richer and most people to get poorer, over the last 100 years in many, many, countries that has been a trigger for social unrest and rioting. It isn't that rioters sit down and say, We'll do it for this reason, but there is a statistical relationship – you can expect trouble when you treat people in this kind of way.[5]

KERRY O'BRIEN: I know you're not saying that this disparity you've measured is evidence of a fundamental failure of capitalism but if it's not, then what kind of challenge does it represent for capitalism?

DANNY DORLING: You have to have widespread consensus agreement that the current level of inequality is wrong, it's bad and it is going to be narrowed and it has to be narrowed and that ostentatious displays of

Figure 25.2: Affluent academic in suit being interviewed, October 2011.

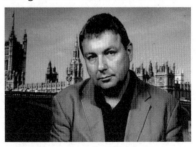

Source: http://www.abc.net.au/4corners/stories/2011/10/04/3331769.htm

---

[3] Editorial Note: Figure 25.2 has been added here to illustrate how television producers tend to choose to switch to more reassuring images of a person in a suit with a fake background superimposed (both background and suit) to imply some kind of authority after showing disturbing images of children living in poverty.

[4] Editorial Note: The work being referred to was Ponticelli, J. and Voth, H.-J. (2011) *Austerity and Anarchy: Budget Cuts and Social Unrest in Europe, 1919–2009*. London: Centre for Economic Policy Research, http://www.voxeu.org/sites/default/files/file/DP8513.pdf.

[5] Editorial Note: See: Lee, C. and Dorling, D. (2011) The Geography of Poverty, *Socialist Review*, October 2011, http://www.socialistreview.org.uk.

wealth and celebrating people getting rich just because they've got rich has become vulgar and you stop doing it.

That's what we did before in Britain, that's what countries which have much lower levels of inequality do. They're not impressed by people showing off that they've managed to make a lot of money, and that's how you get much more civilised countries. There are lots of examples of it happening. It has happened in the past, it's possible to happen again.

But one of the main reasons you may get greater equality again is if people start to look forward to a future without it. ... You're looking at gated estates; you're looking at the people being helicoptered between cities because they're afraid to drive; and you're looking at much, much higher levels of crime and disorder by people who've got very little to lose because they're given so little in the first place.

KERRY O'BRIEN: Danny Dorling, thanks very much for talking with us.

DANNY DORLING: Thank you.

SECTION V
Global inequality

26

Less suffering

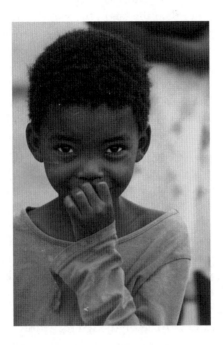

Global inequalities may be rising, and these inequalities often dominate the discussion in many of the chapters in this section, but the key world health inequality target, the global infant mortality rate (IMR), is continuing to fall and to fall quickly. Overall there is a little less suffering in the world with each year that passes, that is, if every premature death is treated as equal. Worldwide, primarily because of the continued falls in infant mortality, life expectancies are rising almost everywhere.

By April 2011 it was reported by United Nations International Children's Emergencies Fund (UNICEF)[1] that globally, in 2009, approximately 42 children died before their first birthday for every 1,000 born alive. Just a year later, in April 2012, the figure for 2010 was released, and we learned then that some 40 children died for every 1,000 born alive (UNICEF, 2012b). A drop from 42 to 40 is a 5% fall in just the space of a year. The global IMR was falling rapidly and was now much less than half that reported in 1975, which was 105 dying for every 1,000 born alive.[2]

---

[1] In their annual publication, *The state of the world's children* (UNICEF, 2012a), 134,754,000 children were reported as born alive in 2010, of whom around 5.4 million did not live out 12 months.

[2] See the data behind maps 261 and 262 on the Worldmapper website (www.worldmapper.org), which in turn relies on the United Nations Development Programme (UNDP) *Human Development Report 2004*, Table 9, the annual rate of infants dying in the first year of life, its source in turn being a combination of UNICEF (2004) UNDP/UNICEF correspondence on infant and under-five mortality rates, March and UNICEF (2003) *The state of the world's children 2004*, New York: Oxford University Press. Data on change since 1970 can be found at www.worldmapper.org/display.php?selected=262

As more contraception is used worldwide, fewer people are becoming parents. This means that despite there being more people who could become parents, fewer are having children, and fewer of those who have children see their children die before their first birthday. Between 1975 and 2010 the fall in the number of parents who lost a child was even greater than the fall in the worldwide IMR.

It is possible to quantify the reduction of suffering more broadly by considering two comparable five-year periods separated by roughly a generation of human life. Between 1970–74[3] and 2005–09[4] the total world human population increased by about two thirds, but the number of children the average woman in the world was giving birth to in her lifetime fell from 4.45 to 2.52, a fall of just over 40 per cent. When the falls in fertility and rises in population are combined, the result is that 28 per cent fewer babies were born in the second period as compared to the first.

As well as having better access to contraception, one reason people worldwide have chosen to have fewer children in recent years, and especially today, is that far more children can be expected to reach adulthood than was the case just a single generation ago. Change in a single year is rapid. Approximately 1,958,000[5] fewer babies were estimated to be born worldwide in 2010 as compared to 2009, despite rapidly growing numbers of young adults who could have become parents. People are choosing to have fewer children because many more of them now have that choice and because many more can expect to see their children outlive them. Their parents' scope of choices and reasonable expectations were often very different.

Today there are much less than half the numbers of grieving parents in the world than there were in the early 1970s, even though the world total population is much larger. This is real progress. Grandparents are not exaggerating when they tell their grandchildren that times have changed greatly. They are also talking of a far wider set of changes than mere access to contraception and improved healthcare – it is not just medical advances that reduce infant mortality; it is more general changes to public health, better economic circumstances and improving attitudes to poverty and inequality. With very few (but very interesting) exceptions,[6] IMRs also tend to be lowest of all in the most equitable of affluent countries.

Assessing progress

How do you measure changing living standards and assess people's impression of how living standards vary? The first chapter to follow in this section (Chapter 27) considers questions that can be asked about living standards in both affluent and poorer countries. Living standards still vary so greatly across the planet that it is hard to think of questions that could be asked of everyone. If you wanted a question on

---

[3] Coincidentally, as it helps to personalise statistics, this was when my younger two brothers were born.
[4] For me this was the period just after my first two children were born. Again it is good to personalise to be able to better understand just how rapid current demographic changes are.
[5] This is the UN's estimate. It will be approximate, but roughly two million fewer children are being born one year as compared to the year before, despite the number of people of childbearing age rising rapidly.
[6] For the most interesting exception, see Chapter 36, this volume, p 322.

healthcare, could that question be: how long do you have to wait to see a doctor, or just to access clean water, or to travel to get to a health clinic?

Talking in generalisations about grandparents' lives being very different from their grandchildren's is easy. Determining specific questions that can be asked to ascertain how living standards vary within a country and over time is more difficult, especially in a context of rising inequalities that makes it harder and harder to ask the same questions in different places.

Chapter 28 shows how inequalities in health have been rising worldwide since a particular point in the early 1980s. It is demonstrated how, despite the picture of aggregate overall improvement concerning rapidly declining infant mortality and birth rates painted above, during early adulthood in the poorest countries of the world life expectancy has often been moving in the opposite, worsening, direction. Although the chapter concentrates on the effects of the AIDS pandemic it is worth pointing out that within Europe, a continent not so badly affected by AIDS, health inequalities also rose. And they rose within Europe with the growing divide between poorer Eastern European countries and the centre of the European Union (EU). Health inequalities within Europe also increased when and where they did partly due to growing divides within one country. In the UK there has been a growing health divide between the southern half of the UK and its western and northern periphery since at least the late 1970s. This growing divide was largely the direct and indirect product of widening wealth and income inequalities within the UK, from the late 1970s onwards.

Most countries within Europe have been less divided than the UK. If people in a country do well economically, that benefit has often spread. When a country hits hard times, the effects are also more widely felt. To emphasise just how unusual the growing health divide within the UK is in a Western European context, along with other ways in which the British are not 'all in it together', it is worth noting how, just over a decade ago, when income inequalities in Europe outside of Britain tended not to be growing, it could be said that:

> ... *the highest SMRs [standardised mortality ratios] in Europe are found in regions in Northern England and the industrial belt of Scotland and these areas are most comparable to East Germany. Other areas in decile 1, in Finland, Portugal and Greece, are peripheral areas containing only a small percentage of the total decile population (the areas of the UK in decile 1 account for 28.4% of the total population on the decile; those in Germany account for 46.2%). Rates are lowest in regions of southern France....* (Shaw *et al*, 2000, p 1053)

In other words, 74.6 per cent of the worst-off tenth of people by health in Western Europe in 2000 lived in the poorest regions of the UK and the eastern regions of Germany. If East Germans were not included in this definition of Western Europe, then a majority of the worst-off people in the 1990s lived in the UK. Furthermore, the widest ranges in European standardised mortality ratios (SMRs) were found within the UK, closely followed by those within Germany across the line of the old iron curtain.

In the years that followed the Shaw *et al* (2000) study, geographical health inequalities in Germany fell while those in the UK rose. The economic crisis of 2008 hurt the peripheral nations of Western Europe most – Greece, Italy, Spain, Portugal, Ireland, Iceland and the peripheral (north western) half of the UK. With increasing income deprivation now across all of peripheral Europe, East and West, it is poorer men who more often die earlier, and the gap between male and female mortality rates grows in Europe as income deprivation increases.[7] But this is not the case worldwide.

In most countries women now live longer than men, especially in the poorer parts of Europe, but not in the poorest parts of the world. Chapter 29 looks at how close we are coming to women living longer everywhere. At the time of writing (2012) the latest World Health Organization (WHO) estimates for 2009 show women outliving men in all countries other than the tiny states of Tonga (males 72 years/females 70 years), Tuvalu (64/63) and the Central African Republic (49/48). An alternative source, the CIA factbook, paints a slightly less uniform picture for its estimates for 2012, with men outliving women not only in the Central African Republic (49/48) but also in Botswana (56/54), South Africa (50/48), Namibia (52/51), Swaziland (49.7/49.1) and Zimbabwe (52/51.7). And also in one area outside of Africa, Montserrat (75/71).[8]

It is generally in Eastern and Southern African countries where life expectancies for women are likely to be lower, and also, according to the data from the UN, where they are most likely to have decreased slightly over recent decades. The social position of women in a society, as summarised by overall life expectancy, might be harmed most greatly in those parts of the world most damaged by disease, inequality and poverty. Chapter 29 was written before the statistics just quoted above were known. Nonetheless, I think it is still worth being positive given the overall progress on infant mortality and the implications that has for women's social position and health.[9] The clearest measure by far of women's position and improving health is when life expectancies for women rise faster than those of men. These rises are not in general caused by men doing worse (although men are, in general, more fragile; see Kraemer, 2000), but they reflect women's position improving on average worldwide, a trend which simultaneously benefits men.

Women's life expectancy began to exceed men's only from the point that childbirth began to become far safer – rather than being the major cause of death of so many women in every country in the world. This has only occurred during the last century.

---

[7] To see how divided the UK now is, see Figure 3 in Bubbico and Dijkstra (2011). On the complexities of measuring inequalities in health across Europe by gender, see Figure 8 in Spinakis *et al* (2011).

[8] The UN's latest estimates, for 2010, published by UNICEF in 2012 (2012b), tend to be more in agreement with the CIA's predictions for 2012, but their estimates show men living longer than women only in Botswana (54/51), Lesotho (50/48), Swaziland (50/49) and Zimbabwe (54/53).

[9] Complications during childbirth are still major killers of young women worldwide, so fewer births of babies also implies fewer younger deaths of women worldwide and rising life expectancy for women overall.

In the most affluent nations of the world women have lived two to ten years longer than men for decades; exactly how many decades depends on which countries are being considered. Chapter 30 shows how, in fits and starts, women's health has in the aggregate improved more quickly than men's across these richest countries that have a total population of over one billion. Interestingly, female life expectancy improves especially quickly with the advent of each major world economic recession. Recessions cause great harm but they can also shake up the status quo.

When viewed from a worldwide perspective the variations in health outcomes within and between affluent nations are just part of a much bigger story. This bigger story is the global tale of those who have most money, who gain the most, who get the most healthcare, who will usually suffer the least and who on average live the longest. Chapter 31 shows how, in general, IMRs are closely related to the rate at which physicians are employed, which often reflects a country's wealth (Cuba being a notable exception). However, Chapter 31 also illustrates the mechanisms whereby the way we look at these graphs, and which scales we choose to view them through, alters our perception. How we see the world and how we see others is inextricably bound up with how we see ourselves.

Changing perspective

To try to illustrate the problem of perspective, several apparently distorted maps and graphs are included in Chapter 31. They are just a few of an almost infinite variety that can be drawn, not just of lands, but also of people. For example, a graphic of the human body can be drawn with the skin area enlarged to be made proportional to nerve endings and sensitivity (a 'sensory homunculus'). Homunculi are almost always drawn of men, but, as Figures 26.1 and 26.2 show, there can be a great deal of subjectivity in what purports to be a scientific picture. A homunculus is any scale model of the human body that, in some way, illustrates physiological, psychological or other abstract human characteristics or functions, not just sensory nerves, although nerves tend to be prioritised in those images that are the most popular.

Figure 26.1: Sensory homunculus I: how strongly different parts of the body are related to the cortex.

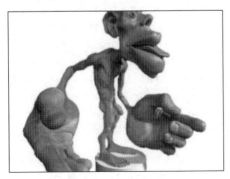

Source: www.cogitoathlete.com/2011/07/sensory_homunculus/

It is worth reflecting on how limited human beings' perceptions are portrayed as being when these diagrams are viewed. Where is the sensation of being hungry or full up, the sensation of feeling tired or energetic? With touch we mainly only register a sensation when something changes. Similarly, this is often the case with registering social evils; it is when life changes and a new evil is imposed that we most notice it (such as the advent of mass unemployment), not when we have lived with it for some time (such as living with class prejudices). Our physical nerve endings grow most dense where this would best protect us individually, for example, from eating food that would harm us, stepping on objects that would lame us; but they do not dictate our current priorities. We need a different perspective to understand what harms us all as a group, a perspective which may not be what we feel individually. It often takes an intellectual and emotional leap to see and tackle what harms us most collectively.

Chapter 32 discusses what the effects of social inequality on health might be at the global scale. It matters how we are influenced by how we think others perceive us. These effects appear not only to be felt within affluent countries, but more widely in the world.[10] In Chapter 32 it is suggested that the adverse effects of living under regimes of greater inequality are greatest on people aged between 15 and 30, and greater for men than for women. In other words, the impact of inequality appears to be greatest at those times and in those places when men (especially) might be competing most strongly for rank position.

It is not *just* better healthcare during childbirth that causes women now to live so much longer than men in most places. Men are harming each other's chances more where there is more conflict between people in general. People are mammals, and social mammals tend to have a rank ordering, which can especially adversely affect males. Social status has health implications that depend as much on the society you live in as on your more personal biology. We cannot ignore either our biology or our society. So much that happens to us is not the aggregate product of our individual actions but is influenced by the biological, social and historical circumstances we find ourselves in.

Many of the effects of our social organisation are subtle and slow-changing. Some are brutal, obvious and result in historical moments with a huge impact. Again, looking at an image can help. Figure 26.3, the map opposite, shows the movement of one family. It shows first the birthplace of a woman, Helene, who was born in an obscure Austro-Hungarian village called Auschwitz in 1909, and next the man

Figure 26.2: Sensory homunculus II: An alternative depiction of the relative sizes of cortex connections.

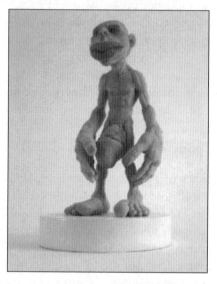

Source: http://commons.wikimedia.org/wiki/File:Homunculus.jpg.

---

[10] See Figure 1.1 (Chapter 1, p 6, this volume), for how inequality in income in just a few of the largest and smallest of the poor countries of the world appears so closely related to life expectancies in each country, and the footnotes in Chapter 48 to see where current thinking on the adverse health impacts of inequality is now heading.

she would later marry, by where he was born, in Crakow, in 1901. It shows how they met, later moved together to Amsterdam and had two children who were born in 1933 and 1938. Next it is revealed how they fled to Lille and then to Malines as the Nazis invaded the Netherlands and France, but how they were then caught and deported, as Jews, to where Helene had been born, three weeks after her 33rd birthday, where she, her children and husband would soon die.

Figure 26.3: The geographical history of the Hirschsprung family, 1901–42.

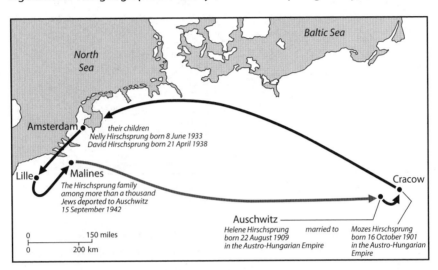

Source: Dorling (1998), redrawn in turn from Gilbert (1982)

Figure 26.3 shows the shortest of geographical summaries of the beginnings, major migrations and ends of four people's lives. The name of Helene's village birthplace is now enough to reveal the end of this particular story and of the hundreds of thousands of sets of stories that all came to be ended there. The map in Figure 26.4 below puts the single set of four stories into the context of tens of thousands of families being loaded onto carriages and cattle trucks in just two weeks in 1942. And, to depersonalise further, the graph in Chapter 33 (Figure 33.1, page 310) puts the millions who were killed in those places in a few years into the context of so many others killed across the world in all the wars, massacres and atrocities that occurred in just one century.

Every time you zoom out, from individuals to family, from family to village, from village to community, to town, to known event, to named era or state, to turbulent decade, to bloody century, to divided country, to war-ravaged continent or to dismal world view, at every step a leap of imagination is being sought and in every case our ability to make those leaps, to see things from different perspectives, alters

Figure 26.4: Deportations to Auschwitz, numbers in two weeks, 16–30 October 1942.

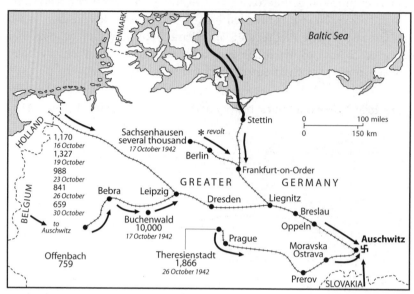

Source: Dorling (1998), redrawn in turn from Gilbert (1982)

and influences our understanding. We get a different point of view at each scale.[11] Individual tragedy can become mass murder, war crime, massacre, genocide and atrocity. We find it hard enough to imagine just an individual tragedy, trapped as we are, with our minds so focused on preserving our own skins with our self-centred ways of thinking. It is quickly overwhelming. It often helps to return to thinking just about how events influence one individual's health and then to try to think of how the world might look from that (other) person's point of view.

Just asking 'How are you?' elicits a response that is strongly influenced by social position and circumstance. It is '... *plausible that in more unequal societies, which are characterized by more status competition, people may more frequently and obviously need to reassure themselves of their strength and wellbeing and their potential to succeed*' (Barford *et al*, 2010, p 497; see also Spinakis *et al*, 2011). Is that why we so often reply, 'I'm doing fine'? Could the way in which so many are living under greater inequality also affect our collective thinking, how we see ourselves, and then also change how we act? Is fascism, with its willingness to kill, acceptance of dictatorship and aggressive nationalism, more likely to rise during an era of greater inequality and desperation

---

[11] Again, it can be very hard to form a perspective, to regard things according to their relative importance, as more and more events enter the picture. I asked my mum to check an early version of this chapter as I write so badly. She told me something I did not know, that before the age of seven, I had briefly gone to the same school as the daughter of the man who drew the maps in Figures 26.3 and 26.4 shown here. Nothing had materially changed but for some reason I felt I knew him a little better even though I have never met him. When we see each other as strangers it is easier to see each other as statistics (Gilbert, 1982; Dorling, 1998).

where a few come to believe, partly because it aids their particular sense of self-respect and self-preservation, that they are strong and will succeed in repressing others whom they fear?

Chapter 35 ends this section with an image of just one aspect of the current arrangement of human life. It shows a map of the planet drawn with countries sized in proportion to the monies their people have collectively lent to the United States (US). The US is the biggest debtor nation in world history. It is not poor countries that have borrowed most, but the (apparently) very richest nation on earth.

The map in Figure 35.1 (on page 319) is an attempt to visualise how people in the US and other debtor nations may come to view their position and readjust their fears of the future. It is an image of how others might begin to resent the levy they pay to the US. Nations and people who currently lend to the US receive interest on the loans they make, but will they ever receive their initial deposits back?

How people around the world react to images like the map in Chapter 35, and whether the thought that US default might one day be possible spreads, might well influence our collective determination to do more that reduces suffering in the world today. More monies are currently spent, worldwide, on loans to keep the US economy afloat than are ever given in aid or used constructively for social policies in the poorest or even average parts of the planet. This should cause people to be angry, but to be angry we need to see the harm, even if just in our mind's eye. We have almost reflex empathy that causes us to squirm when we see others hurt and automatically sense the pain they feel in our own brains, but this is all programmed to mirror another individual's feelings, not the suffering of groups.

Worldwide, far fewer adults today have to experience the death of their child than their parents' generation. The recorded rate of infant mortality has never been lower, nor has there been a faster fall than the 5 per cent with which this chapter began, that reduction from 42 to 40 per 1,000 in one year.[12] On the other hand, deaths caused by perpetuating wars, atrocities and massacres remain at the historic highs of the last century. The majority of humankind can be and is becoming both healthier and more peaceful, but the numbers of victims of violence may also continue to rise for some time. Recent events at an individual level in two of the most affluent but otherwise very different countries of the world, Britain and Norway, have highlighted this.

Harold Frederick Shipman and Anders Behring Breivik's atrocities meant that murder counts rose dramatically in both countries. In different ways both men's arrogant views, that they were superior to their victims, were bolstered by similar views of superiority held by others, which is why Shipman was not declared mad and Breivik was deemed mentally fit enough to undergo trial, and then also declared sane. Although more people may become peaceful, violence can still rise overall. This

---

[12] The previous fastest annual global falls in infant mortality, of just over 3 per cent per annum, were recorded in the early 1960s. The slowest improvement was in the early 1990s, averaging under 1.5 per cent per annum declines. The current rate of improvement is far faster than the predicted rate of about 2 per cent in the 2008 UN revision of its world population estimates. See http://en.wikipedia.org/wiki/Infant_mortality

is inevitable if we do not also moderate all the ideologies we subscribe to which suggest that some people are superior to others, ranging from common everyday elitism to the most pernicious extreme racism.

References

Barford, A., Pickett, K. and Dorling, D. (2010) 'Re-evaluating self-evaluation: a commentary on Jen, Jones, and Johnston (68: 4, 2009)', *Social Science & Medicine*, vol 70, pp 496-7 [reproduced as Chapter 34, this volume].

Bubbico, R.L. and Dijkstra, L. (2011) *The European Regional Human Development and Human Poverty Indices*, Regional Focus No 2, European Union Regional Policy Paper (http://ec.europa.eu/regional_policy/sources/docgener/focus/2011_02_hdev_hpov_indices.pdf).

CIA (Central Intelligence Agency of the United States of America) (2012) *The world factbook* (www.cia.gov/library/publications/the-world-factbook/index.html/).

Dorling, D. (1998) 'When it's good to map', *Environment and Planning A*, vol 30, pp 227-88.

Gilbert, M. (1982) *The atlas of the holocaust*, London: Michael Joseph.

Kraemer, S. (2000) 'The fragile male', *British Medical Journal*, vol 32, pp 1609-12.

Shaw, M., Orford S., Brimblecombe, N. and Dorling, D. (2000) 'Widening inequality in mortality between 160 regions of 15 countries of the European Union', *Social Science & Medicine*, vol 30, pp 1047-58.

Spinakis, A., Anastasiou, G., Panousis, V., Spiliopoulos, K., Palaiologou, S. and Yfantopoulos, J. (2011) *Expert review and proposals for measurement of health inequalities in the European Union – Full report*, Luxembourg: European Commission Directorate General for Health and Consumers (http://ec.europa.eu/health/social_determinants/docs/full_quantos_en.pdf).

UNICEF (United Nations International Children's Emergency Fund) (2012a) *The state of the world's children*, New York: United Nations.

UNICEF (2012b) *Statistics and monitoring* (www.unicef.org/statistics/index_step2.php?justadded=1&sid=63860b8267cde07da3ccfda5fe786c22).

WHO (World Health Organization) (2012) *World health statistics*, Geneva: WHO (http://www.who.int/gho/publications/world_health_statistics/en/index.html).

27

How do the other four-fifths live?[1]

Dorling, D. and Barford, A. (2011) 'How do the other four-fifths live?', *New Internationalist*, vol 442, p 51.

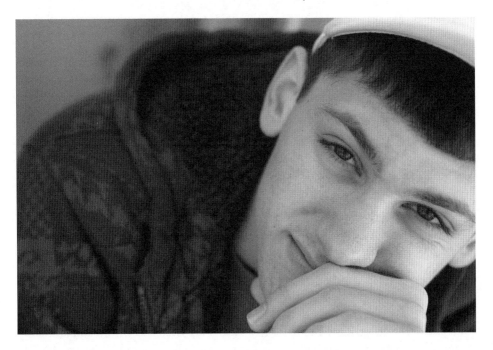

In most of the world today people tend to be segregated, or segregate themselves, mostly along economic lines. This division can block us from meeting and talking with people as equals and can be a barrier to social harmony.

Residential segregation takes place where the well-off buy themselves out of poorer neighbourhoods and rarely visit these places. The poorest often do not even feature in the mental maps which many of the rich hold of their home city. Most people in the poorer half of a city have rarely spent much time in the wealthier quarters and neither do the rich usually know much about the poor.

We have found it useful to divide societies into fifths to talk about inequality. We then ask people to imagine that the population of their country is divided into five groups, ranging from the 'poorest' 20%, to a 'modest' 20%, a 'middle' 20%, an 'affluent' 20% and then to the 'richest' 20%. We find that both rich and poor usually know little of each others' lives nationally as well as locally. The affluent know more of the rich than the poor. Those on modest incomes know more of the poor than the affluent.

---

[1] Editorial Note: A shorter version of this piece appeared in the magazine.

While travelling through for other work, between us in Mexico, the USA, Kenya, New Zealand, the UK, Zanzibar and Japan we have asked people five questions to try to gauge how much variation there is in how much we understand of each other. When we ask these questions we hold up our right hands and point to each of our fingers (and thumb for the rich) to ask for the answer for each quintile groups. We are thus after five answers to the each of the following five questions, concerning the country the interviewee lives in:

1. At what age do you think most people in each group now leave full-time education?

2. How many vacations do you think people take a year in each group? A vacation means a holiday staying away from home for at least one night, not in family or friends' homes.

3. What do you think the typical household income for each group is per year? That is income before tax and including benefits.

4. What is the usual number of cars and vans that most households in each group have and have access to?

5. What age, on average, do you think people in each group live to?

We finish by asking:

6. Which group are you in?

So we get 26 answers in all.

People generally perceive themselves to be average. When David Walker and Polly Toynbee recently asked city high-flyers in London (who are among the top 0.1% of earners) where they stood, many denied they were rich. Most of us tend to know people who are a bit richer and a bit poorer than us. Most of us don't know how many people are very different from us. Thus, from each of our own differing vantage points within every society, it often seems to us that we are average.

When we asked these six questions in half a dozen countries around the world we found a majority of the people placed themselves in the middle quintile. We don't think we accidentally over-sampled from that middle. However, just as it is hard to know where you stand in a country where people don't mix well, in more equitable countries, those countries where social mixing is greater, people are more alike and so it is also harder there to know where you fit.

In Sweden there is almost no difference between the likelihood of relatively poor or rich children staying on to complete their schooling. In Ethiopia twice as many in the rich quintile enrol in school as do those in the poorest quintile.

When it comes to our second question we find from the latest official UK statistics for 2008/9 that in that (financial) year only 61% of British children had least a week on holiday with their family (away from home). Very few affluent people in Britain realise how many British children have no annual holiday.[2]

When it comes to our third question on household incomes, the 'correct' answer in the Czech Republic would be that the richest fifth receive 3.5 times more than the poorest fifth; in China 10.6 times; and in Namibia 56.2 times. But what do you think the answer is for where you live?

It is surprising to find how much most of us don't know of our own countries when we try to provide the 26 answers to even just those $5 \times 5 + 1$ questions posed above. Knowing the answers or even the direction of the gradient is not always easy.

In some countries affluent people do not have to study for as long as poorer people to gain employment, so they don't. In others, like Japan, owning a car (the subject of our fourth question) is something you do in the countryside, not in the city, and so has little to do with economics.

The greatest gulfs are found when we look at what the correct answers should be to the fifth of our six questions. Peru has a 27-year difference in life expectancy between the richest and poorest quintiles, with the richest living, on average, until 80 and the poorest until 53 years old. A much smaller gap is found in Mozambique where there is a five-year difference between the top and bottom quintiles, but no group has a life expectancy of over 45 years old.[3]

Figure 27.1 shows variations in life expectancy between different local districts of the United Kingdom which ranged in 2004–06, from averages of as low as 77 years for women to over 87 years being average in other places. For men the gap ranged from as low as almost 70 to as high as over 83 years. However, for most people they lived in a place which only differed from the national average by a year or two.

Within each place the life expectancy inequalities by social class or between smaller neighbourhoods would have been often as great as those seen across the nation.

Try answering the six questions yourself. Try asking others what they think the answers should be. Try finding out what the answers really are where you live and, if you would not mind, please let us know: send us a postcard.

We just want to know a bit more about the world.

---

[2] If you are British and want to know more about the society you live in, for instance that 82% of the poorest quintile have no home contents insurance while 91% of the richest quintile do, see *Equality Trust Research Digest, #3 The lives of the other four fifths*, http://www.equalitytrust.org.uk/docs/research-digest-quintiles-final.pdf.

[3] For these statistics we relied on Grimm, M., Harttgen, K., Klasen, S., Misselhorn, M., Munzi, T. and Smeeding, T. (2010) Inequality in human development: An empirical assessment of 32 countries, *Social Indicators Research*, 97.

Figure 27.1: Life expectancy at birth 2004–06, females on the left and males on the right. Due to their small populations, data are not supplied for the City of London and the Isles of Scilly. A key map showing some towns and cities is also shown.

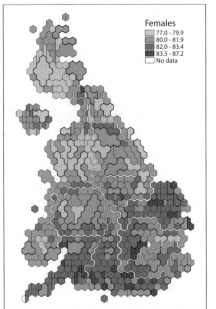

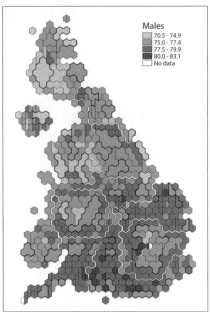

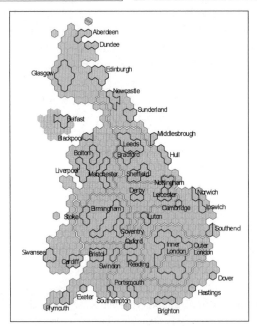

Source: Local authority life expectancy estimates as published annually by ONS (three-year moving average of the years shown).

28

Global inequality of life expectancy due to AIDS

Dorling, D., Shaw, M. and Davey Smith, G. (2006) 'HIV and global health: global inequality of life expectancy due to AIDS', *British Medical Journal*, vol 32, pp 662-4.

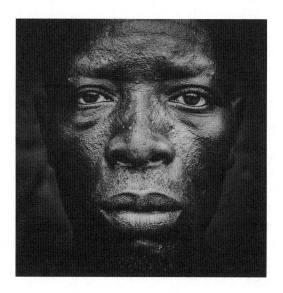

Summary points

- Inequality in mortality between continents reflects the inequality in gross domestic product per capita.
- Inequality of health and wealth between continents began to rise in the early 1980s.
- Africa has been most affected by the widening global inequality in mortality, probably as a result of the AIDS pandemic, which is exacerbated by inequality in wealth.

Global inequality in both health and wealth began to rise worldwide in the early 1980s and has been exacerbated by AIDS in Africa. This trend is not inevitable, and historical trends show that inequality can be reduced.

Inequality in health within the United Kingdom has been widely discussed in medical, health, and social science journals, with the most recent data showing a widening of inequality between areas of the UK.[1] Such inequality is also the focus of several government targets. In other wealthy countries inequality in health is both widely studied and subject to government attention.[2] Recent political events such as the Make Poverty History campaign, the Live8 concerts, the G8 summit in Scotland, the World Trade talks in Hong Kong, and the broader background of 'globalisation' have turned attention towards the global picture. In this article we ask two questions: what is the state of inequality in health and wealth across the globe? and, is inequality increasing or decreasing over time?

Data from the United Nations Organisation can be used to answer the first question,[3] but a suitable measure of inequality is needed to answer the second question. Moser *et al* suggest using a novel measure of dispersion to track trends in the distribution of global mortality over time—the dispersion measure of mortality. They claim that '*the dispersion measure of mortality has advantages over other commonly used summary measures of mortality contrast that only use information from the extremes of the mortality or socioeconomic distribution and do not weight for size of the unit*'.[4] We use another well established measure of inequality, which has the same attributes but is simpler to interpret and compute and is more informative—the slope index of inequality.[5] The index can provide a simple measure of the size of the gap in natural units—in this case—years of life expectancy lost.

Changes over time

Using the UN data, aggregated into six continents (see bmj.com and links from the original article for details), we calculated the slope index of inequality for life expectancy from 1950 to 2005 (Table 28.1). Data for 2001–5 form the central projection used and published by various UN statistical agencies. We calculated the index by continent rather than country for several reasons: we do not have a consistent measure of poverty or wealth to rank all countries at all points in time; data for

[1] Shaw, M., Davey Smith, G. and Dorling, D. (2005) Health inequalities and New Labour: how the promises compare with real progress. *BMJ*, 330, 1016-21.

[2] Mackenbach, J. and, Bakker, M. (2002) *Reducing inequalities in health: a European perspective*, London: Routledge.

[3] United Nations (2005) World urbanization prospects: the 2003 revision population database, http://esa.un.org/unup/; and United Nations (2005) Human development index, http://hdr.undp.org/statistics/data/ (both accessed July 2005).

[4] Moser, K., Shkolnikov, V. and Leon, D. (2005) World mortality 1950–2000: divergence replaces convergence from the late 1980s, *Bulletin of the World Health Organisation*, 83, 202-9.

[5] Low, A. and Low, A. (2004) Measuring the gap: quantifying and comparing local health inequalities, *Journal of Public Health*, 26, 388-95.

Table 28.1: Mean life expectancies across the globe by continent and income inequality, 1950–2005.

		Continent						Indicators of inequality	
		Africa	Asia	Latin America and the Caribbean	Oceania	Europe	North America	Slope index of inequality (95% CI)	North America minus Africa†
	1950-55	38.2	41.1	50.9	60.4	65.6	68.8	41.9 (28.4 to 55.4)	30.6
	1955-60	40.3	44.7	53.8	62.3	68.2	69.6	39.9 (27.9 to 52.0)	29.3
	1960-65	42.4	48.3	56.4	63.7	69.6	70.0	36.6 (26.7 to 46.5)	27.6
	1965-70	44.5	53.8	58.4	64.6	70.7	70.4	30.9 (23.6 to 38.3)	25.9
	1970-75	46.5	56.4	60.5	65.8	71.0	71.5	28.0 (21.9 to 34.1)	25.0
	1975-80	48.5	58.6	62.7	67.4	71.5	73.3	26.1 (21.0 to 31.3)	24.8
	1980-85	50.1	60.3	64.4	69.3	71.9	74.2	24.7 (20.0 to 29.3)	24.1
	1985-90	51.3	62.2	66.2	70.5	73.1	74.7	24.0 (19.0 to 28.9)	23.4
	1990-95	50.5	63.8	67.7	71.5	72.4	75.4	23.7 (16.7 to 30.6)	24.9
	1995-00	49.6	65.4	69.7	72.5	72.9	76.6	25.1 (15.6 to 34.6)	27.0
	2000-05	48.8	67.0	71.0	74.0	73.3	77.4	26.3 (13.9 to 38.7)	28.6
Life expectancy at birth (years 2000-5)	**With AIDS**	50.6	67.7	71.8	74.6	74.3	77.6	25.4 (14.1 to 36.7)	27.0
	Without AIDS	56.9	68.3	72.3	74.6	74.6	77.9	20.0 (13.9 to 26.0)	21.0
	Difference	6.2	0.6	0.5	0.0	0.3	0.3	5.4	5.9
	Error*	1.8	0.7	0.8	0.6	1.0	0.2	-0.9	1.6

CI = confidence interval

*The small difference between the figures calculated from the two different UN sources

†The two most extreme continents in terms of health and wealth

Source: Calculated for this paper from World Health Organization routine data, and the United Nations population and HIV/AIDS wall chart 2005, www.un.org/esa/population/publications/ POP_HIVAIDS2005/ HIV_AIDSchart_2005.pdf (accessed Jul 2005).

countries in war or crisis (or both) are unreliable; the ranking of continents by gross domestic product per capita is constant over time; and a measure of intercontinental inequality in mortality captures most international inequality. Data on gross domestic product before 1950 are unreliable, so our study starts at 1950.

The index was calculated by ranking the six continents in order of increasing life expectancy: Africa, Asia, Latin America and the Caribbean, Oceania, Europe, and North America. The order did not change over the 50-year study period and reflects the average gross domestic product per capita of the inhabitants of each continent. The population of each continent was calculated as a proportion of the world population in each time period. At the start of the study 8.8% of the world's population lived in Africa (the poorest continent) and the median person in Africa was 4.4% along the world population ranking. For the period 1950–5 these cumulative proportions for the ranked continents were: 8.8%, 64.3%, 70.9%, 71.5%, 93.2%, and 100%. The median person in each ranked continent thus stood at 4%, 37%, 68%, 71%, 82%, and 97%. By the end of the study period the median person in Africa reached 7%

along the world population ranking as the population grew. In the years 1950–5 the life expectancies for the ranked continents were 38, 41, 51, 60, 66, and 69 years. The slope index of inequality is the slope coefficient in a simple regression analysis of life expectancy in years against the ranking of the continents (where ranking is expressed as the cumulative proportions of the world population—for example, 0.37 for Asia in 1950–5). Because grouped data are used and heteroskedasticity exists (unequal variance in regression errors) we estimated coefficients by using the transformation proposed by Low and Low.[6] In 1950–5 the coefficient was 41.9 years of life expectancy. This means that the hypothetical poorest person in Africa had a life expectancy 41.9 years shorter than the richest person in North America. The slope index of inequality uses the information for all continents rather than simply comparing the extreme life expectancies.

Figure 28.1: Global life expectancy slope index of inequality (in years).

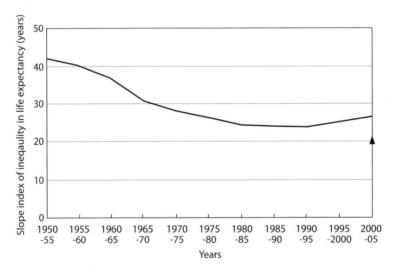

Note: Black triangle shows estimated index in 2000-5 with impact of AIDS removed.

Source: Calculated for this paper from World Health Organization routine data, and the United Nations population and HIV/AIDS wall chart 2005, www.un.org/esa/population/publications/POP_HIVAIDS2005/HIV_AIDSchart_2005.pdf (accessed July 2005).

Figure 28.1 and Table 28.1 show that global inequality in life expectancy fell between 1950 and 1990, but since then it has risen and is now at the same level as in the late 1970s. For the two most extreme continents (see table)—North America and Africa—the gap in life expectancy fell from 30.6 years in 1950–5 to less than 24 in 1985–90 but has since risen to 28.6; it is now almost at the same level as in the 1950s. The slope index of inequality correlates with the dispersion measure of mortality used by

---

[6] See Low and Low (2004), op cit.

Figure 28.2: Life expectancy (in years) by continent, 1950–2005, world.

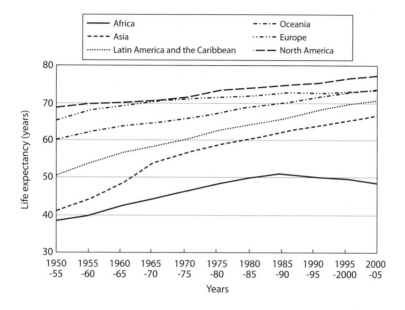

Source: Calculated for this chapter from World Health Organization routine data.

Moser *et al*: both methods show that global inequality in mortality is rising.[7] A plot of life expectancy in the six continents over the study period (Figure 28.2) shows that Africa has been most affected by the widening global inequality in mortality.

Effect of AIDS

The last four rows of Table 28.1 show the effect of AIDS on life expectancy for the six continents. The figures were calculated from a different UN source[8]; the last row (error) shows the small differences between these figures and those cited previously. These alternative figures show that six years of the difference in life expectancy between Africa and North America is accounted for by AIDS. The estimates of life expectancy at birth without AIDS are the average number of years a person would be expected to live in the absence of mortality related to AIDS.[9] Figure 28.1 shows the predicted slope index of inequality for 2000–5 in the absence of AIDS (triangle): global inequality would have maintained a small downward trend. Even without AIDS, global inequality in life expectancy would be more than five times greater than inequality within the UK for a similar period of time. Because of AIDS, global

---

[7] See Moser *et al* (2005), op cit.
[8] United Nations (2005) *UN population and HIV/AIDS wall chart 2005*, www.un.org/esa/population/publications/POP_HIVAIDS2005/ HIV_AIDSchart_2005.pdf (accessed July 2005).
[9] United Nations (2004) *World population prospects: the 2004 revision*, www.un.org/esa/ (accessed July 2005).

Figure 28.3: Average wealth per capita in dollars, corrected for purchasing power parity ($PPP).

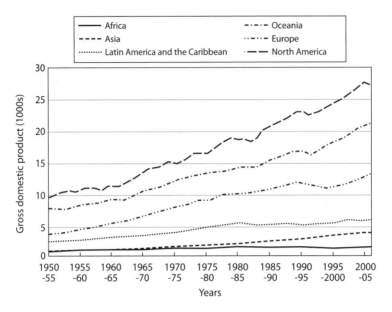

Note: Then: $1 = £0.6, €0.8

Source: UNDP data accessed via www.worldmapper.org.

inequality in life expectancy was seven times greater than within the UK by 2001–4, even though inequality within the UK at that time was the highest ever reported. Figure 28.3 shows average wealth (gross domestic product per capita) for the six continents over the study period and seems to show a continuous widening of inequality since the 1950s.[10] However, Figure 28.4 shows the changes in the relative wealth of continents—the slope index of inequality for log gross domestic product per capita standardised by the world average wealth for each period of time—which removes the effect of inflation. This shows that the global distribution of wealth was becoming more equal from 1950 to 1980, but from the early 1980s onwards it became much more unequal.

Effect of health inequality

Importantly, inequality in mortality between continents began to rise shortly after inequality in gross domestic product per capita began to diverge most clearly. This association could reflect the profound impact of AIDS on one continent, Africa. AIDS is a disease of the poor, and global inequality in wealth will have compounded

---

[10] www.eco.rug.nl/zMaddison/ (accessed February 2005). Site no longer exists but similar data can be accessed via www.theworldeconomy.org/publications/worldeconomy/ (accessed February 2006), and now www.theworldeconomy.org/statistics.htm and www.ggdc.net/maddison/ (accessed June 2012).

the effect of AIDS on Africa by restricting access to effective treatments and means of prevention. Protected trade advantages for pharmaceutical companies in wealthy countries will contribute to both the redistribution of wealth from poor to rich countries and reduced access to effective treatments for AIDS in poor countries, thus exacerbating inequalities in wealth and in death rates. All the data indicate that inequality of health and wealth began to rise worldwide in the early 1980s. Currently the trends towards greater inequality are accelerating, but historic trends can be quickly reversed, as events in the early 1980s showed.

Figure 28.4: Slope index of inequality for global wealth in dollars, corrected for purchasing power parity ($PPP).

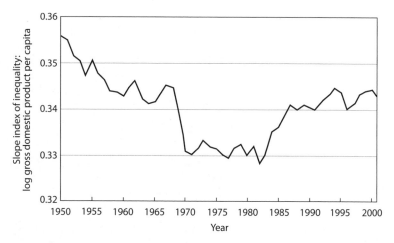

Note: Then: $1 = £0.6, €0.8.

Source: UNDP data accessed via www.worldmapper.org.

29

Life expectancy: women now on top everywhere

Barford, A. Dorling, D., Davey Smith, G. and Shaw, M. (2006) 'Editorial: Women's life expectancy', *British Medical Journal*, vol 332, pp 1095-6.

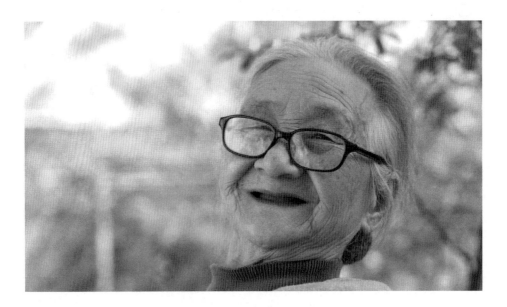

During 2006, even in the poorest countries, women can expect to outlive men.

Women who seek to be equal with men lack ambition. (Timothy Leary, 1920–96)

The year 2006 should not be allowed to pass without at least a quiet celebration that this is the first year in human history when—across almost all the world—women can expect to enjoy a longer life expectancy than men. That the trend is moving in this direction will probably be confirmed this week in the 2006 world health report.

In its world health report of 2002, the World Health Organization, using data for 2001, reported that male life expectancy exceeded female life expectancy in only six countries: Nepal, Botswana, Zimbabwe, Lesotho, Bangladesh, and Swaziland.[1] A

---

[1] World Health Organization (2002) *World health report 2002: reducing risks, promoting healthy life.* Geneva: WHO, www.who.int/whr/2002/en/ index.html (accessed 31 March 2006).

year later, the situation seemed to have reversed in all six countries, with two other countries (Qatar and the Maldives) reporting that men were living slightly longer than women.[2] In its 2004 report the WHO continued to report the same 2002 data and in only those two tiny territories (the Maldives and Qatar) did women die younger than men.[3] In the 2005 report, life expectancy data for 2003 were reported, but only to the nearest year of age, making comparison difficult.[4]

In January this year the US Central Intelligence Agency (CIA) updated its *World Factbook* and reported its estimates for life expectancy in 2005.[5] According to the CIA, in Qatar and the Maldives women now lived longer than men. Elsewhere, however, women's fate had slipped back, by the CIA estimates which do not tally with the WHO data for earlier years. According to the CIA, in Niger women could expect to live a dozen days less than men and in Botswana three dozen days less by 2005, but nearer to two years less in Zimbabwe and Kenya by 2005. The underlying source of the CIA data is vague, as befits a somewhat secretive organisation. We will never know with certainty the exact year in which women everywhere can expect to live on average longer than men, but this year— 2006—is as likely as any.

Almost 30 years ago, amid much fanfare, the eradication of smallpox was announced.[6] But when it becomes certain that women everywhere can expect to live longer than men, also a remarkable achievement, a similar announcement is unlikely. We tend to forget that in many countries of the world women could expect, until recently, to live fewer years than men and that maternal mortality in particular remains a big killer.

The most reliable historical mortality records are in Europe, where states were sufficiently affluent and interested to keep accurate records. In Europe men last outlived women in the Netherlands in 1860 and in Italy in 1889. Elsewhere females' life expectancy has long exceeded males': in Sweden since 1751, Denmark since 1835, England and Wales since 1841 (see Figure 29.1).[7]

But in all western European countries the life expectancy gap between women and men is now narrowing. Except in one aberrant year, 1789, the gap reached its maximum in Sweden in 1978 (6.2 years); in Denmark in 1979 (6.2 years); and in England and Wales in 1969 (6.3 years).

---

[2] World Health Organization (2003) *World health report 2003: shaping the future.* Geneva: WHO, www. who.int/whr/2003/en/index.html (accessed 31 March 2006).

[3] World Health Organization (2004) *World health report 2004: changing history,* Geneva: WHO, www. who.int/whr/2004/en/index.html (accessed 31 March 2006).

[4] World Health Organization (2005) *World health report 2005: make every mother and child count,* Geneva: WHO, www.who.int/whr/2005/en/ index.html (accessed 31 March 2006).

[5] Central Intelligence Agency (2005) *The world factbook, 2005,* www.cia.gov/cia/ publications/factbook/ (accessed 31 March 2006).

[6] Fenner, F. (1988) *Smallpox and its eradication,* Geneva: World Health Organization.

[7] Human mortality database (2005) University of California, Berkeley (www.mortality.org); Max Planck Institute for Demographic Research (www.humanmortality.de); (data downloaded 9 Dec 2005). Editorial Note: Figure 29.1 was not included in the original article but has been added here. It combines all the data from this database, also found at www.mortality.org, that was available in 2005, all of which is for affluent countries. It illustrates how it was at different ages that the gap opened up at different times.

Figure 29.1: Mortality rate by age, men and women, in 1850, 1900, 1950 and 2000, all affluent countries of the world at each point in time.

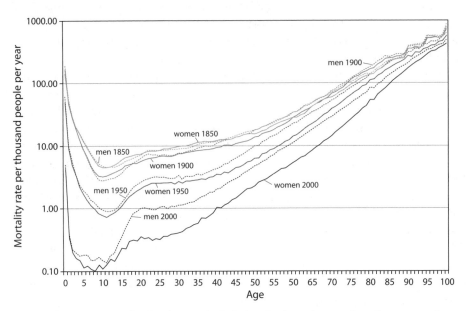

see colour version in plate section

Source: The Human Mortality Database and calculations by the author, see: http://www.mortality.org/

Greater emancipation has freed women to demand better health care and to behave more like men, and most importantly to smoke. A century ago it would have been hard to imagine such changes, or the fact that women now expect to live longer than men almost everywhere. As this transition is so recent, the processes driving it cannot be purely biological: they relate primarily to social change. In a way, women's life expectancy is an indicator of how well everyone can do, akin to the healthy districts identified in the 1850s by William Farr, the British epidemiologist who first reported on health inequalities.[8] In 1990 Amartya Sen, Indian economist and Nobel laureate, concluded from an analysis of unequal rights between men and women and mortality in the developing world that, worldwide, more than 100 million women were missing.[9] The women who were born when Sen wrote this are coming of age in a very different world. We must remember, though, that life expectancy data apply from birth onwards. The picture would be different in some countries if life expectancy from conception was considered: the first doctor to be imprisoned for carrying out sex-selective abortion in India was sentenced on 28 March 2006, which

[8] Lewis-Faning, E. (1930) A survey of the mortality in Dr Farr's 63 healthy districts of England and Wales during the period 1851-1925, *Journal of Hygiene* 30:121-53. doi:10.1017/S0022172400010342
[9] Sen, A. (1990) More than 100 million women are missing, *New York Review of Books*, December, 20:61-6.

may be another landmark.[10] Even securing a higher life expectancy from birth may not be a permanent achievement, given that the largest remaining untapped market for cigarettes in the world is made up of women living in poorer countries.

[10] Srinivasan, S. (2006) Challenges in implementing the ban on sex selection. Info Change Analysis. March 2006, www.infochangeindia.org/analysis121.jsp. Editorial Note: As of June 2012 the article only appeared to still exist in a temporary cache on the web. For possible help locating it in future it begins: 'On March 28, the very first doctor in India was sentenced to two years in prison for violating the Preconception and Prenatal Diagnostic Techniques Act. In the 11 years since the Act was enacted, why have lawbreakers got away? It is more than 11 years since the enactment of the Prenatal Diagnostic Techniques (Regulation and Prevention of Misuse) Act 1994. It is also at least two years since the more comprehensive, amended Preconception and Prenatal Diagnostic Techniques (PNDT) Act, 2003. Yet enforcing the law has proved to be a major challenge.' And ends: 'Opponents of sex selection must face both conceptual and practical tensions. They must ensure women's right to abortion while opposing sex selection. This balance is sometimes difficult to maintain. For example, there have been suggestions that abortion clinics be monitored and the sex ratio of female foetuses be tracked. Such monitoring could threaten the tenuous access to abortion that women have today. There have also been efforts to shift the focus from the medical profession's unethical practices to addressing the social demand for sex selection. One of these is rewarding panchayats [village council's administrative areas] whose sex ratios improve. The problem, as noted by participants at one recent meeting, is that this can encourage the manufacture of data. Second, there are not enough births within a panchayat to monitor for changes in sex ratios – you need a sample of at least 28,000 births to be able to detect changes in the sex ratio, says Dr Bedi. Finally, there is the question of what to do as technology advances to take foetal sex detection beyond regulation. Foetal sex selection using ultrasound has, so far, been doing the damage. But all this may change in the next few years. When the PNDT Act was drafted, ultrasound could not be used for sex selection until very late in the pregnancy. That is no longer true, and this is the technique that is most prevalent today. But the most frightening development, reported by Dr Puneet Bedi at a recent consultation, is a blood test isolating foetal cells from maternal blood, enabling foetal sex detection. This could throw the entire campaign into chaos. "The technology is at a very crude level today," says Dr Bedi. "And even if it becomes accurate, it will be very expensive initially. But in any case, that is a different fight. Today we have to fight the fightable fight." If we don't win this battle, we won't win that one either.'

30

Mortality in relation to sex in the affluent world

Rigby, J.E. and Dorling, D. (2007) 'Mortality in relation to sex in the affluent world', *Journal of Epidemiology and Community Health*, vol 61, no 2, pp 159-64.

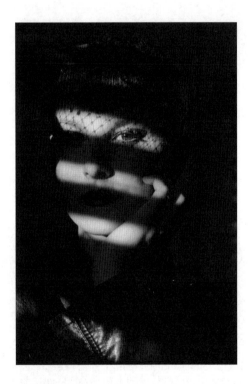

What is already known: It is already widely known that in rich nations, mortality in young males is now several times higher than that in females and that this relative difference has widened as absolute rates have fallen rapidly for both women and most groups of men.

However, almost all studies focus on single-nation states or compare a small number of nations. Few studies group nation states to dramatically increase the sample size and allow more subtle trends to be identified with what is already known. Those subtle trends may produce clues as to why relative inequalities are increasing as they are.

What this paper adds: This study adds the most detailed description of this trend to date in terms of volumes of data involved and hence the clarity of the patterns that result. This allows the second derivative of the trend to be taken—the trend in the trend—and key dates to be identified when it seems that increases in the relative ratios of male to female mortality coincide with cohorts entering world labour markets during more economically depressed times. This study suggests that international socioeconomic factors need to be carefully studied to better understand the recent history of mortality among the most affluent billion people of the world.

Abstract

Background: This chapter explores newly available data for 22 countries with reliably recorded mortality data. The past century saw dramatic falls in mortality for both males and females in the most affluent countries of the world. However, these falls are not consistent for both men and women and the inequalities in the male:female mortality ratios are not well understood.

Design: By aggregating mortality at each year of life for the 22 countries for those years for which reliable data were recorded (during the period 1850–1999), distinct patterns emerge.

Results: In the richer countries of the world, the male:female mortality ratio has been widening for all years of age, particularly for those born from 1942 onwards. Specific cohort effects are clearly identifiable.

Conclusion: Analysis of the emergent trends suggests that economic activity, status and position possibly provide a better overall explanatory model than a purely biomedical approach.

Introduction

Gender differences have been consumed by social change. We are in the midst of an ascent of women matched with an equivalent descent of men.[1]

In the richest fifth of the world, the rate ratio of young men to young women dying per year is 3:1.[2] Among these richest of nations, in recent decades, the mortality of younger women has been falling much more quickly than for men.[3] The demographic and social antecedents of this trend, its historical uniqueness and its potential implications for the future population structure of the rich minority of the

---

[1] Jones, S.Y. (2003) *The descent of men.* London: Abacus, p 260.
[2] World Health Organisation (2004) *World health report 2004.* Geneva: World Health Organisation.
[3] Vaupel, J.W., Carey, J.R., Christensen, K. *et al.* (1998) Biodemographic trajectories of longevity. *Science* 280, 855–860; Waldron, I. (1993) Recent trends in sex mortality ratios for adults in developed countries. *Social Science and Medicine*, 36, 451–462; Kruger, D.J. and Nesse, R.M. (2004) Sexual selection and the male:female mortality ratio. *Evolutionary Psychology* 2, 66–85; Wingard, D.L. (1984) The sex differential in morbidity, mortality and lifestyle, *Annual Review of Public Health*, 5, 433–458.

world are not well understood, and not widely recognised, although many studies have been made of specific aspects of the trends.[4] A new international database, accessible to all researchers, makes the study of 22 countries now possible[5] and the degree of accuracy achieved from amalgamating the data produces new trends for exploration and explanation. The aim of this study is to investigate changes in the male:female mortality ratio over time, and specifically to identify when the trend towards high rates of male/female inequality in mortality began.

Methods

The human mortality database project began in 2000, and is jointly maintained by the Department of Demography, UC Berkeley and the Max Planck Institute for Demographic Research, Rostock, Germany. Countries are included if there is a '*well found belief that coverage of census and vital registration statistics is relatively high*'.[6] Different countries enter the dataset on different dates depending on when their data became reliable: the data have been stringently validated following a strict methods protocol[7] before being accepted for this database. The datasets contain some caveats in terms of data quality, which informed the time period extracted for this work—that is from 1850 to 1999. Thus, the geographical area being considered changes in size over time—but at each point in time the area corresponds to those nations of the world that could record reliable mortality data—in effect to the most economically advantaged nations of the world (countries identified as '*relatively wealthy*'). Clearly, these findings are unlikely to reflect the conditions in the remaining four-fifths of the world, where so much mortality remains attributable to infectious disease and conflict.[8]

The full dataset used here includes some 1.4 billion people: 702 million women and 695 million men living between 1850 and 1999 in the 22 countries shown in Table 30.1. Of these, almost 1 billion are alive now. People 101 years of age or above are not included. Data held include annual live birth counts, annual death counts and population size as on 1 January each year. Hence the data for each country were

---

[4] Conti, S., Farchi, G., Masocco, M. *et al.* (2003) Gender differentials in life expectancy in Italy, *European Journal of Epidemiology*, 18, 107-112; Gjonça, A., Tomassini, C., Toson, B. *et al.* (2005) Sex differences in mortality, a comparison of the United Kingdom and other developed countries, *Health Statistics Quarterly*, 26, 6-16; Guralnik, J.M., Balfour, J.L. and Volpato, S. (2000) The ratio of older women to men: Historical perspectives and cross-national comparisons, *Aging Clinical and Experimental Research*, 12: 65-76; Pampel, F.C. (2002) Cigarette use and the narrowing sex differential in mortality, *Population and Development Review*, 28, 77-104; and Verbrugge, L.M. and Wingard. D,L. (1987) Sex differentials in health and mortality. *Women Health*, 12, 103-145.

[5] In spring 2005 a 23rd country, Belgium, was added to the database which is omitted from the study here. It almost certainly had no effect.

[6] Human Mortality Database (2005) University of California, Berkeley (USA), and Max Planck Institute for Demographic Research (Germany); available at www.mortality.org, or www.humanmortality.de (data downloaded on 20/11/2004; last accessed on 12/09/2005).

[7] Wilmoth. J,R., Andreev. K., Jdanov, D., *et al.* (2006) Methods Protocol for the Human Mortality Database; available at www.mortality.org, last accessed on 24/03/06.

[8] World Health Organisation (2006) Mortality Database; available at http://www.ciesin.org/IC/who/MortalityDatabase.html, last accessed on 24/03/06.

Table 30.1: Years of data available for places forming the 'affluent world', 1751–2002.

	Data available at time of access	Population 1999 (millions)
Sweden	1751-2002	8.9
England and Wales	1841-1998	52.6 (1998)
Norway	1846-2002	4.5
Italy	1872-2000	57.6
Switzerland	1876-2002	7.1
Finland	1878-2002	5.2
France*	1899-2001	58.5
Spain	1908-2001	40.3
Canada	1908-1996	29.8 (1996)
Denmark	1921-2000	5.3
Bulgaria	1947-1997	8.3 (1997)
Austria	1948-1999	8.1
Czech Republic	1948-2001	10.3
Hungary	1950-1999	10.1
Japan	1950-1999	125.3
Netherlands	1950-1999	15.8
E. Germany	1956-1999	15.3
W. Germany	1956-1999	66.8
Latvia	1959-1999	2.4
USA	1959-1999	272.5
Lithuania	1960-2001	3.5
Russia	1970-1999	146.3

Note: * Territorial changes during World Wars I and II

Source: The Human Mortality database, accessed in 2006.
See: http://www.mortality.org/

used to produce counts of deaths by age and sex for each year, and thus to calculate the mortality for each year of life. The male: female mortality ratio was calculated by dividing the male mortality by the corresponding female mortality. The work did not require ethical approval.

It is extremely difficult to visualise changing rates, let alone rate ratios by age and cohort, in our imagination; a map of mortality trends is worth 15,000 numbers.

Figure 30.1: Sex ratio of mortality (male : female rate) for the richer countries of the world, 1850–2000.

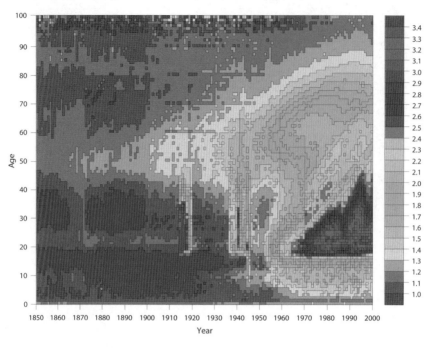

Source: The Human Mortality Database and calculations by the authors, see: http://www.mortality.org/

Hence, to assist with interpretation, Figures 30.1 and 30.2 depict Lexis maps[9] of the ratio of male to female mortality by single year of age and year, and of the first derivative of change in that ratio (by age). The x axis (or easting) represents time, showing the years from 1850 to 2000. There are thus 150 columns of data. The y axis (or northing) represents age, from <1 to between 99 and 100 years. There are thus 100 rows of data and 15,000 cells in all. Each cell is coloured according to the mortality rates of women and men in each specific year of each particular age. Thus, the top right-hand cell refers to the mortality of people in their 100th year of life living in the calendar year 1999.

The cells in the Lexis map are coloured according to the ratio of male : female mortality. For example, the top right cell in the colour plate of Figure 30.1 (p x) is given a shade of orange that corresponds to a ratio between 1.1 and 1.2 on the key to the right of the diagram. This means that for every 1000 men, between 10% and 20% more died in the year 2000 before their 100th birthday than did women of the same age group during the same time period. To distinguish between shades

---

[9] The software used to draw the Lexis maps was Lexis 1.1, written by Kirill Andreev and named after the German demographer Wilhelm Lexis; available from www.demogr.mpg.de (software at http://www.demogr.mpg.de/books/odense/9/cd/default.htm).

of colour, locate the darkest red in the diagram. This refers to mortality ratios of <1 (in which case more women died than men). Note that the 'ratio surface' on the Lexis map is quite smooth. Areas of time and age where rates were <1 tend to be surrounded by areas where rates were between 1.0 and 1.1, and so on up to the few cells in time and by age where >3.4 men died for every woman who died.

Figure 30.2: First derivative of sex ratio of mortality, showing change in the ratio for the richer countries of the world, 1850–2000.

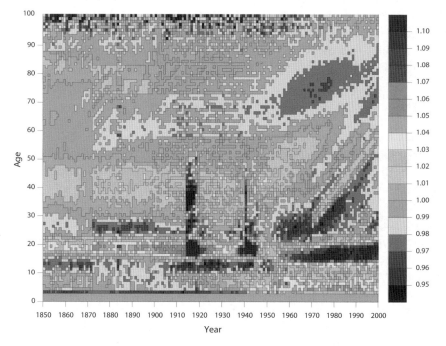

Source: The Human Mortality Database and calculations by the authors, see: http://www.mortality.org/

The quality of the data allows a single year of age first derivative (a measure of change) to be calculated for the first time. This shows the increase or decrease in any calendar year of mortality ratios comparing one cohort with that aged one year older (Figure 30.2). Here, we are looking at the change in slope by age, so for each cell, we divide its value by the value in the cells below it, relating to people aged one year younger. If there is a sudden increase or decrease in the smoothness of the Lexis map's surface, it becomes evident by showing this first derivative. Note that we have smoothed the first derivate surface by taking a 5-year moving average by age. The average is actually the geometric mean for 2 years younger, one year younger, the age group being considered, one year older and 2 years older. The geometric mean is calculated as the product of the five ratios (of ratios (of rates)) to the power of a fifth. We only smooth vertically (by age) and calculate the derivative by age, as we would expect some breaks of slope by time as new territories are introduced over time. Therefore, we do not calculate the first derivative over time. We interpret the maps by looking for specific features—for example, diagonal lines of colour will show cohort effects, where vertical chimneys show a situation in a particular year: the World Wars are good illustrations of such period effects. In the colour plate of Figure 30.2 these chimneys appear strongly in blue, but much of the remainder of the diagram before 1950, for the ages between 20 years and 70 years, is green—corresponding to around 1 on the legend, and indicating a relatively stable change as males and females age by one year at a time. However, where we see diagonal lines of colour are apparent, for example in dark blue from 1970, the diagonal highlights a cohort of people as they age year by year, and the colour indicates the rate of change: so blue indicates that, year on year, the rate of male mortality is worsening compared with that of women. This is explored in more depth in the next section.

Results

Mortality has fallen rapidly over time in the rich world. In the first half of the 20th century, much of this was attributable to continued public health interventions to supply clean water, sanitation and improved housing quality. In addition, improved healthcare and nutrition were reflected in dramatic falls in maternal and infant mortality.[10]

Before turning to the relative mortality of men to women, trends in each warrant consideration. These are summarised in Table 30.2, which shows the total male and female mortality for the data at approximately 10-year time intervals across the 20th century. From this summarised information, we can see how the rates for males and females fell over the 20th century, but not at the same pace. For specific ages, the figures are particularly noticeable (see Figure 30.4 shown later).

For 10-year-old girls, rates fell from just under 5 per 1000 in 1850, to 4 in 1867, halving repeatedly to 2 in 1925, to 1 in 1947, 0.5 in 1955, 0.25 in 1975 and being approximately 0.125 now. For 10-year-old boys, rates were similar in 1850 and the first milestone (<4/1000 deaths/year) was reached in 1867, but subsequent milestones were attained later than for girls (1926, 1949, 1961 and 1996, respectively); mortality for 10-year-old boys is currently approximately double that for girls of that age.

There has been only one outstanding worldwide single-year period effect in the rich countries between 1850 and 1999. Girls aged 10 years in 1918 experienced a mortality equal to that in women aged 40 years during the years either side of 1918. This shows the historic magnitude of the influenza pandemic of 1918.[11] For men, the First World War raised mortality in general from 1914 to 1920, but rates in 1918 were still twice those of earlier and later years for all ages between 1 and 40 years.

The peaks in mortality are more evident for men. These occur at 30 years of age in 1853 at 10.6/1000, falling then and rising again to 10.3 in 1871, falling then and

---

[10] Loudon, I. (1991) Maternal and infant mortality 1900–1960, *Social History of Medicine*, 4, 29–73.

[11] Cliff, A.D., Haggett, P. and Ord, J.K. (1986) *Spatial aspects of influenza epidemics*, London: Pion.

Table 30.2: Overall female and male mortality rates at time intervals for the 'affluent world', 1910–90.

Year	Female mortality rate per 1000	Male mortality rate per 1000	Comment
1910	16.76	18.28	
1919	16.44	18.76	Influenza pandemic
1930	12.44	13.84	Beginning of Great Depression
1940	12.65	15.17	Early World War II in Europe
1950	9.99	11.25	Beginnings of regeneration
1960	8.63	10.59	Stability and prosperity
1970	8.56	10.33	Widespread contraception
1980	8.81	10.18	Periods of recession
1990	9.01	9.83	Onset of Japanese recession; AIDS

Source: The Human Mortality Database, accessed in 2006, see: http://www.mortality.org/

rising through the First World War to peak at 31.6 in 1918, then alternately falling and peaking at the times of the Wall Street Crash in 1929 (5.4), the depression in 1936 (5.2), reaching 9.8 in 1940 during the start of World War II, then falling rapidly to a low of 1.6/1000 in 1967. These rates then rose and fell repeatedly, with peaks coinciding with economic depressions[12] in 1970 (2.3), 1981 (2.1), 1994 (2.4) and ending with rates of 1.9 in 1999, higher than those in 1958, 40 years earlier. Conversely, mortality for women aged 30 years halved from 1.3/1000 in 1958 to 0.7/1000 by 1999.

The Lexis maps show trends hinted at by previous studies,[13] but with a degree of accuracy achievable only when the sample size exceeds 1 billion, which has not been achieved previously, and is possible only if this (albeit expanding) area of the globe is considered as a single areal-unit of study.

Figure 30.1 shows the changing ratio of male to female mortality in these rich countries of the world by single year of age each year from 1850 to 1999. Hence, the greater the scale value, the greater the proportion of men dying as compared to women. Before 1940, at many ages, slightly more women died per 1000 per year than men. The main exceptions were for younger men during the First World War and for those aged 50–60 years from the 1870s onwards, with maximum inequalities being recorded as mortality up to a third higher than for women in particular years at particular ages. For men aged 21 years, mortality was 20% higher than women of the same ages in 1934, 31% higher in 1936, 60% higher in 1938 and 300% higher in 1940. Although falling again after the war, the ratio never fell back to its 1934

---

[12] Webber, M.J. and Rigby, D.L. (1996) *The Golden Age Illusion: rethinking postwar capitalism*. New York: Guilford Press.

[13] See footnote 3 on p 277 above.

level. It rose steadily again from 1950 to reach 113% in 1959, 216% in 1974, to end by peaking at 251% in 1995. By then, for every 100 women dying aged 21 years, some 351 men were dying at that age each year in the rich world.

As Figure 30.1 shows, the recent fortunes of 21-year-old men were part of a general trend that began around 1950 for men aged around 20 years, included all those aged 20–30 years by 1960, extending to 40 years of age by 1970, 50 years by 1980, 70 years by 1990 and covering the ages of 20–80 years by 2000, for whom it became normal to die at almost twice the rate of women per year. Although this triangle has been identified previously, it has not been mapped in as much detail as here and that detail provides more clues as to its possible origins. At the heart of this triangle, for men in their 20s in particular years in the 1980s and 1990s, rates of mortality three times those of women became normal. This is an unprecedented level of inequality in the richest countries of the world. While deaths attributable to AIDS in younger men might contribute to this phenomenon, the contribution is relatively small, particularly for the youngest ages most affected (early 20s) and in the period in which inequalities became the highest (1990s), before antiretroviral treatment became effective.

Figure 30.2 shows the first derivative of change in Figure 30.1 by age. Clearly, the increases in the ratios which have occurred over time are cohort-led—that is, from around 1950 onwards diagonal trends appear in the change in rate ratios. The first of these trends is for men aged around 80 years in 2000 who would have entered the labour market in the 1930s; the second for men aged 68 years in 2000 who were 15 years old in 1947; the third for men aged 58 years in 2000 (aged 15 years in 1957); the fourth for men aged 37 years in 2000 (entered labour market in late 1970s or early 1980s); the fifth for men aged 24 years in 2000 (entry in early 1990s); and the sixth for men entering the labour market around 2000. Each of these cohorts is of men who had to compete for work more than was normal (as compared with men born slightly earlier or later), both as a product of when they were born and of subsequent economic circumstances. For later cohorts that competition has also been increased as women have entered competing (rather than separate) labour markets in increasing numbers.[14] Figure 30.1 also shows how, in terms of changes to the ratios, the worse years of the two world wars are similar regarding effect of social change since 1960.

Figure 30.3 shows male : female mortality by age for successive 10-year cohorts from 1850, exploring the trends over time. The lowest line in the figure and the first cohort is of all people born between 1850 and 1859. For this cohort, ratios at all ages were near 1, and the same proportion of men and women died each year as they aged. For successive cohorts, the flat lines of risk rise slowly and then more rapidly until, for men born in the 1930s, their chances of dying between ages 40 and 65 years were twice those of women born in that decade. This rise in male mortality

---

[14] Rogot, E., Sorlie, P.D. and Johnson, N.J. (1992) Life expectancy by employment status, income and education in the National Longitudinal Mortality Study, *Public Health Reports*, 107, 457-461.

Figure 30.3: Male: female mortality ratio by age in the rich world by 10-year cohort, 1850--1990.

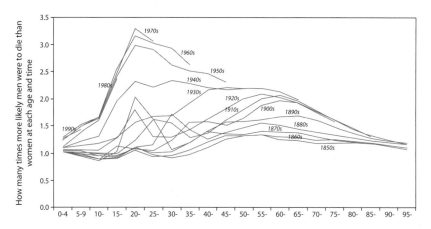

Source: The Human Mortality Database and calculations by the authors, see: http://www.mortality.org/

see colour version in plate section

in middle age coincides with the rise in smoking (originally more among men).[15] For men born before the turn of the century—cohorts in the 1880s and 1890s—ratios rise at the age they would have been during the First World War. There are shallow peaks for those born in the 1910s and 1920s at the ages they would have been most likely to have been fighting in the Second World War.

From the cohorts of those born in the 1940s onwards, the peak age of inequality quickly becomes the early 20s and there is little subsequent rise in inequalities at older ages. By the time the members of the 1970s-born cohort reached their early 20s, male:female mortality inequalities had exceeded 3:1, and both the 1980s-born and 1990s-born cohorts were following similar trajectories. On analysing Figure 30.2 it can be discerned that the trend changed the fastest for those children born in 1942. Men born in this year in the rich world were the first to be twice as likely to die as women, each year, from the age of 18 years onwards.

Discussion

Manhood tells a social tale as much as one written in nucleic acids. It must, with all that it implies be constructed, and once its foundations are laid, what rises from them has little to do with DNA.[16]

For those born since 1942, by the age of 18 years, men have been twice as likely to die per year as compared to women. Their relative chances then exceed this until they

[15] Pampel, F.C. (2002) Cigarette use and the narrowing sex differential in mortality, *Population and Development Review*, 28, 77–104.
[16] Jones, S.Y. (2003) *The Descent of Men*. London: Abacus, pp 239–240.

reach their 50s, when again they are twice as likely to die per year. Below 20 years and above 50 years of age inequalities between men and women have been stable over the course of more than four decades. Between the ages of 20 and 50 years, subsequent cohorts of men have experienced successively poorer relative mortality as compared with women. At times, male mortality rises in absolute terms for men of these ages, whereas for women it relentlessly falls. What has changed since 1942 to create these new trends?

In 1942, the rich world was in turmoil. The United States had joined the war a few weeks before the start of the year. Stalingrad was held, with huge losses, by the Russians, and at El Alamein, the course of the war changed in the autumn of that year. However for those born during the height of this war, it was the social changes that came later that most influenced their lives. When they turned 18 years in 1960, the contraceptive pill was first marketed in the United States, coming a year later to Germany.[17] Women born in rich countries around 1942 were among the first in the world to have substantial control over both their bodies and social destinies. As Jones succinctly phrases it, the changing social relationships between men and women were what led to the current descent of men.[18]

No single medical, biological or 'lifestyle' explanation can account for why young men's mortality is improving so much more slowly than that of young women across all the richer nations of the world. Unlike the early rise in inequalities at older ages, there is no obvious agent such as the introduction of mass-produced cigarette sales being clearly biased towards men, and no small group of causes accounting for the majority of inequality. The work of Gjonça et al makes a very useful contribution to identifying social and biological factors when comparing England and Wales with France, but does not explore the crucial history of their economic contexts.[19] Given the history of epidemiology and public health, it is not surprising to find the predominance of biological explanations frequently suggested and indeed we may be witnessing the outcomes of some evolutionary processes that are only just emerging. However, any mechanical explanation has to encompass the whole growth in relative inequalities from 10 to 80 years of age from the middle of the past century to the start of this one. No single biological explanation can account for why a 10-year-old boy is half as likely again to die as a girl of that age in any given recent year, likewise for an 80-year-old man compared with an 80-year-old woman.[20] In 1912, their chances were almost equal. Although aspects of high-risk behaviours (reflected in road accidents, suicides and lethal drug misuse statistics) feature in explanations of higher mortality for young male adults, such explanations are hardly applicable for boys aged 10 years.

---

[17] Foster, P. (1995) *Women and the health care industry*, Buckingham: Open University Press.
[18] Jones (2003) op cit.
[19] See footnote 4 on p 278 above.
[20] Owens, I.P.F. (2002) Sex differences in mortality rate, *Science* 297, 2008-9; Moore, S.L and Wilson K. (2002) Parasites as a viability cost of sexual selection in natural populations of mammals. *Science*, 297, 2015-18.

Figure 30.4 shows the mortality separately for males and females, for the single ages of 10 and 30 years. The influenza pandemic, and for males the First and Second World Wars, and post-war economic depressions, are all evident. It is also clear that the male:female rates for 10-year-olds begin to diverge at the same time as those for 30-year-olds, from the mid-1940s.

Figure 30.4: Mortality rates in the 'affluent world', selected single years for ages 10 and 30, male and female, 1841–2000.

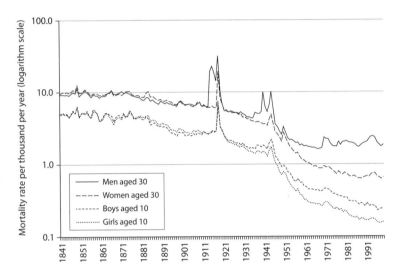

see colour version in plate section

Source: The Human Mortality Database and calculations by the authors, see: http://www.mortality.org/

The recent collection of reliable, validated historical mortality data from around the world allows both the patterns at large to be studied and individual countries' trajectories to be compared. There may well be clues in the fluctuations to the general trend that point to its origins and likely future. Ratios improved slightly more slowly for women under the rule of Mussolini in Italy and Franco in Spain, for instance. Between the ages of 5 and 14 years, many more girls died in 1918, for all years studied, than did boys. Did fascist regimes perhaps hold back women's emancipation enough to slightly influence relative mortality? Were boys perhaps valued so much more than girls that in times of stark deprivation (during war and pandemic in 1918) more brothers were kept alive than their sisters? The variations between the fortunes of men joining the increasingly global labour market at dates determined by their birth (listed above) provide more clues, through the coincidence of events, of the underlying processes at play. It may just be coincidence that men suffer more biological effects during recessions, benefit from recessive regimes and die less in childhood in one unique year. Alternatively, perhaps all these signs point to the growing importance of social context in terms of sex equality and most importantly, female emancipation in the rich world.[21]

If women's emancipation is the driving force of this global trend, then the prospects for men's future are not good, as in almost all rich countries the economic and social position of women still has a long way to improve to reach that of men. Fourfold and fivefold mortality inequalities are not hard to imagine at particular ages in the near future, especially in particular countries (the ratio already exceeded 3.5 in 1995 for men aged 21 years). Just as the causes of these inequalities are not medical, nor will the solutions be.

Clearly, this study is limited to the findings from the data available—that is, those countries that had the infrastructure to supply the human mortality database with population and mortality data, which met its stringent requirements. All available countries were included at the time this paper was written. There are other, affluent countries that are not in the database, but their populations are unlikely to be large enough to affect the trends discussed. We also acknowledge that the historical events incorporated in the discussion are, although persuasive, clearly subjective and influenced by our UK perspective.

In the richer nations of the world, the lives and social roles of young men and women only vaguely resemble those of their grandparents. If the same order of change were to occur in the next two generations, then perhaps the relative descent of men could decelerate. As yet there is no strong evidence for that. It can, however, be seen that the step changes in Figure 30.1 start to shift direction in the upper age ranges (over 70 years) from about 1990; this convergence might reflect the 'rounding off' of the middle-aged bubble. This study suggests that international socioeconomic factors need to be carefully studied to better understand the recent history of mortality among the most affluent billion people of the world.

---

[21] Sen, A. (1990) More than 100 million women are missing, *New York Review of Books*, 37, 61–66.

31

Anamorphosis: the geography of physicians, and mortality

Dorling, D. (2007) 'Anamorphosis: the geography of physicians, and mortality', *International Journal of Epidemiology*, vol 36, no 4, pp 745-50.

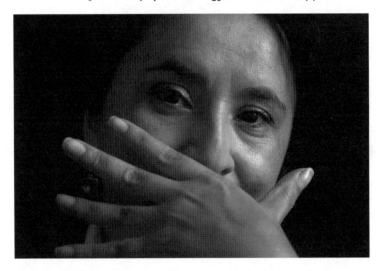

Visual images can have an impact that is different and often more immediate than the written argument or reported statistical effect. Photographs are especially effective and, hence, the photo essay.[1] But serendipitous intuition can also be fostered with schematic diagrams. However, we quickly become immune to the distortion of some forms of graphic; for instance, oblivious to distorted scaling of traditional maps,[2] or to the ubiquity of the log scaling required to squeeze all extremes of life within one inequitable planet onto the square of the graph; dispassionate to the implications of moving an inch to the left or up graphs such as that shown in Figure 31.1.

The five figures that follow take the same data as shown in Figure 31.1 but show parts of it—recombined in different ways.[3] They illustrate how simply showing the

---

[1] Darwell, J. (2006) Photoessay, Legacy: inside the Chernobyl exclusion zone, *International Journal of Epidemiology*, 35, 827–31.

[2] Dorling, D. (2007) Worldmapper: The Human Anatomy of a Small Planet, *PLoS Medicine*, 4, 1: e1, doi:10.1371/journal.pmed.0040001 (published: 30 January 2007) [reproduced as Chapter 37, this volume].

[3] All these graphics save the last are taken from spreadsheets and images made available on the website www.worldmapper.org (the last is the same as the first without the log scaling and was derived from them). More than three hundred related distributions are depicted in graphical and map form there and also over one hundred maps of death attributable to different causes will appear there early in 2007. Editorial Note: There are now roughly 1,000 maps on www.worldmapper.org including 117 on cause of death distributions.

Figure 31.1: Physicians per head and child mortality (aged 1 to 4), countries of the world, 2002.

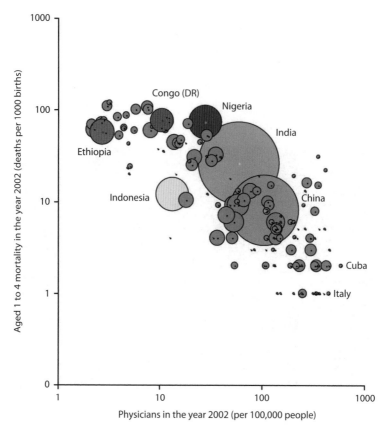

Note: Territories of the world drawn as circles with area in proportion to births. Both axes are drawn with a log scale here.

Source: www.worldmapper.org

absolute numbers the rates are based on (Figures 31.2 and 31.3), reveals information not apparent from the rates (compare with Figures 31.4 and 31.5); and how showing both the absolute numbers and the rates makes visible yet more, despite the geography being lost (Figures 31.6 and 31.7).

Images have a long history in medicine and politics, as does both deliberate and hidden distortion, hidden meanings and signs (Figure 31.8). In the end is shown (Figure 31.9) how simply turning off one of the most common distortions—the log option—and re-scaling again . . . reveals a very different image again—an anamorphosis: '*an unconventional way of seeing*'[4]:

---

[4] An image that is painted in a way that makes it appear distorted unless viewed from a specific viewpoint or using a cylindrical or conical mirror, or a different world view. See also http://www.anamorphosis.com.

Figure 31.2: Territories of the world drawn with area in proportion to deaths at ages 1–4, 2002.

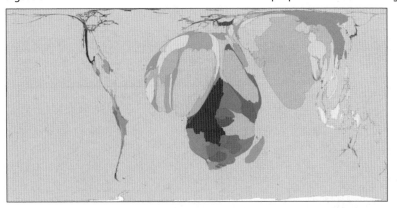

Note: This image is of the world as shaped when drawn in proportion to the more than 3 million children who die each year aged between 1 and 4 (inclusive) almost all from superficially easily preventable causes. In most cases their death is not simply due to the lack of intervention of a trained physician. However: 'There are more nurses from Malawi in Manchester than in Malawi and more Ethiopian doctors in Chicago than Ethiopia', Kinnock, G., 4 April 2006, Strasbourg: http://www.welshlabourmeps. org.uk/gk/gk_press/healthbudget04.04.06.htm.

Source: www.worldmapper.org

Figure 31.3: Territories of the world drawn with area in proportion to physicians, 2002.

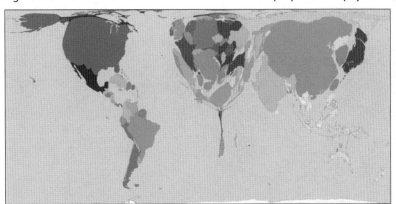

Note: There are more than two working physicians for every child that dies aged 1 to 4 worldwide each year. A traditional map in which territories are shaded according to the ratio of the population to physicians gives the reader little real impression of just how geographically concentrated physicians are: most into just a few territories worldwide.

The proof that a map of this kind could be drawn was made in 1975 when A.K. Sen published 'A theorem related to cartograms' (in *American Mathematics Monthly*, 82, 382-385). The first fully working practical realisation of that proof did not emerge until 30 years later and the latest version at time of writing is: Newman, M. (2006) Cart: Computer software for making cartograms [online]. University of Michigan. Available from: http://www-personal.umich.edu/%7Emejn/cart/ [accessed 5 July 2006].

Source: www.worldmapper.org

Figure 31.4: Territories of the world drawn with area in proportion to population, 2002.

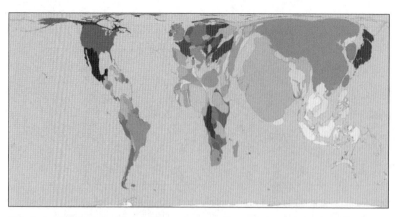

Note: Some 200 territories of the world are ranked according to their populations' weighted average score on the United Nations Development Programme's Human Development Index for 2002. That ranking is then used to determine the original colours used in these maps, from the poorest in red, through the rainbow shades, to the country with the highest index, Japan, in violet [see colour version]. 2002 is also the year from which the world population is drawn that is used to scale each territory according to its area.

Figure 31.5: Territories of the world drawn with area in proportion to land area.

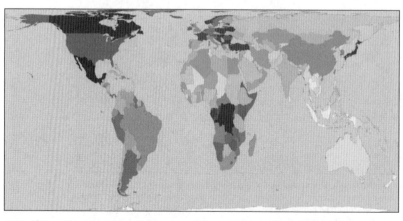

Note: This equal area projection appears very similar to that reproduced by Arno Peters and adopted by many parts of the United Nations as a more equitable projection than traditional world maps. However, this, and Peter's projection, give most prominence to where there is most land – not most people. 'Africa's population density of 249 people per 1,000 hectares is well below the world average of 442. However, a great deal of the total destruction of the natural environment is occurring in the region. Poverty is a major cause and consequence. The area of Africa on the population cartogram is roughly half what the continent is on the equal land area map as a result of population density across Africa being almost half the world average.' (United Nations Population Fund, The State of the World Population 2001; Chapter 2: Environmental Trends: http://www.unfpa.org/swp/2001/english/ch02.html).

Source: www.worldmapper.org

Figure 31.6: Territories of the world drawn with rectangular area on this graph in proportion to physicians, 2002.

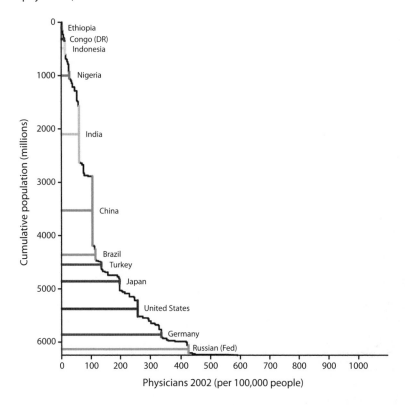

Note: On this graph the area of each territory is proportional to the number of physicians who work there, as also in Figure 31.3 above, but here information on geographical location is lost so that territories can be ordered by rates. The area to the left of the line is thus proportional to absolute numbers. This image is another example of an anamorphosis where area is drawn in proportion to a count, in this case numbers of physicians.

Source: www.worldmapper.org

Figure 31.7: Territories of the world drawn with rectangular area on this graph in proportion to deaths at ages 1–4, 2002.

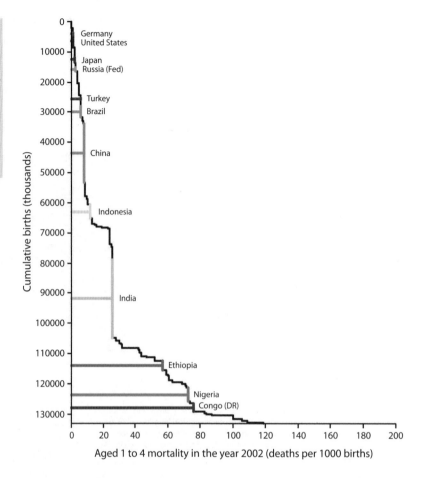

Note: All territories of the world are shown in this image and thus there is a minute space to the left of the line to represent the death of each child aged 1 to 4 that occurred in this one year. Worldwide 3,200,000 are estimated to have died, give or take well over 100,000 as recording is so poor. Some dozen territories that are home to over half the world's population have been labelled as, unlike on a map, it is far from obvious where places are on a graph.

Source: www.worldmapper.org

Figure 31.8: Anamorphosis in medicine and politics, from anatomy to subterfuge.

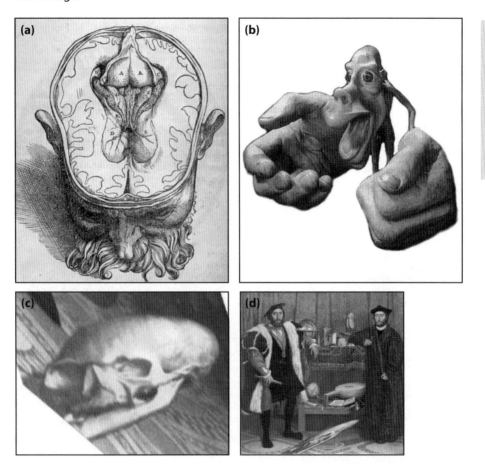

see colour version in plate section

Note: Ambassadors engage in diplomacy in the interest of their country but, not necessarily, in the interest of others.

Sources: (a) Dissecting the cortex: taken from Vesalius' De humani corporis fabrica, 1543 [On the Fabric of the Human Body] now published online: http://vesalius.northwestern.edu/. This image sourced from: http://pages.slc.edu/~ebj/iminds01/notes/L1-Descartes-bats/s8-vesalius.html
(b) Homunculus, taken from http://wwwppeda.free.fr/progressions/3/homunc_sens_grand.jpg
(c) Detail of skull, transformed with photo software and derived from Holbein's 'The Ambassadors'
(d) From http://www.dodedans.com/Eholbein.htm, accessed 26 October 2006

> *We prefer an ordered world, regular patterns, familiar forms, and when flaws or distortions occur, provided they are not too gross, our mind's eye tidies them up. We see what we want or expect to see …* [5]

---

[5] Wright L. (1983) *Perspective in Perspective*, London: Routledge and Kegan Paul Books Ltd, p 27; unread and referenced in turn at end of page on: http://www.anamorphosis.com

Figure 31.9: Physicians per head and child mortality (aged 1 to 4), countries of the world, 2002.

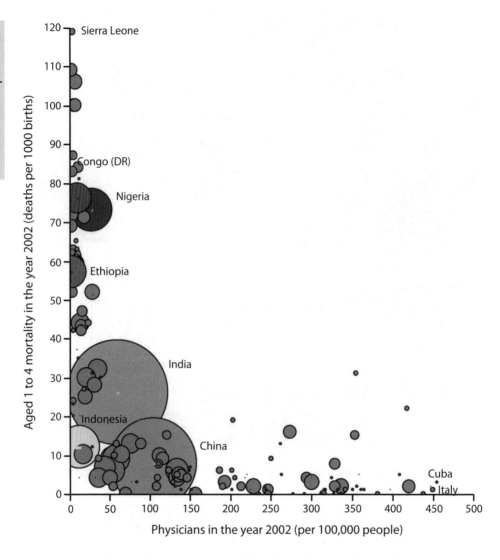

Note: Cuba is the most easterly circle, Sierra Leone the most northerly, and the most prominent circle to the south west extreme of the distribution is Malaysia. Here the territories of the world are drawn as circles with area in proportion to births. Both axes are drawn with a linear scale.

Source: www.worldmapper.org.

The final graphic (Figure 31.9) is identical to the first (Figure 31.1) other than that the scales used to place the circle representing each territory on the page are no longer log-based. There no longer appears to be a simple relationship between physicians per person and the very premature deaths of young children when the world is looked at like this.[6]

> *It is difficult to escape the conclusion that this loss of infant life is in some way related to the social life of the people.*[7]

---

[6] Only two territories of the world have been promoted out of the poorer groups into a richer category in the last three decades: Malta by geographical inevitability and South Korea by invitation; Babones, S.J. (2005) The country-level income structure of the world-economy. *Journal of World-Systems Research* 2005; XI, 1, 29–56. Millions of skulls are hidden beneath the illusion of development.

[7] This observation was not made of the graphs shown here but of very similar rates of infant mortality found within England almost exactly a century ago. Source: Newman, G. (1906) *Infant Mortality: A Social Problem*. London: Methuen and Co., p vi.

32

The global impact of income inequality on health by age: an observational study

Dorling, D., Mitchell, R. and Pearce, J. (2007) 'The global impact of income inequality on health by age: an observational study', *British Medical Journal*, vol 335, pp 873-5.

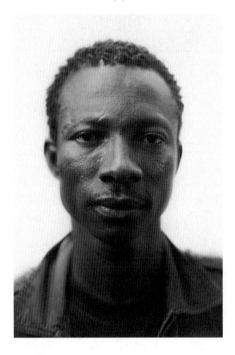

What is already known on this subject: Mortality falls as incomes rise, and this relation holds both between and within countries. Among affluent nations, this relation is tempered as income inequalities increase: the health gains from increases in income are less in more unequal nations. There is some evidence that these effects are more pronounced at different ages.

What this study adds: High inequalities in income are closely associated with higher mortality in both poor and rich nations of the world. This is particularly apparent when the effects are studied by age: worldwide, income inequality is most strongly detrimental to health in young adulthood.

Abstract

Objectives: To explore whether the apparent impact of income inequality on health, which has been shown for wealthier nations, is replicated worldwide, and whether the impact varies by age.

Design: Observational study.

Setting: 126 countries of the world for which complete data on income inequality and mortality by age and sex were available around the year 2002 (including 94.4% of world human population).

Data sources: Data on mortality were from the World Health Organization and income data were taken from the annual reports of the United Nations Development Programme.

Main outcome measures: Mortality in 5-year age bands for each sex by income inequality and income level.

Results: At ages 15–25 and 29–39 variations in income inequality seem more closely correlated with mortality worldwide than do variations in material wealth. This relation is especially strong among the poorest countries in Africa. Mortality is higher for a given level of overall income in more unequal nations.

Conclusions: Income inequality seems to have an influence worldwide, especially for younger adults. Social inequality seems to have a universal negative impact on health. Humans are social animals and are not well constructed physiologically to survive in uncooperative surroundings—particularly during the prime of life.

Introduction

Many studies of the potential impact of inequalities in income on health outcomes have been undertaken in recent years.[1] Some have claimed that the apparent association between greater income inequality in a nation with higher mortality

---

[1] See references in footnotes 3, 6, 7, 8, 10 and 13 and also: Hales, S., Howden-Chapman, P., Salmond, C., Woodward, A. and Mackenbach, J. (1999) National infant mortality rates in relation to gross national product and distribution of income, *Lancet* 354, 2047; Lynch, J., Davey Smith, G., Harper, S. and Hillemeier, M. (2004) Is income inequality a determinant of population health? Part 2. US National and regional trends in income inequality and age- and cause-specific mortality. *Milbank Quarterly*, 82, 355-400; Chiang, T. (1999) Economic transition and changing relation between income inequality and mortality in Taiwan: regression analysis, *British Medical Journal*, 319, 1162-5; and Weatherby, N., Nam, C. and Isaac, L. (1983) Development, inequality, health care, and mortality at the older ages: a cross-national analysis, *Demography*, 20, 27-43.

may be an artefact,[2] but the weight of recent evidence has pointed towards it being a real effect.[3] In rich nations, the most prominent hypothesis is that the psychosocial stress of being in a relatively low position within a social and economic hierarchy leads to physiological harm.[4]

Most studies of this relation have focused on wealthier nations. In such nations, being among the poorest in society is usually no longer a situation adverse enough to threaten life directly through mechanisms such as malnutrition, poor sanitation, and poor shelter— as is often the case in poorer nations of the world. However, it has recently been suggested that the effect of social inequalities on health is important worldwide, not just in affluent nations.

If psychosocial stress is a key mechanism by which inequality is damaging to population health in affluent nations, we should expect the impact of inequality to vary over the life course.[5] This is because how we are viewed by our peers is thought to matter more at some ages than others. However, international studies of the effects of income inequality on mortality across the life course are rare. A study of 22 countries in the third wave of the Luxembourg income study (1989–92) found that the effect of income inequality was strong among infants but decreased with age and reversed for those older than 65.[6] Similarly, a study of 13 countries in the Organisation for Economic Cooperation and Development (OECD), using data from the 1970s to the early 1990s, found that the association between income inequality and mortality weakened after the age of 25.[7]

The age-specific relation between income inequality and mortality is well studied in the United States. The weight of evidence suggests that income inequality is a significant predictor of mortality among infants,[8] [9] but this relation is weaker or

[2] Wagstaff, A. and van Doorslaer, E. (2000) Income inequality and health: what does the literature tell us? *Annual Review of Public Health*, 21, 543-67.

[3] Ram, R. (2006) Further examination of the cross-country association between income inequality and population health, *Social Science and Medicine*, 62, 779-91.

[4] Marmot, M.G. (2004) *The status syndrome: how social standing affects our health and longevity*, London: Bloomsbury.

[5] Davey Smith, G. (2003) *Health inequalities: lifecourse approaches*, Bristol: The Policy Press.

[6] Lynch, J., Davey Smith, G., Hillemeier, M., Shaw, M., Raghunathan, T. and Kaplan, G. (2001) Income inequality, the psychosocial environment, and health: comparisons of wealthy nations, *Lancet*, 358, 194-200.

[7] McIsaac, S. and Wilkinson, R.G. (1997) Income distribution and cause-specific mortality, *European Journal of Public Health*, 7, 45-53.

[8] Kaplan, G.A., Pamuk, E.R., Lynch, J.W., Cohen, R.D. and Balfour, J.L. (1996) Inequality in income and mortality in the United States: analysis of mortality and potential pathways, *British Medical Journal*, 312, 999-1003; Lobmayer, P. and Wilkinson, R.G. (2002) Inequality, residential segregation by income, and mortality in US cities, *Journal of Epidemiology and Community Health*, 56, 183-7; Brodish, P.H., Massing, M. and Tyroler, H.A. (2000) Income inequality and all-cause mortality in the 100 counties of North Carolina, *Southern Medical Journal*, 93, 386-91; and Lynch, J.W., Kaplan, G.A., Pamuk, E.R., Cohen, R.D., Heck, K.E., Balfour, J.L. *et al.* (1998) Income inequality and mortality in metropolitan areas of the United States. *American Journal of Public Health*, 88, 1074-80.

[9] Duleep, H.O. (1995) Mortality and income inequality among economically developed countries. *Social Security Bulletin*, 58, 34-50.

disappears[10] among people older than about 65. In all age-specific studies, income inequality exerted the greatest influence on mortality at some point between the ages of 15 and 64 years. Thus, inequalities seem to be most damaging to health during working adult ages.

In this study we have explicitly examined variation by age in the relation between income inequality and mortality and, more importantly, have extended such analyses to countries not included in previous studies. This has been made possible through the use of recently released (and independently validated) secondary data which cover nations other than the richest that are members of the OECD. Thus, not only can we explore variation in the relation between income inequality and mortality by age, we can explore it in a truly global dataset.

Methods and data

We report results based on 126 countries for which complete data on income inequality and mortality by age and sex were available around the year 2002, and which include 94.4% of the world's population. We obtained the mortality data from the World Health Organization.[11] These data enable us to calculate mortality by age group (<1 year, 1–4, 5–9, and 5-year bands up to 95–99) and sex (see Table 32.1 for details). We used a consistent measure of wealth that is well known and available for most countries in the world—the log of gross domestic product (GDP) per capita adjusted to ensure purchasing power parity. We also used a widely published measure of inequality from the same United Nations Development Programme source—the Gini coefficient.[12] The mean and median (range) values for these two measures respectively are $9348 and $4955 ($521–$68,000), and 40.1 and 38.0 (24.4–70.7).

We treated whole countries as units in a natural experiment. This approach assumes that the nation state is the level at which the effects of material wealth and income inequality should be most apparent. The nation state is arguably the key unit of social, political, and economic systems which produce both wealth and inequality.[13] All countries were thus weighted equally in the results shown here. Results of analyses in which countries were weighted by population (not shown) did not differ greatly.

[10] Daly, M,C., Duncan, G.J., Kaplan, G.A. and Lynch, J.W. (1998) Macro-to-micro links in the relation between income inequality and mortality, *Milbank Quarterly*, 76, 303-4, 315-39; and Ross, N.A., Wolfson, M.C., Dunn, J.R., Berthelot, J.M., Kaplan, G.A. and Lynch, J.W. (2000) Relation between income inequality and mortality in Canada and in the United States: cross sectional assessment using census data and vital statistics, *British Medical Journal*, 320, 898-902.

[11] Lopez, A., Ahmad, O., Guillot, M., Inoue, M. and Ferguson, B. (2001) *Life tables for 191 countries for 2000: data, methods, results*. Geneva: World Health Organization (GPE discussion paper No 40).

[12] United Nations Development Programme (2004) Table 14 (Gini index of income inequality). In: *Human development report 2004*. Geneva: UNDP.

[13] Wilkinson, R.G. and Pickett, K.E. (2006) Income inequality and population health: a review and explanation of the evidence, *Social Science and Medicine*, 62, 1768-84.

Table 32.1: Summary statistics for annual mortality per 100,000 people worldwide by age and sex – global summary.

Sex and age (years)	Mortality per year per 100,000 people	
	Mean	Median (range)
Males		
<1 year old	5608	3147 (304-30 093)
1-4	446	187 (12-2819)
5-9	126	60 (7-798)
10-14	82	58 (11-368)
15-19	150	131 (29-465)
20-24	309	220 (67-1281)
25-29	491	241 (58-3098)
30-34	703	304 (71-5229)
35-39	824	395 (95-5723)
40-44	947	541 (148-5545)
45-49	1141	787 (236-5150)
50-54	1407	1153 (375-4507)
55-59	1865	1740 (613-3865)
60-64	2648	2653 (1023-4780)
65-69	3908	4018 (1759-6553)
70-74	5890	5942 (2839-9828)
75-79	8835	9000 (4524-13 322)
80-84	13632	13757 (7624-22 229)
85-89	20448	21269 (11 580-34 015)
90-94	29702	30948 (16 875-47 586)
95-99	41839	43264 (24 675-60 000)
Females		
<1 year old	4759	2575 (246-23 775)
1-4	475	168 (10-3201)
5-9	120	50 (4-831)
10-14	79	39 (8-496)
15-19	167	65 (16-872)
20-24	337	87 (22-2615)
25-29	516	106 (24-4753)
30-34	626	129 (26-5966)
35-39	607	186 (60-5059)
40-44	615	277 (90-4170)
45-49	659	426 (144-3117)
50-54	826	632 (221-2729)
55-59	1134	928 (306-2712)
60-64	1625	1491 (460-3213)
65-69	2580	2371 (745-4860)
70-74	4160	4026 (1234-7665)
75-79	6677	6643 (2248-10 670)
80-84	10856	11369 (4307-15 644)
85-89	17138	18112 (7986-25 757)
90-94	26076	27680 (13 722-41 719)
95-99	38176	40043 (21 620-58 196)

Source: Calculated by authors from data provided by: Lopez, A., Ahmad, O., Guillot, M., Inoue, M. and Ferguson, B. (2000) *Life tables for 191 countries for 2000: Data, methods, results*. Geneva: World Health Organization, 2001. (GPE discussion paper No 40).

Statistical analysis

We modelled the extent to which relations between health and income, and between health and income inequality seemed to vary across each of the age bands. We used linear regression to measure the association between mortality as the dependent variable and log of adjusted gross domestic product per capita as the independent predictor. We took a similar approach for the Gini coefficient.

We compared the predictive power of each of the independent variables by means of standardised coefficients for each variable, derived from each separate age-group model. These regression coefficients are those obtained by first standardising all variables to have a mean of 0 and a standard deviation of 1. We used Stata v9.2 to run the models. We also performed a two-tailed test and found with $p < 0.05$ support for the hypothesis that the coefficients varied with age.

Sensitivity analyses

Many facets of modelling can have a significant effect on the outcome—such as the weighting used, the countries included, dates to which data refer, whether to control for other aspects of the nature of societies; whether to treat all national societies as separate entities; and the source of inequality measure used. We therefore undertook extensive sensitivity analyses, and ran models to include an extra 70 or so countries without complete data, using estimates to fill the gaps. These countries tend to have small populations and contain only about 5% of the world population. We also tested alternative measures of income inequality,[14] weighting each country for population size, and examined each continent independently.

Results

Figures 32.1 and 32.2 show the strength of the relation between each variable and age-specific mortality for both sexes combined (a larger coefficient indicates a stronger relation). A statistical test that the coefficients varied with age suggested that the correlation with the standardised Gini coefficient was −0.559 ($p < 0.01$), but the relation between age and log of income coefficients was not significant (0.334, $p > 0.05$). We find that income inequality had the greatest influence on mortality between the ages of 15 and 29 in OECD countries (Figure 32.1), and between the ages of 25 and 39 worldwide (Figure 32.2). The strength of the worldwide relation was reduced when we omitted countries in Africa (results not shown). The worldwide result is thus partly a product of processes operating most strongly in this continent, not simply a reflection of those operating within OECD countries.

The figures suggest that the strength of the association of inequality with mortality varies inversely with that for the association of affluence with mortality— that is,

---

[14] Babones, S.J. (2005) The country-level income structure of the world economy, *Journal of World Systems Research*, XI(1):29-58 (http://jwsr.ucr. edu/archive/vol11/number1/index.php?art3=&).

as inequality reaches its maximum influence, affluence reaches its minimum. This is a new finding which may have important implications for debates on the likely causal mechanisms.

Figure 32.1: Association of income inequality and affluence with mortality in the 30 countries of the OECD, around the year 2000.

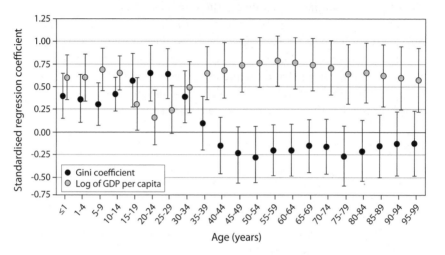

Note: Income inequality measured as the Gini coefficient, and affluence as the log of gross domestic product (GDP) per capita adjusted to ensure purchasing power parity. A higher regression coefficient indicates a closer correlation with mortality rates of either log GDP or Gini at those particular ages. Only data for 30 affluent countries are used here and GDP alone only comes to have a significantly greater effect than inequality after age 40. A higher correlation implies that the possible link is stronger, and that the influence of the factor is greater at those ages.

Source: Calculated by authors from data provided by: Lopez, A , Ahmad, O., Guillot, M., Inoue, M. and Ferguson, B. (2001) *Life tables for 191 countries for 2000: data, methods, results.* Geneva: World Health Organization (GPE discussion paper No 40) and United Nations Development Programme. Table 14 (Gini index of income inequality). In: *Human development report 2004.* Geneva: UNDP, 2004.

Secondary analyses

We obtained similar results when we studied the two sexes separately (results not shown). Inequality seemed to matter slightly more for males than females, but the shape and nature of the associations with age were not fundamentally altered. Similarly, the factors included in our sensitivity analyses had little impact on the results. A further concern that we were not able to address was the effect of using only nation-state data (Figure 32.3). If it were possible to use data on subdivisions of India and China, say, rather than treating those countries as two homogeneous observations, that might well be worthwhile.

Figure 32.2: Association of income inequality and affluence with mortality in all countries worldwide, around the year 2000.

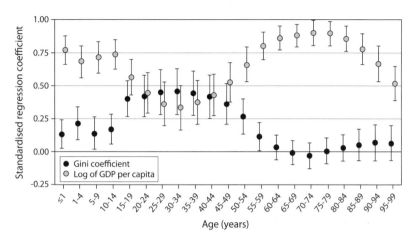

Note: Income inequality measured as the Gini coefficient, and affluence as the log of gross domestic product (GDP) per capita adjusted to ensure purchasing power parity. A higher regression coefficient indicates a closer correlation with mortality rates of either log GDP or Gini at those particular ages. Data for almost 200 countries are used here and GDP is seen to matter more at younger and older ages, but even with so many poor countries included inequality has a clear influence between ages 15 and 50.

Source: Calculated by authors from data provided by: Lopez, A., Ahmad, O., Guillot, M., Inoue, M., Ferguson, B. (2001) Life tables for 191 countries for 2000: data, methods, results. Geneva: World Health Organization, (GPE discussion paper No 40) and United Nations Development Programme. Table 14 (Gini index of income inequality). In: *Human development report 2004*. Geneva: UNDP, 2004.

Figure 32.3: The world's countries shaped with area in proportion to the number of people living on ≤$10 a day, 2002.

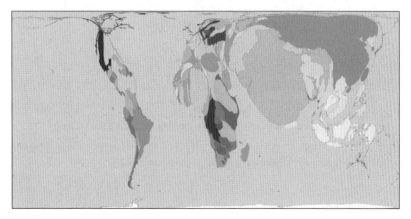

Note: In 2002, some 3.5 billion people, then more than half the world population, survived on the equivalent, or less, of what $10 in the United States of America would buy a day.

Source: From Worldmapper, www.worldmapper.org/display.php?selected=153.

305

Discussion

Our results prompt a series of hypotheses that we think are worth further investigation. Firstly, that the much disputed impact of income inequality on health is real, but that, because the impact varies with age, studies that have not accounted for this can show wide variation in the association of inequality with population health. Future studies should consider outcomes for different age groups.

Secondly, there is an age-related mechanism that results in higher mortality being experienced in societies where there is greater social competition, all else being equal. Higher rates of income inequality tend to reflect more competitive rather than more cooperative societies. Whatever the mechanism that results in harm from competition (or protection from cooperation), it has its strongest effects in early to middle adulthood.

Thirdly, in the nations with the lowest child and infant mortality, the importance of income inequalities will often be most obvious. This might be why the influence of income inequalities has been found most strongly in studies of all-age mortality in OECD countries (Figure 32.4).

Figure 32.4: The world's countries shaped with area in proportion to the gross domestic product per capita of people adjusted for purchasing power parity, 2002.

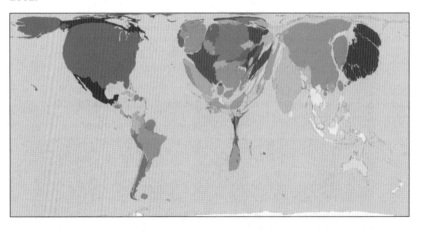

Note: In 2002 roughly $50 trillion was 'earned' a year worldwide, $7800 per person, or $21 on average a day, as measured in dollars given what a dollar then bought in the United States of America.

Source: Worldmapper, www.worldmapper.org/display.php?selected=170.

Fourthly, given the importance of African countries in providing evidence of a relation between inequality and mortality worldwide, high mortality from AIDS, armed conflict, and other causes common in more unequal and very poor countries might be a factor in explaining the observed relation.

Lastly, social inequalities as reflected through unequal incomes are damaging to health for those living in both rich and poor nations and the direct mechanisms for such damage are likely to vary by area (Figure 32.5). Psychosocial stress is unlikely to be the only route by which income inequality damages health. However, the underlying mechanism may be similar—that, because humans are social animals, human health is best protected when people cooperate.

Figure 32.5: The world's countries shaped with area in proportion to the deaths of adults aged 25–29 years inclusive, 2001.

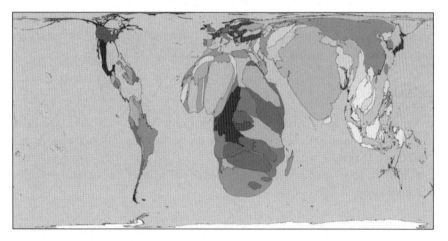

see colour version in plate section

[Editorial Note: Some 1.5 million adults of these ages die every year. The original version of this figure had shown the map for children aged 1 to 4, but that map was shown earlier in this book as Figure 31.2 on p 291 of Chapter 31, so an older age group is shown here.]

Source: Worldmapper, www.worldmapper.org/display_extra.php?selected=535.

Our finding that, as inequality reaches its maximum influence on mortality, affluence reaches its minimum influence may have important implications for debates on the likely causal mechanisms. Although some hypotheses are consistent with this finding, others would predict the opposite. It may well be the case, for example, that greater equality mitigates the need for greater affluence to be present for health to improve (as reflected in lower mortality).

Future research

More detailed studies are needed to consider mortality and psychological morbidity by age and sex in relation to social inequalities between people. Furthermore, time trends should be studied where possible. Do changes in mortality and morbidity over time correlate well at particular ages with increases or decreases in social (reflected by income) inequality for particular age cohorts and not for others? Patterns in the prevalence of mortality by cause, age, and sex should be studied to infer the possible biological processes at play and the extent to which external injuries and accidents are particularly important. Lastly, the possible protective effects of old age and of young age (if not actual infancy) need to be further studied to ascertain why no strong relation is observed between income inequalities and mortality at these ages.

It has been argued that estimates of the potential impact on mortality of a narrowing of inequalities are useful in promoting policies to preserve life. This has been attempted in countries where a great deal of detailed evidence has been amassed.[15] Such data are not available worldwide. Our exploratory analysis found that the simplest of models suggest that, at the most affected ages, up to a quarter of deaths might be avoided were the most unequal of countries to become more equal. However, such simple models may well overestimate or underestimate the benefits of improved equality in the complexity of the real world.

Conclusion

Income inequality is associated with higher mortality levels in all nations worldwide, not just affluent ones, but the effects are more pronounced at different ages. Although the direct mechanisms that operate are likely to be different between different countries, there does not seem to be a beneficial impact of social inequality on health anywhere.

[15] Mitchell, R., Dorling, D. and Shaw, M. (2000) *Inequalities in life and death: what if Britain were more equal?*, Bristol and York: Joseph Rowntree Foundation.

33

Wars, massacres and atrocities of the 20th century

Dorling, D. and Coles, P. (2009) 'Featured graphic: wars, massacres, and atrocities of the 20th century', *Environment and Planning A*, vol 41, no 8, pp 1779-80.

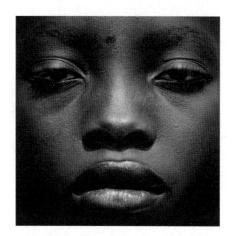

In Figure 33.1, measured by the scale shown to the left, the heights of the twelve stacked histograms depict how many millions of people were killed each year in selected wars, massacres, and atrocities worldwide 1900–1995. From the 1930s to the 1980s a year in which less than a million people were slaughtered was uncommon.

To the right, the stacked shaded bars show a cumulative estimate of the deaths attributable to war, decade by decade, as recorded from 1960 onwards. They counter any illusion of a tapering off that the histograms might suggest. By the end of the century atrocities were taking place in far more countries, involving far more wars, than the twelve groups individually identified here.

The 20th century began with orchestrated massacres in Africa, where Europeans first practised the genocide they later carried out at home (Goldberg, 2009). The mid-century was dominated by wartime killing, and the Soviet and Chinese atrocities that also took place both under the fog of world war, and later under the threat of nuclear war. The century ended with half the worldwide war-deaths since 1960 having been suffered in Africa. Table 33.1 shows where risk of death from war has been highest since 1945.

Reference

Goldberg, D.T. (2009) *The threat of race: Reflections on racial neoliberalism*, Oxford: Wiley-Blackwell.

Figure 33.1: Wars, massacres and atrocities of the 20th century.

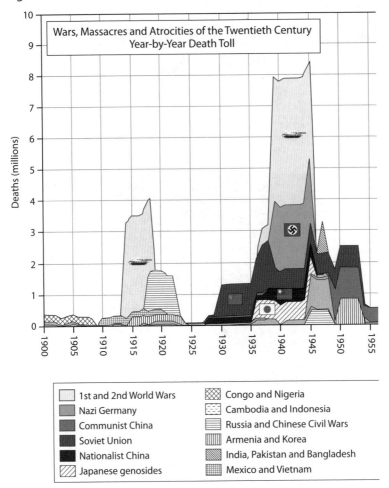

Table 33.1: Highest proportion of people killed by war, whole population, 1945–2000.

Rank	Country	Value*
1	Cambodia	16.1
2	Timor - Leste	14.4
3	Angola	12.9
4	Rwanda	10.3
5	Democratic People's Republic of Korea	10.0
6	Afghanistan	8.7
7	Sudan	8.4
8	Burundi	7.6
9	Democratic Republic of Congo	5.9
10	Mozambique	5.0

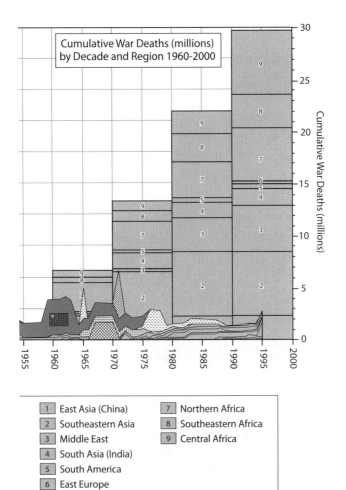

Cumulative War Deaths (millions) by Decade and Region 1960-2000

Cumulative War Deaths (millions)

1	East Asia (China)	7	Northern Africa
2	Southeastern Asia	8	Southeastern Africa
3	Middle East	9	Central Africa
4	South Asia (India)		
5	South America		
6	East Europe		

Sources of data: Redrawn from Matthew White's Historical Atlas of the 20th Century web pages (http://users.erols.com/mwhite28/) with cumulative war death estimates made from many sources documented at www.worldmapper.org (see map 287, technical notes).

11	Republic of Korea	4.7
12	Vietnam	4.7
13	Iraq	4.6
14	Western Sahara	4.4
15	Lebanon	3.7
16	Algeria	3.5
17	Liberia	3.1
18	Uganda	2.8
19	Congo	2.8
20	Somalia	2.7

*War deaths 1945–2000 as percentage of population 2000.

Source: Worldmapper, www.worldmapper.org (Map 287).

34

Re-evaluating self-evaluation: a commentary on Jen, Jones and Johnston[1]

Barford, A., Dorling, D. and Pickett, K. (2010) 'Re-evaluating self-evaluation. A commentary on Jen, Jones, and Johnston', *Social Science & Medicine* (2010) vol 70, pp 496-7.

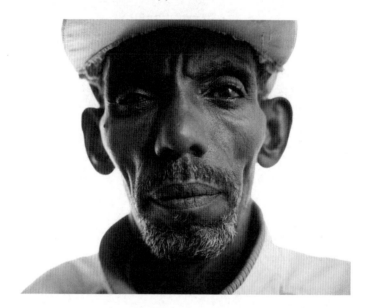

Introduction

In a paper recently published in *Social Science & Medicine*, "Global variations in health: Evaluating Wilkinson's income inequality hypothesis using the World Values Survey', and one in another journal, Jen, Jones and Johnston provided analyses of self-rated health, using data from the World Values Survey (Jen, Jones and Johnston, 2009a, 2009b). They showed that income is significantly associated with self-rated health; higher incomes being related to better health. Although they found that self-rated health varied between countries, they did not find an independent effect of income inequality on self-rated health. The authors concluded that their analyses provided a test, and refutation, of what they described as the 'Wilkinson hypothesis'.

Briefly stated, the 'Wilkinson hypothesis' is that population health in rich countries tends to be better in societies where income is more equally distributed. There are now more than 200 analyses of the nature of this relationship, and reviews of these

---

[1] Editorial Note: For an earlier related article see Chapter 22, this volume.

studies have come to conflicting interpretations of the evidence, with researchers disagreeing over methodological issues, such as the scale at which inequality is measured, whether or not various control variables should be interpreted as confounders or mediators, and the appropriateness of various statistical models (Lynch *et al.*, 2004, Macinko *et al.*, 2003, Subramanian and Kawachi, 2004, Wilkinson and Pickett, 2006).

In the context of this controversy[2], do Jen *et al*'s (2009a, 2009b) analyses put a final nail in the coffin of the 'Wilkinson hypothesis'? In this paper, we consider the relationship between 'health' (the outcome in the Wilkinson hypothesises to be affected by income inequality) and 'self-rated health' (the outcome analysed by Jen and colleagues). We argue that 'health' and 'self-rated health' cannot always be assumed to be proxies for one another. We also suggest that if, as Jen *et al.* find, average levels of self-rated health tend to be higher in more unequal societies, that this has something to tell us about the psychosocial effects of living in unequal societies (see Figure 34.1)[3].

Rating our health

What are we actually measuring, when we ask people to rate their own health? Self-rated health might reflect a 'spontaneous assessment', which incorporates many elements of a person's health into an overall or global statement about health status. Alternatively self-rated health might be thought of as reflecting a person's 'enduring self-concept' which remains stable over time, often with independence from changes in health (Bailis, Segall and Chipperfield, 2003, pp 205–207). The data on self-rated health collected in the World Values Survey fits into the first typology, a global assessment of health that amalgamates all aspects of one's health into a single statement. The question to which respondents replied was:

> '*All in all, how would you describe your state of health these days? Would you say it is excellent, very good, good, fair, poor or don't know?*' (Jen *et al.*, 2009b, p 645)

In a review of 27 studies, Idler and Benyamini (1997) found that self-rated health was generally predictive of mortality (Idler and Benyamini, 1997, Table 1 and p 34), this paper is referenced by Jen *et al.* to support their use of self-rated health as a measure of actual health (Jen *et al.*, 2009a, 2009b). Only one of the 27 papers reviewed by Idler and Benyamini was a cross-country study – which included the cities of Kaunas in Lithuania and Rotterdam in the Netherlands; all the others were national or sub-national studies. Self-rated health measures within a single country might

---

[2] Editorial Note: See Chapter 22, footnote 2, on p 225, for the controversy. As far as I know this particular argument ended here.
[3] Editorial Note: Figure 34.1 has been added to this chapter to help illustrate the generally well-established relationship between income inequality (variously measured) and poor mental health (as measured by the World Health Organisation and work of a similar standing for samples of national populations).

Figure 34.1: Prevalence of mental illness by income share of best-off 1% and by quintile income ratio.

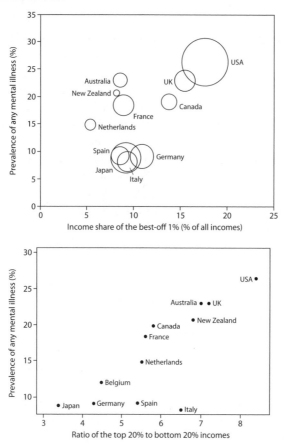

Note: Areas shown in proportion to population. The mental health data are from The World Health Organisation (WHO) except for Australia, the UK and Canada for which national surveys have been used. The figures are for prevalence of any mental illness in the previous 12 months, adults, 2001-3, Demyttenaere, K., *et al.* (2004) , Prevalence, severity, and unmet need for treatment of mental disorders in the World Health Organization World Mental Health Surveys. *JAMA*,291(21): pp 2581-90.
Wells, J.E., *et al.* (2006), Te Rau Hinengaro: the New Zealand Mental Health Survey: overview of methods and findings. *Aust NZ J Psychiatry* 40(10): pp 835-44. Office for National Statistics (2001) Psychiatric morbidity among adults living in private households, 2000. HMSO: London.
Australian Bureau of Statistics (2003), National Health Survey, Mental Health, 2001. Australian Bureau of Statistics: Canberra. WHO International Consortium in Psychiatric Epidemiology (2000) Cross-national comparisons of the prevalences and correlates of mental disorders. *Bulletin World Health Organisation*, 78(4): pp 413-26.

Source: Wilkinson, R.G. and Pickett, K.E. (2007) The problems of relative deprivation: Why some societies do better than others, *Social Science and Medicine*, 65, 9, 1965-1978. Inequality data from the Paris School's World Top Incomes Database: http://g-mond.parisschoolofeconomics.eu/topincomes/ (excluding Tanzinia where only data to 1970 were included). Note all 11 countries for which there are data are included (12 countries for the lower diagram).

be reasonably assumed to be unaffected by factors that might affect cross-country measures, such as cultural, institutional and political heterogeneity.

International differences in self-rated health

Jen *et al.* found that self-rated health is better in more unequal countries, despite the fact that numerous studies find that life expectancy is lower in more unequal countries. If self-rated health is not correlated with actual health in a cross-country comparison, then how can we interpret the measure of self-reported health? Jen *et al.* acknowledge the possibility that responses are 'cultural constructs' rather than true reflections of health, but argue that compromises to validity and reliability of responses due to the cross-cultural nature of this research have been reduced through careful survey design (Jen *et al.*, 2009b, p 645).

Studies show that people's ratings of their health are affected by social position, choice of referent group and gender (Idler and Benyamini, 1997, p 26). Is it possible that the level of inequality within a society has a direct impact on the way in which people perceive and report their health? If relative social position is an important influence on self-rated health, then in more equal societies, fewer people occupy extreme positions in the social hierarchy and each person's frame of reference for comparing their health to other people's is likely to be wider/include more people (see Figure 34.2).[4]

It also seems plausible that in more unequal societies, which are characterized by more status competition, people may more frequently and obviously need to reassure themselves of their strength and wellbeing and their potential to succeed. Asserting that one has excellent or very good health might be part of maintaining one's self-image. A Nepalese saying, which probably works better in English than in Nepali, is that 'health is wealth'. The connection between health and wealth is, of course, bi-directional. If you are healthy you can work, and if you are wealthy you can afford a healthier lifestyle.

An alternative, and equally plausible explanation, might be that people in more equal societies are less inclined to rate themselves at the top of a scale. Perhaps growing up in a more egalitarian society, where the quality of social relationships between people is better, means that people are less likely to label themselves as 'the best' or 'excellent'. Among the countries included in Jen *et al*'s analyses (Jen *et al.*, 2009a, 2009b), Japan had the lowest level of self-rated health, but it has the highest life expectancy among rich developed countries. In Japan, it is much less common to report that one is happy than in the United States, where it is expected that people at least say they are happy (Ballas, 2006). Cross-country comparisons of happiness are widely believed to be affected by cultural differences in expressing

---

[4] Editorial Note: Figure 34.2 has been added to this chapter to help illustrate the very close relationship between the share of income held by the top 1% of earners in a country and overall inequality in each country as reported by the Gini statistic (these both can be compared to quintile ratios in Figure 34.1).

Figure 34.2: Income share of best-off 1% and overall income inequality (Gini coefficient), all countries included in both source datasets.

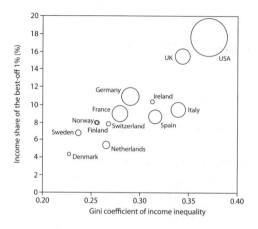

Gini	1%	Country (survey date)
0.37	18	United States (2008)
0.34	15	United Kingdom (2007)
0.29	11	Germany (1998)
0.31	10	Ireland (2000)
0.34	9	Italy (2009)
0.28	9	France (2006)
0.32	9	Spain (2008)
0.26	8	Norway (2008)
0.26	8	Finland (2002)
0.27	8	Switzerland (1995)
0.24	7	Sweden (2009)
0.27	5	Netherlands (1999)
0.23	4	Denmark (2005)

Note: Area of circles is drawn in proportion to population.

Source: World top income database (Paris), and Luxembourg income data study statistics as of June 2012. Note that Japan is not included in the Luxembourg data study.

happiness, and the same cultural influences seem to be affecting how people express their feelings of health.

Interpretation and inference

Jen *et al.*'s (2009a, 2009b) studies of income inequality, income and self-rated health have produced more intriguing questions than answers. Instead of being a test of the 'Wilkinson hypothesis' they suggest new hypotheses and rich possibilities for future research on the influence of status hierarchies on self-perception.

References

Bailis, D.S., Segall, A., and Chipperfield, J. G. (2003) Two views of self-rated general health status, *Social Science & Medicine*, 56, 203–217.

Ballas, D. (2006) Geography, economics and happiness, World Universities Network – Horizons in Human Geography series, Virtual seminar: Bristol, Leeds, Manchester, Sheffield, Southampton, Madison–Wisconsin, Illinois–Urbana Champaign, Penn State, Oslo.

Idler, E.L. and Benyamini, Y. (1997) Self-rated health and mortality: a review of twenty-seven community studies. *Journal of Health and Social Behaviour*, 38, 21–37.

Jen, M.H., Jones, K. and Johnston, R. (2009a) Compositional and contextual approaches to the study of health behaviour and outcomes: using multi-level modelling to evaluate Wilkinson's income inequality hypothesis. *Health and Place*, 15, 198–203.

Jen, M.H., Jones, K. and Johnston, R. (2009b) Global variations in health: evaluating Wilkinson's income inequality hypothesis using the world values survey. *Social Science & Medicine*, 68, 643–53.

Lynch, J., Davey Smith, G., Harper, S., Hillemeier, M., Ross, N., Kaplan, G.A., *et al.* (2004). Is income inequality a determinant of population health? Part 1: A systematic review, *Milbank Quarterly*, 82(1), 5–99.

Macinko, J.A., Shi, L., Starfield, B. and Wulu, J. T., Jr. (2003) Income inequality and health: a critical review of the literature, *Medical Care Research and Review*, 60, 407–52.

Subramanian, S.V. and Kawachi, I. (2004) Income inequality and health: what have we learned so far? *Epidemiologic Reviews*, 26, 78–91.

Wilkinson, R.G. and Pickett, K.E. (2006) Income inequality and population health: a review and explanation of the evidence, *Social Science & Medicine*, 62, 1768–84.

35

America's debt to the world[1]

Hennig, B.D. and Dorling, D. (2011) 'In focus: America's debt to the world', *Political Insight*, vol 2, no 3, p 34.

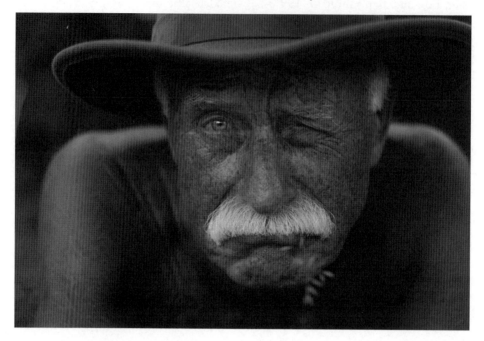

The ongoing global financial crisis gained new momentum in early August [2011]. As Europe struggled to find a sustainable solution for its debt crisis, a downgrade in the US credit rating pre-empted a worldwide slump in stock markets.

But the current American debt level did not appear overnight. It started piling up long ago, as a look at the development of US amassed debt over the last decade reveals: today, the total national debt of the United States is $14.3 trillion, up from $5.8 trillion in 2001. Particularly interesting for global markets is the external debt that America owes to foreign holders outside the country; George W. Bush took over approximately $1 trillion in foreign debt from the Clinton administration (Bill Clinton managed to reduce national debt levels in his second term). After a short period in which this downward trend continued, foreign US debt started to rise after September 2001. In 2009, George W. Bush handed over more than $3 trillion of national debt to Barack Obama. There has been a considerable trend upwards

---

[1] This article was jointly written in collaboration with Ben Hennig for the back cover of the journal.

since the financial crisis hit the nation in 2008. Only recently has this upward trend started to level off slightly, and US foreign debt is now just below $4.5 trillion.

Figure 35.1: Map of the world with countries resized according to the total amount of US treasury securities that were held in each place, July 2011.

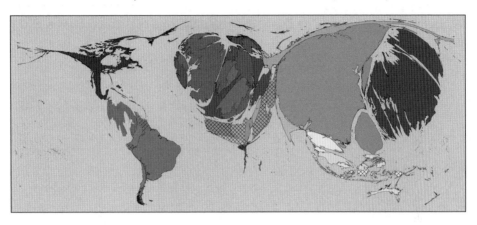

see colour version in plate section

Source: Figures published by the US Treasury. Map created by Ben Hennig. See text for why some parts are dotted and some shaded with a criss-cross pattern.

Looking at the distribution of US debt (Figure 35.1) provides interesting insights into the complex interdependencies that developed over almost a decade of increasing external liabilities. China is the largest single holder of foreign US debt, with $1,159.8 billion, but the total liabilities are much larger and more spread around the globe. Despite itself being in great debt, Japan comes second in the ranks of US creditors with $912.4 billion. A considerable amount of credit has been extended to the US by some of the other highly indebted economies such as the United Kingdom (the European country with the largest external debt) with $346.5 billion.

Looking at this complex cobweb of debt emanating from the world's – still – largest economy, it is not hard to imagine that the other large economies have equally diverse interdependencies of their own (very high) foreign liabilities, making one wonder how long this system can continue to work without considerable adjustments. The political world has already started to change because of this new and emerging picture: China increasingly finds a political voice, its leaders' official publications giving bold advice and seeing the crisis as removing its possible last obstacle of being the world's new superpower. The changing economic world may be slowly leading us towards a new political world order. Figure 35.1 shows the countries of the world resized according to the total amount of US treasury securities that are held in each country as of July 2011 and as published by the US Treasury.

All countries holding less than $12.3 billion (which equals Australia's share as the smallest single country included in the data) are not included in Figure 35.1. Their securities are $202.5 billion, less than 4.5% of the total foreign debt in total. Furthermore, foreign liabilities for some countries are only published as a merged single figure. These are the oil-exporting nations (Ecuador, Venezuela, Indonesia, Bahrain, Iran, Iraq, Kuwait, Oman, Qatar, Saudi Arabia, the United Arab Emirates, Algeria, Gabon, Libya and Nigeria) and the Caribbean banking centres (Bahamas, Bermuda, Cayman Islands, Netherlands Antilles, Panama and the British Virgin Islands). For both categories the respective countries were merged and treated as one homogeneous region in the map transformation. The distribution of US debt within those countries may therefore differ slightly from the representation in the map. The regions are marked on [the colour plate of] the map with the red and yellow outlines and the crisscross/dotted pattern [the colour version is shown on p 9 in the plate section].

SECTION VI
Thinking, drawing and counting

36

It's the way that you do it[1]

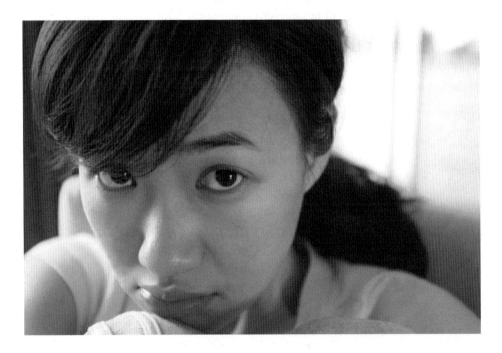

In studying inequalities in health it is not always what you do but how, when and where you do it that matters. The maps first published in 2007 in the paper reproduced as Chapter 37 remain a particularly effective way of showing who has most and who has least around the world, but there are many things that such depictions miss. For example, when a country has a relatively small population, as in the case of Singapore, and when it appears to be doing very well, when its population appear to enjoy very good health and what looks like adequate health spending, then it is easy to decide to ignore it and concentrate more on where things are obviously going wrong.

Preventing infant mortality

Singapore doesn't feature in the map of early neonatal deaths shown in Figure 37.4 (Chapter 37) as its rate of early neonatal mortality is so low. The rate used is taken from Table 36.1. This suggests that people in Singapore enjoy the lowest rate of such

---

[1] Apologies for borrowing from the lyrics of Bananarama and the Fun Boy Three's 'It ain't what you do (it's the way that you do it)', from 1982 although they were, in turn, covering Oliver and Young's 1939 calypso song and it is sung to an old tune.

suffering in the world, ranking top, along with Japan. But before celebrating this 'fact', consider the denominator. Who were the 'people' being measured?

Japan and Singapore are jointly ranked first among 200 countries as having had the lowest recorded early neonatal mortality rate in the world in 2000. While this is not surprising in the case of Japan, given what else is known about that country, it is odd that in Singapore, a country with a much lower overall life expectancy than

Table 36.1: Deaths in the first week of life per 1,000 live births, highest and lowest rates by country, 2000.

Rank	Territory	Value
1	Mauritania	52
2	Liberia	48
3	Iraq	46
4	Afghanistan	45
5	Cote d'Ivoire	44
6	Sierra Leone	42
7	Nigeria	40
7	Mali	40
7	Angola	40
10	Pakistan	38
185	France	2
185	Germany	2
185	Rep. of Korea	2
185	Italy	2
185	Spain	2
185	Belgium	2
185	Sweden	2
185	Czech Republic	2
199	Singapore	1
199	Japan	1

Note: Fourteen territories reported two early neonatal deaths per 1,000 live births (Austria, Norway, Finland, Iceland, Monaco and San Marino are not shown); four reported 38 deaths per 1,000 births (Ethiopia, Guinea and the Central African Republic are not shown). Those with the most births are shown in the top 10 and bottom 10 on the Worldmapper website, map 250 (early neonatal deaths). Because of the tie, the two lowest-ranking countries are given rank 199. For more details see: www.worldmapper.org/posters/worldmapper_map260_ver5.pdf

Japan, and very high income and wealth inequality, infant health should appear to be so good. In 2009, for every 1,000 infants born alive in Singapore, only two died before their first birthday.[2] Singapore reports the lowest rate of infant mortality in the world today. To begin to discover why Singapore appears to do so well, you have to delve beneath the headline statistics. The key is to look at the denominator, what the rate is calculated as a proportion of. Here the denominator is 'live births'. If a birth never occurs then it is not included in the statistics, but not all the women living in Singapore are free to give birth in Singapore.

Some of the poorest people in Singapore are the maids. These are the servants who work for around one in five of all middle-class households. They act as personal cleaners, shoppers and childcarers. Most are guestworkers. They are not citizens but come from abroad, and as guestworkers they have no right to remain in Singapore. In more economically unequal countries, like Singapore, the poor tend to have fewer legal rights. Every six months these maids must take a pregnancy test; if they are found to be pregnant, they are deported.

Maid employer's nightmare – Asia One News, Tuesday, 23 December 2008

(verbatim)

Under Singapore law, if a maid gets pregnant, she will get repatriated immediately or employers stand to lose their $5,000 security deposit.

However, for Madam W.L. Lim's maid (Nina), regular medical tests failed to indicate her pregnancy and eventually she gave birth to a premature baby boy.

In the local newspaper report, Madam Lim was shocked when she was rang [sic] up by the police who told her Nina just gave birth. It did not occur to her that this is possible given that the doctor cleared her tests just two months ago. But nothing prepared her for the size of the hospital bill.

The sizeable bill of $5,500 for her maid's Caesarean delivery on Dec 11, ballooned to $67,000 for the hospitalisation of Nina's 27-week old premature baby boy, now warded at the KK Women's and Children's Hospital (KKH) Intensive Care Unit.

It was like a maid employer's nightmare come true. According to Dr Juliana Abu-Wong, a gynaecologist and obstetrician with more than 10 years' experience, the pregnancy tests currently administered comprise a urine check and an abdominal examination which are 90 to 95 per cent accurate. "So how is it that the doctor failed to detect my maid was four months pregnant?" Madam Lim questioned.

A blood test for pregnancy would have been more accurate. Blood testing is not made mandatory to keep costs down for employers. But to Madam Lim, this added cost is a small price to pay to avert the 'stress' now brought about by Nina's birth.

---

[2] In 2002 it was three per 1,000, on a par with Iceland, Sweden and Japan.

In Madam Lim's defense, lawyer Mr Mark Goh said that the undertaking was signed by Nina's friend Ms Shushma, a maid. "Though the rules require the employer to bear the full cost of the maid's medical care, nowhere does it say the employer should bear the medical cost of her kin," said Mr Goh.

The hospital's stance is clear as it will not pursue Ms Shushma for payment.

Said Mr Johnny Quah, KKH's chief financial officer, "Part of the admission process includes financial counselling. As the staff was unable to contact Nina's employer, she explained the estimated charges to Nina's friend and the signature obtained was more as an indication that she understood the charges and would convey it to Nina's employer."

Source: www.asiaone.com/News/AsiaOne%2BNews/Singapore/Story/A1Story20081223-110002.html

In total, migrant workers make up about a quarter of the population of Singapore and are mainly at the bottom of the income range, where you would expect infant mortality to be highest. This section of the population is effectively removed from the picture by deportation and the threat of it.[3] Poorer women trying very hard not to become pregnant are one way in which infant mortality can be reduced. Those babies who would have a greater chance of dying are never actually born (or are born abroad and count as a death abroad if they die). This is the reason IMRs in Singapore are so low, but for every baby that statistically would die, at least another hundred that would live are not brought into the world, against the choice that these women may have made were they free to do so.

There is some good news. In March 2012 it was announced that there was a plan in place to try to at least allow the 200,000 domestic workers of Singapore a few hours off work a week. This could be the start of the long slow process that would eventually, after many more apparently minor and then more major victories are won, see their human rights to pregnancy and medical care begin to be recognised. Currently 88 per cent of the maids in Singapore are forced to work seven days a week (Hodal, 2012). Their pay ranges from between 20p and 60p an hour in a country where, by 2010, average (mean) GDP per capita was over US$40,000 (Google, 2012). The arithmetic average income means very little in a very unequal country just as do, as it turns out, the apparently extremely low IMRs. It is no wonder Singapore does not boast about this apparent achievement.

Statistics such as a national average cannot be taken at face value. Chapter 38 considers how statistics can be used to describe and explore data in general. It contains some warnings but none as dark as that just given about why Singapore now reports the lowest infant mortality statistics in the world. It contains the two

---

[3] Around 100 of the maids are deported a year (out of a total of 196,000 in 2000. It is likely that more leave without being deported and thousands more avoid becoming pregnant or have abortions to avoid deportation. 'Some others ask friends or relatives back home to mail them abortion-inducing drugs ahead of their half-yearly checkups, said one maid agency' (HanQing, 2010).

classic equations for estimating confidence limits around a mortality rate, but before applying them you need to be sure that the rate was not being manipulated by deportation and the threat of deportation or other forms of intimidation. You need to be wary when looking at any health or related social statistics.

Reducing unemployment

Consider the case of unemployment and health in Britain. It is generally well known among health researchers that mortality rates tend to roughly double among people who are unemployed and that compulsory youth training schemes could be *'almost as detrimental to psychological good health as unemployment itself'* (Dorling, 2012, p 244). So we should expect a reduction in general improvement in health as unemployment rises following the onset of a recession. But what if the rise in unemployment is artificially curtailed?

Figure 36.1 compares the magnitude of the major recessions that have hit the UK in the period following the 1929 crash. It shows the current recession to have been almost as deep and now certainly lasting longer than all the others that preceded it. There are no comparable figures for before 1929. In fact it is debatable, given that national accounts were only devised post–Second World War, whether the 1930s monthly estimates can be that reliable. Nevertheless, bar a little uncertainty, the current 'great recession' has been a more prolonged recession than even the depression of

Figure 36.1: Comparison of the five major UK recessions/depressions, 1930–2012.

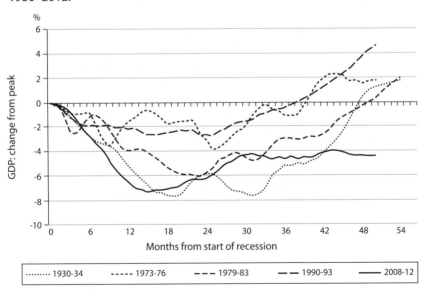

Source: National Institute of Economic and Social Research. Monthly GDP estimates, found here as of April 2012: www.niesr.ac.uk/gdp/GDPestimates.php

the early 1930s. So why has unemployment not yet surpassed the levels it reached in the 1930s?

At the start of 2012 it was widely recognised that the economy was still shrinking, four years on from the start of the prolonged 2008 slowdown:

> *Yesterday we discovered that the national debt has climbed above £1 trillion for the first time. It will almost certainly never fall below that figure ever again – the Office for National Statistics has just published the latest GDP figures, and it's not good news. In their first estimate of GDP growth (admittedly prone to revision), the ONS reckons that output shrank by 0.2 per cent in the fourth quarter of 2011. The economy is shrinking.* (Knowles, 2012)

Unemployment can be prevented from rising if people are not allowed to be officially unemployed. In Britain during February 2012 it was announced that over 10,000 people had started a Skills Conditionality training placement and almost 30,000 had been moved on to a Skills Conditionality Next Step placement (DWP, 2012). These numbers may not sound very high but hundreds of thousands of other people have had their freedoms (not to be forced to work for little or no reward) curtailed by the threat of being put on these placements. Such multiplier effects are not unlike the wider impact of the 100 or so maids being deported from Singapore each year.

Here are some examples of employers recognising the wider detrimental effects that flow from the introduction of forced labour schemes:

> *Sainsbury's, one of the UK's largest retailers, confirmed to* The Guardian *that it has stopped branch managers from taking on jobseekers under the work experience scheme. The move follows that of Waterstones book chain, which last week announced it had pulled out of the scheme because it did not want to 'encourage work for no pay'. Under the work experience scheme, hundreds of thousands of largely young jobseekers will work in charities and private businesses for 30 hours a week, for eight weeks, without pay, and can have their benefits removed if they withdraw. The government has also introduced a plethora of other schemes, such as mandatory work activity, sector-based work academies, and the community action programme, which can force jobseekers to take unpaid work for up to six months as a condition of their benefits. The schemes are in operation at more than a dozen well-known chains, such as Boots, Tesco, Asda, Primark, Argos, TK Maxx, Poundland and the Arcadia group of stores run by billionaire Sir Philip Green, which includes Top Shop and Burton.* (Malik, 2012)

Knowing that you might be put on a Skills Conditionality placement if you do not take any work you can, no matter how demeaning or badly paid, may make people take desperate measures, which can include begging from relatives and friends for a meagre living rather than claiming the £9 a day Jobseeker's Allowance that is the basic UK unemployment benefit. The result is that the overall official unemployment rate rises more slowly or even appears to fall. Skills Conditionality schemes came to be called 'slave labour' in the UK press in early 2012 because people were not just *unpaid* for the work they did, but they could also face destitution, with benefits being stopped initially for three months:

> *Skills Conditionality makes attendance at skills provision compulsory for some claimants and introduces a benefits sanction for those who fail to turn up.* (DWP, 2012)

The decision of so many large companies and charities to no longer collude with such 'slave labour' may have had a beneficial effect in allowing people to admit to being unemployed when there are not enough jobs to go round.[4] However, the most significant way in which unemployment numbers in the UK are kept low, in comparison with the recessions of the 1980s and 1990s, is that unemployment benefits are now so much lower compared to the cost of living. The lower the levels to which a government can reduce unemployment benefits, the lower unemployment will be. No one is officially unemployed in countries where no unemployment benefits are paid.

Some don't realise that reducing the official count of the unemployed by reducing unemployment benefits is not clever or productive; instead, they think that 'slave labour' and reducing benefits to below a survival minimum is just fine, if not essential, and call it *'going the extra mile'*.

> *Slave labour they call it. Well that's just insulting to some great companies who are helping young people get a job, not to mention the young people benefiting from placements. They just don't understand that in today's world, things don't come on a plate … people have to go the extra mile if they want to succeed.* (Chris Grayling, Employment Minister, May 2012, quoted in Wintour, 2012)

Helping troubled families

Chapter 39 shows that, in general, in Britain, the poorer an area is, the more 'insults' of every kind people will tend to suffer and the earlier people will, on average, die. However, the greatest variation in death rates is found among the poorest tenth of all areas, and the greatest variations in life chances are found between areas within the poorest group of places. It is affluent areas that are far more predictable and uniform. Thus, within the poorest tenth of British parliamentary constituencies are those places that have the highest (census measured) rates of unemployment among men and also the highest mortality rates (see Table 39.2, Chapter 39, page 356).

The lowest mortality rates among the poorest tenth are, perhaps unexpectedly, found where overcrowding within homes is highest, the general population density

---

[4] As far as it is possible to tell, the scheme has not been abolished, so smaller institutions that did not get publicly shamed are probably still employing such 'slave labour'; just as no one can be precisely sure how many maids in Singapore have avoided pregnancy or even had abortions to avoid deportation, so, too, the numbers of people forced to work for a pittance or who face destitution through benefit sanctions in the UK are not known.

is highest, more people are from black and other minority ethnic groups and where there has been a high population turnover in recent years – in other words, in London, which is a strangely different place, quite different in these respects from what might be thought of as other similar metropolises. Children in the poorest tenth of wards within London, for example, achieve higher GCSE results, on average, than the children of entire English towns not considered to be deprived.[5]

As more and more factors adversely influencing chances of an early death are added to the model, not having a car appears to become more important than being unemployed (see Table 39.3, Chapter 39, page 357). Statistics can be confusing. Not having a car cannot directly make you more likely to die. In fact, it is when you are driving in a car that you are usually at most risk of dying during a typical day. When statistics are about averages for areas it is often the more indirect links between influences on communities and individual health that are being revealed.

Having hope, moving to London with parents with the get-up-and-go to have done that, is, it turns out, 'protective' of health. Health-'protective' events are the opposite of health 'insults'. However, that hope can then be dashed by prolonged exposure to being valued as worthless, being unemployed. In areas outside of London the level of car ownership is a good distinguisher of the very poorest from the rest of the poor. Within London, car ownership is more of a luxury than a necessity. Given all these things to consider, it is hardly surprising that so many researchers, policy makers and politicians balk at trying to understand statistics. To explain how and why statistics are often used to try to confuse, we need one final example, but this time of deliberate obfuscation rather than simple complexity.

Take, for instance, the current Coalition government's so-called Troubled Families programme (CLG, 2012), where it is claimed that there are 120,000 such families in trouble that *'cause serious problems, such as crime and anti-social behaviour'* and where *'[i]t is unacceptable to leave the children in these families to lead the same disruptive and harmful lives as their parents'*.

The figure of 120,000, in fact,

> ... *derives from a 2007 Cabinet Office analysis of data from the 2004 Families and Children Study. It refers to families with five of these characteristics: no parent in the family is in work; the family lives in overcrowded housing; no parent has any qualifications; the mother has mental health problems; at least one parent has a long-standing limiting illness, disability or infirmity; the family has low income (below 60% of median income); the family cannot afford a number of food and clothing items. None of these constitute behaviours that need government intervention to prevent reoffending. There is no evidence in the analysis of any link to offending. Government rhetoric makes a quite illegitimate and cynical slide from families who undoubtedly have troubles, through troubled families, which suggests they are somehow dysfunctional as families, to families who cause trouble.*

---

[5] See the capped GCSE average point scores for pupils at the end of Key Stage 4 in maintained schools (referenced by location of pupil residence) based on ward-level data for 2010 (GLA, 2011).

This is yet another example of government misuse of research and demonisation of the poor and the sick. (Levitas, 2012)

Conclusion

This penultimate section of the book ends with a short book review (Chapter 40) that largely concerns one of the most celebrated supposed uses of spatial statistics in health research and epidemiology, Dr John Snow's plotting of deaths from cholera in 19th-century London (see Chapter 2 of this book for more details).

Just as in modern-day London we continue to argue over the causes and consequences of premature mortality, so, too, some of us are still arguing about the statistics of death from when those distinctive circular black dots were first plotted on maps of streets to try to determine precisely why so many were dying young at very similar times and in much the same places.

The enduring fame of Dr Snow's reports is not so much because of what he did as the way in which he presented it, and the simplistic way in which others have presented his story since. A reply from Tom Koch, the author of the book being reviewed, *Disease maps: Epidemics on the ground*, is included as a textbox in Chapter 40 to illustrate just one example of how debate progresses.

The truth may be simple, but it may be a very different truth from that which we have been led to believe and which the preliminary examination of statistics can initially suggest. Women in Singapore do not enjoy the lowest chances of their babies dying worldwide. More are forced not to have babies, or to have abortions, or to have their babies abroad. Similarly, real unemployment in Britain is not lower than in past recessions; it only seems so because today more people in Britain are forced into demeaning, underpaid work. More jobs need to be available that people want to do, just as women in Singapore need to be able to choose to have babies and maids should not be forced to work seven days a week.

Poor areas and poor people are not all the same; in fact they vary far more than affluent estates and affluent people. Cars do not make you healthy no matter how significant any apparent correlation between high car ownership and low mortality may be. Cars reduce people's fitness, reduce sociability, increase fear and mistrust, pollute lungs and occasionally kill or maim, although they are useful for shopping and going on holiday. Similarly the world is not so black and white that there are some 120,000 'troubled families' in Britain. And simply taking the handle off a water pump did not end one particular cholera outbreak in Soho, London, just over a century-and-a-half ago, but it did help direct thinking in the right direction. It was not so much what Dr Snow did, but the way that he did it, that got results.

References

CLG (Department of Communities and Local Government) (2012) *What is a troubled family?*, 11 April (www.communities.gov.uk/communities/troubledfamilies/).

Dorling, D. (2012) 'Unemployment and health', in D. Dorling (ed) *Fair play: A reader on social justice*, Bristol: The Policy Press, Chapter 32.

DWP (Department for Work and Pensions) (2012) *Pre-work programme and Get Britain Working official statistics* (http://statistics.dwp.gov.uk/asd/asd1/pwp/pwp_gbw_feb12.pdf).

GLA (Greater London Authority) (2011) *Ward profiles 2011* (http://data.london.gov.uk/datastore/package/ward-profiles-2011).

Google (2012) 'GDP per capita in current US$' (www.google.co.uk/publicdata/explore).

HanQing, L. (2010) '100 pregnant maids sent home a year', *The Straits Times*, 29 September (www.healthxchange.com.sg/News/Pages/100-pregnant-maids-sent-home-a-year.aspx).

Hodal, K. (2012) 'Singapore's maids to get a day off', *The Guardian*, 6 March (www.guardian.co.uk/world/2012/mar/06/singapore-maids-one-day-off-a-week).

Knowles, D. (2012) 'The economy is shrinking again – what does a double dip recession mean?', *Telegraph* Blog of Assistant Comment Editor, 25 January (http://blogs.telegraph.co.uk/news/danielknowles/100132455/the-economy-is-shrinking-again-what-does-a-double-dip-recession-mean/).

Levitas, R. (2012) 'The riots' deeper roots in poverty and alienation', Letter, *The Guardian*, 29 March (www.guardian.co.uk/uk/2012/mar/29/riots-deeper-roots-poverty-alienation).

Malik, S. (2012) 'Unions call on UK high street giants to halt unpaid work schemes', Public Interest Lawyers news report (www.publicinterestlawyers.co.uk/news_details.php?id=224) [based in turn on an article in *The Guardian*, 10 February 2012 (www.guardian.co.uk/business/2012/feb/10/unions-shops-unpaid-work-schemes)].

Wintour, P. (2012) 'Employment minister Chris Grayling rails at "Polly Toynbee left"', *The Guardian*, 18 April (www.guardian.co.uk/politics/2012/apr/18/chris-grayling-polly-toynbee-left).

37

Worldmapper: the human anatomy of a small planet

Dorling, D. (2007) 'Worldmapper: the human anatomy of a small planet',
PLoS Medicine, vol 4, no 1, pp 13-18

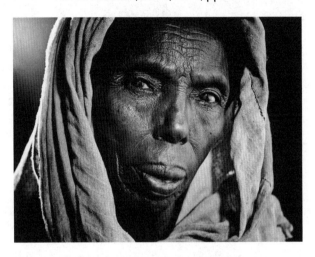

The challenge: understanding global inequalities

Throughout the world, people who are vulnerable and socially disadvantaged have less access to health resources, get sicker, and die earlier than people in more privileged social positions. Health equity gaps are growing today, despite unprecedented global wealth and technological progress.[1]

You can say it, you can prove it[2], you can tabulate it[3], but it is only when you show it that it hits home[4]. There is a long history of using illustrations to help spread new medical scientific ideas. Anatomical imagery, for example, is at least 500 years old[5].

[1] Irwin, A., Valentine, N., Brown, C., Loewenson, R., Solar, O. *et al* (2006) The Commission on Social Determinants of Health: Tackling the social roots of health inequities, *PLoS Medicine* 3: 749–751. doi:10.1371/journal.pmed.0030106.

[2] Dorling, D., Shaw, M. and Davey Smith, G. (2006) HIV and global health: Global inequality of life expectancy due to AIDS, *British Medical Journal*, 332: 662–664. doi:10.1136/bmj.332.7542.662. [Reproduced as Chapter 28, this volume.]

[3] World Health Organization (2006) *The world health report 2006: Working Together for Health*. Geneva: World Health Organization. Available: http://www.who.int/whr/2006/en. Accessed 29 December 2006

[4] Anonymous (2000) *Seeing is believing: 700 years of scientific and medical illustration*. The New York Public Library exhibition. Available: http://seeing.nypl.org/. Accessed 29 December 2006 [and 5 June 2012].

[5] Vesalius, A. (1543, 1555) *De humani corporis fabrica* [On the fabric of the human body]. Available: http://vesalius.northwestern.edu/. Accessed 29 December 2006 [and 5 June 2012].

That imagery allowed us to look inside human beings and, among much else, showed us just how much of the brain was dedicated to visual understanding.

We now know that good health relies as much on the anatomy of society as on the anatomy of our bodies (Figures 37.1 and 37.2). And we are just beginning to

Figure 37.1: Public Health Spending: Worldmapper Poster 213.

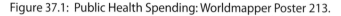

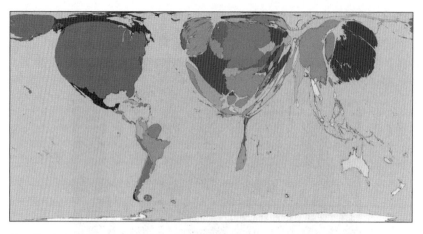

Note: The figure shows a cartogram in which territories are drawn with their area in proportion to the values being mapped. Territories are shaded identically on all cartograms here to aid comparison with the world cartograms shown in Figures 37.2 to 37.6 which employ identical shading. For detail on shading see http://www.worldmapper.org.

Source of data used to create map: United Nations Development Programme, Human Development Report 2004.

Figure 37.2: Private Health Spending: Worldmapper Poster 214.

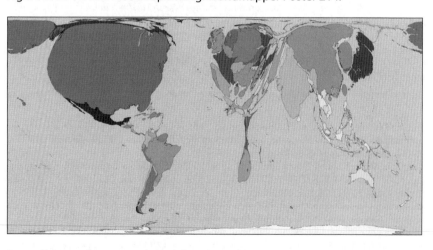

Source of data used to create map: United Nations Development Programme, Human Development Report 2004.

learn that an unequal human world is also more likely to be a sick world[6]. How, though, can we better understand the distribution of health resources around the world, and of where most people are sick and die early as compared to people in more privileged positions? How can we fathom the extent to which health equity gaps are growing despite unprecedented global wealth and technological progress? Drawing images is one way to engage more of our imagination to help understand the extent and arrangement of world inequalities in health (see Figures 37.3 and 37.4).

Medical mapping

The science of the make-up of world human anatomy—cartography—has a similar history to that of anatomical drawing. Gerardus Mercator's wall maps of 1569 were produced just 14 years after the second edition of Andreas Vesalius' *humani corporis fabrica*. And just as Vesalius' images helped guide the scalpel through flesh, Mercator's maps helped guide ships across the oceans. But these products of the enlightenment were not just simple guides. The images they produced helped change the way we thought about the world. In the long run they helped us learn to be less superstitious, but also presented a very mechanical, inhuman image of both person and planet.

Mercator's projection is the one you still see when the weather is described on television and it, or a near equivalent, is the one used in most medical mapping (for example depicting the world geography of malaria[7]). The Mercator projection is a useful projection to carry with you if you wish to sail around the planet. It is not, however, that useful for showing how a disease such as malaria is spread amongst the population. To show such spread, a world population cartogram is a far better base map[8].

The Mercator projection is the worst of all the well known global map projections to use to depict disease distributions because it stretches the earth's surface to the most extreme of extents and hence introduces the greatest visual bias. On a Mercator projection area is drawn in ever expanding proportion to how near territory is to the poles. Thus, on such a projection, India appears much smaller than Greenland, whereas India is in land area alone over seven times larger than Greenland. The world distribution of malaria shown on a conventional map gives the impression that the global distribution of clinical episodes of Plasmodium falciparum malaria is confined to a much smaller proportion of the earth's surface than is actually the case. However, even if the distribution of a disease such as malaria had been drawn on an equal land area map it would still give the impression that malaria was only confined to a small portion of the world's land. Malaria is, however, a disease of people, not of

---

[6] Wilkinson, R. (2005) *The impact of inequality: How to make sick societies healthier.* New York: The New Press. Summary available at: http://www.pohg.org.uk/support/downloads/ukhealthwatch-2005.pdf. Accessed 29 December 2006.

[7] Snow, R.W., Guerra, C.A., Noor, A.M., Myint, H.Y. and Hay, S.I. (2005) The global distribution of clinical episodes of Plasmodium falciparum malaria. *Nature* 434: 214–217. doi:10.1038/nature03342. Available: http://www.nature.com/nature/journal/v434/n7030/full/nature03342.html. Accessed 29 December 2006.

[8] Webb, R. (2006) Cartography: A popular perspective, *Nature*, 439: 800. doi:10.1038/439800a.

Figure 37.3: People dying over age 100: Worldmapper Map No 550.

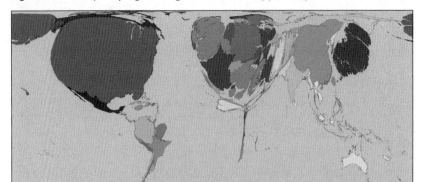

Note: The map shows the number of all 100-plus-year-olds who died in 2001. The estimates come from the World Health Organization's Burden of Disease Estimates, published in 2006.
For further information on these mortality estimates (first made for 1999), see http://whqlibdoc.who.int/hq/2001/a78629.pdf

Source of data used to create map: Lopez, A., Ahmad, O., Guillot, M., Inoue, M. and Ferguson, B. (2001) *Life tables for 191 countries for 2000: data, methods, results*. Geneva: World Health Organization (GPE discussion paper No 40).

Figure 37.4: Early Neonatal Mortality: Worldmapper Poster 260.

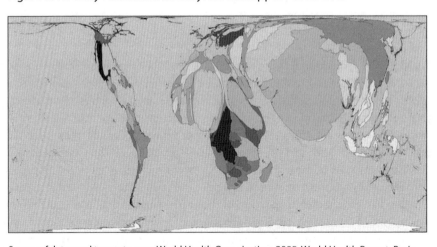

Source of data used to create map: World Health Organization, 2005, World Health Report, Basic data.

land. A better base-map (had it been available) upon which the distribution could have been drawn would have been the population cartogram. My aim here is not to specifically criticise the depiction of the distribution of malaria on a conventional map. Such depiction is simply representative of what is accepted as normal in much

see colour version in plate section

see colour version in plate section

medical mapping, even by authors with access to software that allows them to produce non-unique cartograms.[9]

The solution: creating maps of inequalities

The new world population cartogram published in *Nature* in 2006 was produced by Mark Newman[10] and shows the world with land area drawn in proportion to the population. Unlike previous cartograms, this cartogram is produced by software which approximates to the best unique world cartogram (that which distorts the least on the surface of the sphere whilst still scaling areas correctly). One criticism of older algorithms has been that they produce an 'area correct' but somewhat arbitrary solution with an end result that often reflects the initial projection used. For any given distribution there are an infinite number of cartograms that can be drawn with area in proportion to that distribution, but only one which also minimises distortion. That first shown in *Nature* (see footnote 8 above) is just such a cartogram. Put most simply, if rates of malaria were drawn upon the equal population map, then the area shaded as being affected by malaria on that map would at least relate to the number of people living at risk of malaria—and not to land area.

Newman's new projection required the adaptation of a previously working computer algorithm to allow it to produce a cartogram on the surface of the sphere. Once adapted for world mapping the algorithm could be used to show much more than simply population distribution. Furthermore, unlike its predecessor projections, Newman's does not reflect the arbitrary choice of initial projection[11] (for instance it joins East–West unlike any other equal population projection). Newman's algorithm produces an image that approximates a unique least distorting solution. This means that the reader has only one new projection to learn should they wish to map upon population rather than land. But for the more imaginative of readers, why just stop at one?

The human eye–brain system is far better equipped to judge the relative values of objects by the size of the area that each object occupies rather than to translate shades of colour into rates and then imagine what they imply. An example of the effectiveness of rescaling area to show value from medical illustrations is the traditional homunculus upon which the skin of a human is rescaled in proportion to even out number of nerve endings. See, for example, http://en.wikipedia.org/wiki/Homunculus; what you see is that our hands and lips are large, and our genitals are much smaller, in terms of sensitivity, than many of us may have imagined.

---

[9] Hay, S.I., Guerra, C.A., Tatem, A.J., Noor, A.M. and Snow, R.W. (2004) The global distribution and population at risk of malaria: Past, present, and future, *Lancet Infectious Diseases*, 4, 327–336.

[10] Newman, M. (2006) *Cart: Computer software for making cartograms online*. University of Michigan. Available: http://www-personal.umich.edu/%7Emejn/cart/. Accessed 29 December 2006.

[11] Dorling, D. (2006) New maps of the world, its people and their lives. *Society of Cartographers Bulletin* 39: 35–40. Available: http://www.sasi.group.shef.ac.uk/publications/papers.htm. Accessed 29 December 2006.

The homunculus presents an image that is not easy to forget[12]. In that tradition then, consider some maps of the world rescaled to show the areas of territories drawn in proportion to the amounts of monies spent publicly and privately on health (Figures 37.1 and 37.2), and drawn in proportion to the number of people surviving beyond age 100 (Figure 37.3). Or consider the world rescaled to show the almost wholly avoidable annual deaths of 3 million infants in their first week of life (Figure 37.4), the millions currently living with HIV/AIDS (Figure 37.5), of whom 3 million died [in 2006], and the tens upon tens of millions of people who experience malaria each year (Figure 37.6).

Figure 37.5: HIV/AIDS Prevalence: Worldmapper Poster 227.

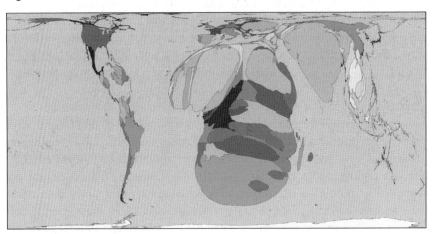

Source of data used to create map: United Nations Development Programme, Human Development Report 2004.

Details of the sources of data for these maps are given in brief beneath each figure, and in greater detail on the Worldmapper website (http://www.worldmapper.org). Note, however, that the choice of map projection and even of specific cartogram algorithm usually has a far greater effect on what you see, as compared to most ambiguities over data estimation. In the case of malaria especially, different estimates of risk (rather than the number of cases) produce very different images[13].

Worldmapper is a collaboration between researchers at the Social and Spatial Inequalities Research Group of the University of Sheffield, United Kingdom, and Mark Newman, from the Center for the Study of Complex Systems at the University of Michigan in the United States. During the course of 2006, the project aimed to create 365 new world maps, embed them in explanatory posters, and provide raw data and technical notes on many of the most prominent of the world major datasets

---

[12] Editorial Note: Two are shown in Figures 26.1 and 26.2, this volume, pages 255 and 256.
[13] Guerra, C.A., Snow, R.W. and Hay, S.I. (2006) Mapping the global extent of malaria in 2005, *Trends in Parasitology*, 22: 353–358.

Figure 37.6: Malaria Cases: Worldmapper Poster 229.

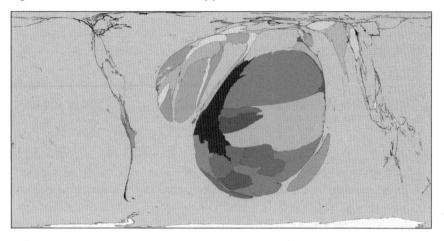

Source of data used to create map: World Health Organization and UNICEF, World Malaria Report 2005.

published mainly by various United Nations organisations. This information is all provided open-access through the website. Only a minority of the maps concern issues of medical services, diseases, and ill health—but these are related to almost everything else that is mapped. By the end of October 2006, over 893,000 hits were already recorded on the then far from complete website[14].

As a species we are just beginning to learn that unprecedented global wealth and remarkable technological progress does not result in the reduction of inequalities in health, nor in a decline in human suffering, nor in an enlightened and glorious new age. An anatomically correct technical image of the planet or the human body is not enough for us to learn how to better live with each other, nor to see other individuals or distant large groups of people as human. But new ways of depicting the world and people can change how both it and we are seen; possibly for the better. Traditional illustrative anatomy, just like scientific cartography, can dehumanise. The human body was first clearly laid bare in ink for the beginnings of modern surgery in 1543 and the coastlines of the continents were first consistently exposed on paper for crude mercantile trade in 1569. For almost all of the last five centuries these 'scientific' human and world views have shaped our thinking in one particular direction. They have suggested purely technical fixes, implied we were enlightened, and reinforced a world view that progress simply requires more detailed understanding rather than re-thinking, new imagination, and greatly expanded empathy. The maps in Worldmapper are part of a much wider attempt to see and think differently.

---

[14] Editorial Note: A year later the Worldmapper website recorded 13 million hits within 12 months; by 2011 the site was receiving 26 million hits a year despite much of the information beginning to be dated. It is easy to underestimate how much interest there is in global images.

Next steps

Currently the maps in the Worldmapper project are two-dimensional and are not particularly interactive. It is possible to spin them around the sphere and allow viewers to zoom in and out of the globe and query where they were looking—to find out more about each place, to learn more, more quickly, and even to see one image morph into another. We are hoping to create such 3-D images, and by the time you read this article, the Worldmapper website may well have such spinning globes[15].

We also hope to create further global health maps early in 2007 beyond those already shown in the 365 created in 2006. One plan we have is to produce over 100 extra maps of all major causes of death based on new estimates for the year 2002 recently released by the World Health Organization. We aim to work on these 100 maps in spring 2007, after the first 365 new world maps have all been put on the web. Worldmapper maps 368 to 484 will show the global distribution of all major world diseases, self-inflicted deaths, and aggregations of the two. Further, it is planned that maps 485 to 528 will show images of the world resized according to the numbers of people who die, for subgroups of both sexes in 22 age groups. Finally, in this new section of the Worldmapper site, map 367 will show what a more equal world would look like by sizing territory in proportion to the numbers that would be expected to die in each territory were mortality rates by age and sex equal worldwide. When map 367 is seen, and compared to map 368—of the numbers observed that actually die in each place in each year—the extent of world health inequalities will hopefully be made clearer still. In contrasting these two images, those inequities masked by the much younger age profile of the poorer majority of the world's population will be revealed[16].

One of many limitations to the project is the fact that currently only 200 territories are mapped by Worldmapper[17]. These are the member states of the United Nations and a few dozen other territories and areas that contain many people or that cover a large area, and for which values are sometimes provided by international organisations, or can be estimated. Incidentally, trying to estimate the number of countries in the world's human anatomy is rather like trying to count the number of bones within a single human body—the number varies depending on your point of view and the age of the subject.

Looking further into the human anatomy of this small planet, in addition to adding more subjects to map, we could begin to think of how to fly in, to look at variation within the borders of the state as well as between territories, and to move beyond the nation-state as our means of categorising people. There is much more that could

---

[15] Editorial Note: It still doesn't have spinning globes, but it has several animations and some very different ways of viewing individual countries than those we imagined six years ago. To see how it has changed, see: www.worldmapper.org

[16] Editorial Note: We managed to achieve this. The cause of death and death by age maps are now all available on the website.

[17] For a solution to allow mapping of many tens of thousands of smaller areas, see Ben Hennig's: http://www.viewsoftheworld.net/.

be done. However, what I think matters most are the new ways of thinking that we foster as we redraw the images of the human anatomy of our planet in these ways. What do we need to be able to see—so that we can act?

Acknowledgments

I am grateful to my colleagues Graham Allsopp, Anna Barford, Ben Wheeler, and John Pritchard at the University of Sheffield and to Mark Newman at the University of Michigan for their collaboration with this work. I also thank Simon Brooker at the London School of Hygiene and Tropical Medicine and another anonymous reviewer for their helpful comments on an earlier draft.

Figure 37.7: Equal population cartogram of the UK[18]

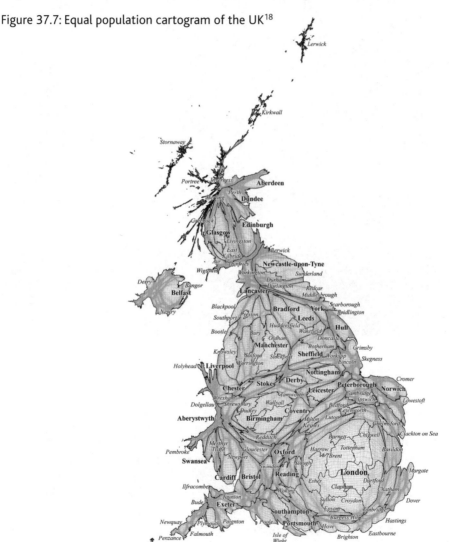

---

[18] Editorial Note: Figure 37.7 was not included in the original paper but illustrates how cartograms have developed in recent years. It shows the UK as an inset of a highly detailed world population cartogram. Drawn by Ben Hennig.

38

Using statistics to describe and explore data

Extract from: Dorling, D. (2009) 'Using statistics to describe and explore data',
Key methods in geography, London: Sage Publications, chapter 21

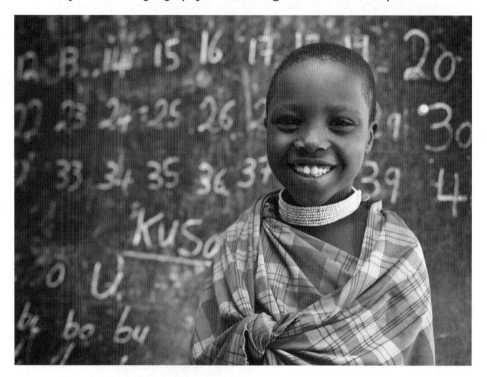

...

Introduction

Statistics are duller than ditch water. In and of themselves they tend to be of interest only to people who are not very interesting. To me, it is only when statistics are set in a wider context that they begin to come to life. In geography this wider context obviously also varies widely[1]. Suppose you are swamped by a series of floods and want to know how likely they are to happen again and how large they could be. Statistics give you techniques to make good guesses – guesses that don't necessarily rely on you knowing much about floods. Suppose you are interested in poverty and

---

[1] Editorial Note: This chapter was originally written with geographers in mind, but it may appeal to any group of readers not that interested in statistics, but forced to use them, and it uses examples from health.

how poverty rates compare between countries. Poverty rates are statistics. You need to understand the statistics if you are interested in the issue of poverty. You could, of course, ignore the statistical study of floods or poverty while still being interested in either subject. Were you to do this, however, you would be missing out on a great deal that has been learnt about these things. Statistics on floods might miss out the nature, causes and meaning of floods. Similarly, statistics on poverty may dehumanize suffering. But if you are concerned about getting wet or about why higher levels of poverty persist in some places and not others (and hence one key aspect of what reduces poverty – variation in, say, policies that influence poverty), you are unlikely to get far without the numbers and methods which make up statistics.

Statistics are dull because they are so general – because so many different things can be turned into a percentage; because similar techniques can be used to study so many different processes. The generality of statistics is also their main weakness as well as being a strength. Often issues and problems in geography are shoe-horned into a question that can be addressed, perhaps answered, statistically. A researcher turns an interesting research question into a series of dull hypotheses, the answer to none of which quite gets to address his or her original question. It is, for instance, much easier with classical statistical tests to suggest that certain things are (probably) not true – rather than to assert what is true. Statistics can also have the disadvantage that many students have built up a resistance to them, an inherent dislike of their use and feel a chill wind travel down their spine when the word is mentioned. Ask yourself this (assuming you are a student studying for a geography degree): what proportion of your fellow students are likely to be reading this book and, of those, what proportion would skip this chapter? Are you in a minority of a minority to have got this far? Perhaps I am wrong, but hopefully if you read a little further I will try to show you that statistics are not quite as painful as they may be thought to be – particularly if you only use them when you need to.

There is at least one other probable reason why you may have got this far through this chapter. You bought or read this book a year or so ago when you were first being introduced to methods in geography. You read about the interesting ones, the novel and the new, but you skipped this chapter. Later, in a seminar or tutorial, someone asks 'what statistics are you using?' for your research project. That feeling of panic returns. Or you referred to some statistic in an essay and your marker irritatingly scribbled 'explain!' next to it. In this short chapter I am going to show you only one statistical method (calculating and interpreting a confidence limit). No statistical test and no actual statistics – of the '95% of statistics are wrong' variety. Instead I'll follow this introduction with five simple rules for using statistics in geography and then talk a little about the origins of statistics, give some common misinterpretations of statistics and end with possibilities for the future use of statistics in geography.

Five rules

1. Often there is little point in using statistics

All too often statistics are included in a study or student essay to try to show that the writer or student had been working hard. An essay on the geography of employment in Britain might begin: 'Thirty million people work in Britain today.' So what? Statistics in and of themselves are dull (unless dull things excite you!). 'There are thirty million people working in Britain and forty million jobs' would be a little more interesting – many people would have to have two jobs – but that is only interesting if it is new to you as a reader. 'There was a positive correlation between the number of people working in each county and the number of jobs' – hardly surprising, and what's your point? Perhaps what you were trying to say was:

> More people are working then ever before at more and more tasks in Britain and at even more in the USA. Work, rather than removing human drudgery, has added to it. As we work harder we have created more work. Huge numbers of people have to work at two or three jobs a week compared to our labours in the recent past. The proportion of both children and the 'retired' who work has risen. For the affluent, childcare and housework are increasingly subcontracted as work for others, as for many is cooking (when we eat out). It is difficult to see a smooth end to the apparent unstoppable commodification of human time. Work turns time into money. We now have both more money and less time.

Only the very crudest of statistics were used in that argument. Things had simply gone up or down – were more or less. It would have helped the argument if I had listed some sources for this information. It is probably not all true and what is described is certainly not true for many people. However, the argument did not need numbers or tests to strengthen it. There is a time and place for statistics.

2. If you do use statistics make sure they can be understood

Most people, including a majority of human geography lecturers and a fair share of physical geography lecturers, are innumerate – as are most students of geography. By innumerate I do not mean innumerate in the sense of 'could not get an A grade at GCSE maths'. By innumerate I mean do not have an innate feel for numbers, mathematics and simple algebra in the same way that the minority of students who are dyslexic do not have an innate feel for words and their spelling. Because dyslexia is a minority condition it is given a name. Because innumeracy is the norm in America, Britain and most of the western world, we do not call it as such but save the word for people with almost no ability to handle numbers. If you are in the innumerate majority you may have thought you had some weakness and everyone else could understand maths and statistics and did not need to learn examples by rote as you did. You are wrong: you are normal. If you are in the numerate minority (that is, you could walk into an exam and get an A in maths without trying) you have a problem – many people (including often those reading or marking your work) might not understand you because they do not think like you. Statistics in geography are primarily a form of communication – a way of trying to convey information convincingly. You will only convey information convincingly if, to begin with, the person you are conveying that information to can understand the language you are using.

3. Do not overuse statistics in your work or methods

How many facts should there be to the page? Occasionally a great many simple statistics all pointing to the same things or suggesting a trend is going one way using many examples can be a powerful tool in making an argument. Generally, however, I'd try to stick to two or three facts on a page unless you are writing a reference book. You are trying to build up a picture in the mind of the reader/marker – explaining an argument through an essay. Similarly, how many numbers should tables of statistics contain? Part of the history of geography has been that multiple regression was a favoured statistical technique for several decades. Multiple regression allows dozens of variables to be entered into a model to predict an outcome. Each variable can have numerous parameters associated with it – for example, its 'effect', 'significance', 'error' and so on. When computers first began to be used in geography, a huge amount of work was required to enter the data and variables to undertake the work required to make use of the new techniques. One result was that huge tables of 'results' were often printed in papers which in fact only referred to a few of the numbers in the tables of sometimes hundreds of figures. Have a look at a journal like *Environment and Planning A* in the 1970s and 1980s for these giant tables. The tables give the impression of thoroughness, but if you want people to read the numbers in your tables I'd aim to have only a dozen numbers there. Finally, concerning tests and techniques, there should be little need to use more than one statistical test or technique on a set of data. If you are using more than one, the chances are that only one is appropriate.

4. If you find a complex statistic useful then explain it clearly

Sometimes, for some problems, only a complex statistical method or complex statistics get to the heart of the issue you are interested in – and it is the issue rather than the method that we are interested in. A typical case in geography might be that you have access to a whole series of river–water samples and know the level of a particular pollutant in each sample. You also know whether the sample was taken from water near the surface of the river or near its bed, whether from a pool in the river, a riffle, or a bend and what both the slope and velocity of the river were at each sample point. You want to know whether some rivers are more polluted than others or whether they just appear to be so because of the nature of the way the samples of water were collected from each river. Your data are arranged in at least two geographical levels: that of the river and that of geographical location within each river. Each individual sample point also has a number of characteristics you want to keep taking into account. There are a number of techniques you could use to study these data. They range from various types of ANOVA (analysis of variance) tests to MLM (multi-level models). The one you are likely to choose will depend most on what you have been taught and remembered, or perhaps on what you have read. My recommendation is that, when using a complex technique in a complex situation like this, explain every step simply – but above all understand why you are using these techniques. The above techniques are interesting for their abilities to identify 'interactions'. Within a particular set of rivers you might expect more pollution in riffles than in pools and vice versa in another set of rivers. If you are not interested in interactions, why are you using these complicated techniques? Furthermore, check first that there is not a very simple pattern in your data that simple statistics could uncover more persuasively. For example: *'Pollution levels are on average ten times higher in the pools of rivers than when measured at any other point.'*

5. Recognize and harness the power of statistics in geography

Statistics have a political power across much of geography. In physical geography their use implies you are (or are becoming) a competent 'scientist'. Many scientific (and, in particular, medical) journals use statisticians to referee papers before publication as well as referees who understand the substantive subject of the paper. Statistics has become a language of scientific credibility – rather like Greek, and then Latin, was the language of religious credibility in the Christian church for most of its history. Languages are used both for their ability to communicate and to exclude the uninitiated. The power of statistics (in particular, statistical methods) in human geography has fallen in recent years. This fall was partly the result of researchers seeing through the way statistics have been used to exclude and also partly because fewer numerate human geographers choose to teach (or research) geography than once did. However, within human geography, statistics placed carefully can still add authority to an argument that, without them, appears little more than a considered rant. This is particularly true when you are arguing against the generally accepted case. As I argue (or rant!) below, statistics are increasingly used in general debates outside of geography. It is possible both to appreciate the weaknesses of statistics and to use them with effect. But it helps first to know where they have come from.

...

Three statistical examples

Hopefully this chapter has given you some food for thought about the use of statistics in geography today. Rather than list a series of techniques and refer you on to books about their use, I've tried to give you a more personal view about one of the supposedly most impersonal of subjects taught within geography. My view may be a little odd: I use numbers but believe they are deadly dull; I like both to undermine them and use them in the arguments I make. I think our legacy of complicated statistical techniques in geography is more of a historical accident of what was found to work at certain times than a particularly useful set of tools – at least where the study of the geography of society is concerned. I'd like to end this chapter, however, with three examples of how statisticians think differently – which, hopefully, show some things to be learnt from statistics.

Example 1: a simple prisoner's dilemma

You are playing a quiz game on TV. In front of you are three doors. Behind one door is the prize and behind the other two doors – nothing. You pick a door. The quiz host then picks another door. If you picked the right door the host picks a wrong door; if you picked a wrong door the host picks the right door. You then have a chance to change your mind over which door you enter. Which do you go through?

The answer is relatively simple, or it is if you find this kind of thing easy: you pick the door the host picked. Your chance of winning the prize is 2 out of 3. Why? Because 2 out of 3 times you will have initially picked the wrong door. Why does this matter to a geographer? Well, go back to where we started this chapter. There's been a large flood and you are interested in the probability of another large flood happening. The fact that you are suddenly interested in the probability of the flood is not independent of the flood occurring. In fact, the chance of the flood having occurred after the event was 100%. You cannot say 'that was the 1-in-100-year flood', just that 'this is what it would be like' (or perhaps, better, might be like!). Probabilities are usually conditional. In geography we often make simple statistical mistakes as geographers learnt most of their statistics during the discipline's classical phase (when statisticians didn't worry about conditional probabilities so much).

Example 2: another conditional probability

You are worried you have a disease. One per cent of students have the disease. You take a test for the disease. For people who have the disease the test is accurate 95% of the time. The test is positive for you. What is the chance you have the disease?

As you might have guessed, the answer is not 95%. There are two possibilities: either you have the disease and tested positive or you didn't have the disease but the test gave you a false positive. Take 10 000 students. Of the 100 who had the disease, 95 would test positive. Of the 9900 who did not have the disease, 495 (5%) would test false positive. Thus the chance of you having the disease, having tested positive for it, is 95/(95 + 495) or roughly 1 in 6. You are unlikely to have the disease. Note that almost 6% of students would think they had the disease had they all taken the test. Of course, if you think there was a particular reason for you to be worried and could quantify that, more conditional probabilities would be introduced!

Now, substitute for disease and students, heavy metal pollution and soil samples. You are working in the labs and have a test for heavy metal pollution in a sample of soil that is 95% accurate. About 6 of your 100 soil samples appear to be polluted after you have tested them. Three of these are located in the same village – have you found a cluster? (Answer: no, probably not.)

Example 3: classical confidence limits

There is only one even mildly complicated statistic I now work out on a regular basis and even that has a more complicated interpretation than is usually taught to geography students. I often work out rates in areas – comparing how many things have happened in an area compared to how many you might have expected to have happened in that place given certain assumptions. Most commonly, this is how many people died in an area compared to how many you would have expected to die there given the ages and sexes of the people living there and national mortality rates. Given these things I might work out, for instance, that 120 people died in an area where you would expect 100 people to have died (this is called the indirect method of standardizing rates). Thus it looks as if 20% more people have died than could have been expected. However, it might just have been a bad year in that place. So with what confidence can I say that 20% more people died there? The equations to approximate the confidence limits for this statistic are as follows:

Given a standardized rate of $100 \times O/E$, where O = the number observed and E = the number expected:

Lower confidence limit (95%) = $100 \times O \times (1 - 1/(9 \times O) - 1.96/(3 \times \sqrt{(O)}))^3/E$

Upper confidence limit (95%) = $100 \times (O+1) \times (1 - 1/(9 \times (O+1)) + 1.96/(3 \times \sqrt{(O+1)}))^3/E$

Thus our standardized rate is $100 \times 120/100 = 120$ with a lower confidence limit of approximately:

$100 \times 120 \times (1 - 1/(9 \times 120) - 1.96/(3 \times \sqrt{(120)}))^3/100 = 120 \times (1 - 1/1080 - 1.96/32.86)^3 = 99.49$

And an upper confidence limit of approximately:

$100 \times (121 \times (1 - 1/(9 \times 121)) + 1.96(3 \times \sqrt{(121)}))^3/100 = 121 \times (1 - 1/1089 + 1.96/33)^3 = 143.49$

So what does this say? That we can be 95% sure that the real death rate in that area lies between 99 and 143? That we can't be 95% sure that the death rate in that area is not average (100)? What it actually says it that given, say, lots of years of data, 95% of the time the true death rate of that area will lie within these limits – so that if we were to work out confidence limits for the Standardized Mortality Ratio (SMR) of an area each year for 20 years, on average the true rate would lie within those limits for 19 of those years. This assumes there is an unchanging 'true' rate – that something about the area raises or lowers the mortality rates of the population living there. But, of cause, that rate itself will change over time (see Table 38.1[2]).

Given this, these classical confidence rates do not tell us what we thought they told us. It is not the case that the true mortality rate of this area lies between 99 and 143 with 95% certainty. This has not, however, stopped researchers, including myself, from labelling areas on maps as 'significant' if their lower confidence limits exclude 100, but strictly speaking we have little idea what level of significance applies! (For more on this, see Congdon, 2001.) …

References

Breslow, N. and Day, N.E. (1980) *The Analysis of Case-control Studies.* Lyon: International Agency for Research on Cancer.

Congdon, P. (2001) *Bayesian Statistical Modelling.* Chichester: Wiley.

Dorling, D. and Simpson, S. (eds) (1999) *Statistics in Society: The Arithmetic of Politics.* London: Arnold.

Playfair, W. (1800) *A Geographical, Historical and Political Description of the Empire of Germany, Holland, the Netherlands, Switzerland, Prussia, Italy, Sicily, Corsica and Sardinia: With a Gazetteer of Reference to the Principal Places in those Countries, Compiled and Translated from the German: To which are Added, Statistical Tables of all the States of Europe,* London: J. Stockdale.

Tanur, J. (1989) *Statistics: A Guide to the Unknown* (3rd edn), Pacific Grove, CA: Wadsworth.

---

[2] Editorial Note: This table was not included in the original chapter, but has been added here to illustrate how the underlying mortality rates of groups of people do appear to change. The confidence limits around these SMRs will be very small given that a tenth of the population aged under 65 is included in each calculation. If you can estimate that, you can use the equations above to calculate those limits for this table. Note also that I ignore here my own suggestion of including only a few numbers in a table. Sometimes it can help to see more detail,

Table 38.1: Standardised Mortality Ratio by areas sorted into deciles by mortality ratio, ages 0-64, Britain, 1921–2006.

Decile	1921-25	1926-30	1931-35	1936-39	1950-53	1959-63	1969-73	1981-85	1986-89	1990-92	1993-95	1996-97	1999-2001	2002-04	2004-06
1	141.1	136.7	135.5	154.8	131.0	135.5	131.2	135.0	139.2	144.3	148.9	152.6	151.3	150.4	149.1
2	123.9	121.7	120.0	121.8	118.1	123.0	115.6	118.6	120.9	122.1	121.7	123.0	123.9	124.1	123.4
3	114.0	111.8	112.0	110.7	112.1	116.5	112.0	114.2	113.9	112.8	113.5	114.9	115.6	115.2	116.3
4	107.8	107.3	105.7	105.1	107.0	110.7	108.1	109.8	106.9	106.8	106.8	109.0	108.0	108.0	108.7
5	102.5	102.8	102.1	100.5	102.5	104.5	103.0	102.1	102.2	99.6	98.4	98.3	99.7	100.2	100.8
6	95.6	97.0	97.2	94.4	98.6	97.4	96.9	95.7	95.6	93.7	93.7	94.2	94.7	94.7	95.5
7	89.7	89.9	90.2	87.8	93.1	90.9	91.8	91.6	91.9	90.7	90.6	90.7	90.1	90.7	89.7
8	83.9	82.9	83.7	82.1	88.7	87.6	88.9	89.3	89.1	86.0	85.4	85.1	83.0	82.3	82.8
9	77.3	79.0	80.5	77.9	85.7	83.1	87.0	84.3	83.0	79.6	78.7	76.8	77.2	76.7	76.0
10	70.0	74.7	73.9	68.7	81.8	77.1	83.0	79.2	78.1	74.6	72.3	70.7	69.7	70.2	69.7
Ratio	2.02	1.83	1.83	2.25	1.60	1.76	1.58	1.70	1.78	1.93	2.06	2.16	2.17	2.14	2.14
RII	2.64	2.41	2.35	2.89	1.96	2.25	1.92	2.12	2.22	2.49	2.64	2.80	2.85	2.83	2.84

Note: The time periods vary due to data limitations; in particular, there is a large gap between 1939 and 1950. For 1990 (included in 1990– 92), 1991 population figures were used. For 2006 (included in 2004– 06), 2005 mid-year estimates (the latest available at small area geography) were used. Note that the final column does not follow on but overlaps; it is the latest 3 years for which mortality data were available for all of Britain at the time of writing the paper this table is taken from. RII stands for Relative Index of Inequality. It is a more sensitive measure than the ratio between the mortality ratios of the best-off and worst-off tenth of people by area (which is also shown above).

Source: Table 4.3 in Dorling D. and Thomas, B. (2009) Geographical inequalities in health over the last century, in Graham, H. (ed) *Understanding health inequalities*, Open University Press. pp 66-83.

39

Socio-demographic diversity and unexplained variation in death rates among the most deprived areas in Britain

Tunstall, H., Mitchell, R., Dorling, D., Gibbs, J. and Platt, S. (2012) 'Socio-demographic diversity and unexplained variation in death rates among the most deprived areas in Britain', *Journal of Public Health*, vol 34, no 2, pp 296–304.

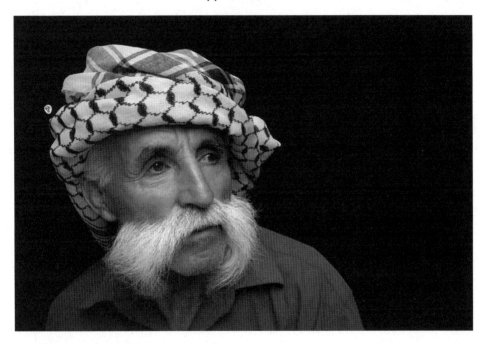

Abstract

Background: There is considerable unexplained variation in death rates between deprived areas of Britain. This analysis assesses the degree of variation in socio-demographic factors among deprivation deciles and how variables associated with deaths differ among the most deprived areas.

Methods: Death rates 1996–2001, Carstairs' 2001 deprivation score and indicators, population density, black and minority ethnic group (BME) and population change 1971–2001 were calculated for 641 parliamentary constituencies in Britain. Constituencies were grouped into Carstairs' deciles. We assessed standard errors of all variables by decile and the relationship between death rates and socio-demographic variables with Pearson's correlations and linear regression by decile and for all constituencies combined.

Results: Standard errors in death rates and most socio-demographic variables were greatest for the most deprived decile. Death rates among all constituencies were positively correlated with Carstairs' score and indicators, density and BME, but for the most deprived decile, there was no association with Carstairs and a negative correlation with overcrowding, density and BME. For the most deprived decile multivariate models containing population density, BME and change had substantially higher R^2.

Conclusions: Understanding variations in death rates between deprived areas requires greater consideration of their socio-demographic diversity including their population density, ethnicity and migration to and from them.

Keywords: geography, mortality, socio-economics factors

[*Note – all references in this chapter are numbered and are listed at the end.*]

Introduction

A strong relationship between rates of deprivation and death in areas of Britain has been demonstrated in numerous studies.[1–3] Analyses of the relationship between area deprivation and death rates commonly group together areas with 'similar' levels of deprivation into quintiles and deciles of deprivation. However, several studies have indicated that among the most deprived group of areas in Britain, there is considerable unexplained variation in death rates.[4–16] This variation in death rates raises questions regarding how similar the most deprived areas are to one another, whether different factors underlie death rates in deprived areas and less deprived places and whether factors other than deprivation are important to understanding health in the most deprived areas. This study explores the hypotheses that the large variation in death rates between deprived areas in Britain reflects their socio-demographic diversity and that there are differences in the associations between sociodemographic characteristics and death rates among these areas compared with less deprived places.

Methods

Areal units: This study analyses death rates in the 641 Westminster parliamentary constituencies in Britain, as at 1997–2001. Constituencies were used in the analysis as their populations are similar in size and sufficient to allow the calculation of death rates (~89,100 on average in the 2001 Census), and they have boundaries which fragment urban areas.

Deprivation deciles: The Carstairs 2001 deprivation index, selected to measure deprivation in this study, is one of the most widely used deprivation indices in analysis of deprivation and health.[17] The index is based upon four measures from the 2001 Census: the proportion of economically active males aged 16 and over who are unemployed, residents in households with no car, residents in households with an economically active head of household in social classes IV–V (approximated from NS-SEC) and residents in households with at least one person per room (including kitchens, living rooms and other non-bedrooms) – overcrowding. The Z-scores of each indicator were combined to create the Carstairs scores. Constituencies were grouped by Carstairs score into deciles containing equal numbers of areas (64–65).

Socio-demographic variables: The socio-demographic variables were the Carstairs score, the Carstairs component deprivation indicators, population density (persons per hectare), proportion of the population in a black and minority ethnic group (BME) and proportion change in population 1971–2001. These variables were based upon 2001 Census data from the Office for National Statistics (ONS) and the General Register Office for Scotland (GROS) and 1971 Census data from the Linking Censuses Through Time (LCT) website.

The Carstairs component indicators were selected as commonly used measures of deprivation and to allow further assessment of the operation of the Carstairs index. Preliminary analysis demonstrated that the association between overcrowding and death rates varied significantly between the most deprived decile and all constituencies combined. The variables population density, BME population and population change were selected because they were likely to be associated with overcrowding and death rates, to explore these relationships further.

Death rates: Death rates for constituencies were based upon death registrations from ONS and GROS. This data set includes year, age and postcode of residence at death. Average all-cause death rates were calculated for the time period 1996–2001 using denominators based on straight-line (linear interpolation) estimates from Census data for 1991 and 2001. All 2001 Census data were obtained from ONS and GROS and 1991 Census data, 'corrected' for undercount, from LCT. Age- and sex-standardized death rates were calculated using age groups 0–4, 5–9, 10–14, 15–19, 20–24, 25–29, 30–44, 45–59, 60–64, 65–74, 75–84 and 85 and over years.

Analytic strategy: Standard errors for death rates and the socio-demographic variables were compared between deprivation deciles groups. Then Pearson's correlations between death rates and the socio-demographic variables were assessed for each of the deprivation decile groups and all constituencies combined.

Finally, four linear regression models were used to assess the relationship between the dependent variable, death rates and the independent socio-demographic variables for all of the constituencies combined and each of the decile groups separately.

The independent variables were in the first model; Carstairs score and the component indicators of the Carstairs index in the second model; in the third the Carstairs score, population density, BME population and population change; and, in the fourth, the component indicators of the Carstairs index, population density, BME and change.

Results

When the parliamentary constituencies were split into deciles by Carstairs score, the most deprived decile contained 18 London, 10 North West England, 10 Scotland, 10 Yorkshire and Humber, 8 West Midlands, 5 East Midlands and 3 North East England constituencies.

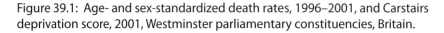

Figure 39.1: Age- and sex-standardized death rates, 1996–2001, and Carstairs deprivation score, 2001, Westminster parliamentary constituencies, Britain.

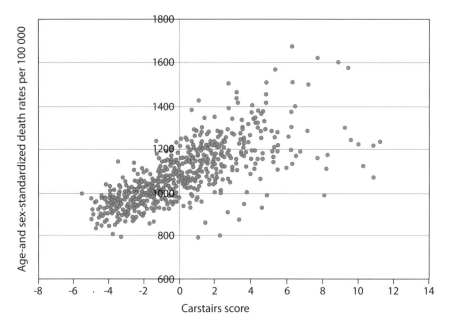

Note: Average all-cause death rates were calculated for the time period 1996–2001 using denominators based on straight-line (linear interpolation) estimates from Census data for 1991 and 2001. 2001 Census data were obtained from ONS and GROS and 1991 Census data, 'corrected' for undercount, from LCT. Age- and sex-standardized death rates were calculated using age groups 0–4, 5–9, 10–14, 15–19, 20–24, 25–29, 30–44, 45–59, 60–64, 65–74, 75–84 and 85 and over years.

Source: Death rates for constituencies were based upon death registrations from ONS and GROS. This data set includes year, age and postcode of residence at death. Carstairs scores were calculated from 2001 Census data provided by those same two bodies.

Figure 39.1 demonstrates that the relationship between age- and sex-standardized death rates and Carstairs score has a 'splaying pattern' among the most deprived constituencies. This illustrates the wider variation in death rates, Carstairs scores and the associations between them among the most deprived areas.

Standard errors: Standard errors by decile in Table 39.1 demonstrate that there is the greatest variation in death rates, Carstairs scores, Carstairs' component deprivation indicators, population density and BME population among the most deprived decile. However, standard errors for population change were similar in most of the decile groups.

Table 39.1: Standard errors of age- and sex-standardized death rates and socio-demographic variables by deprivation decile, Westminster parliamentary constituencies, Britain, 2001.

Carstairs decile	Age and sex standardized death rates (per 100 000)	Carstairs score	Male unemployment (%)	No car (%)	Social classes IV and V (%)	Over-crowding (%)	Population density (per hectare)	Black and minority ethnic group (%)	Population change (%)
1 - least deprived	6.22	0.06	0.08	0.43	0.19	0.03	1.22	0.35	2.27
2	7.39	0.03	0.09	0.36	0.23	0.05	1.22	0.44	2.10
3	7.64	0.02	0.10	0.49	0.24	0.06	1.51	0.55	5.12
4	8.27	0.03	0.10	0.51	0.32	0.08	1.73	0.83	1.85
5	8.46	0.03	0.10	0.50	0.26	0.08	1.62	0.72	2.69
6	8.98	0.03	0.14	0.70	0.34	0.10	2.46	0.95	2.16
7	13.23	0.03	0.14	0.69	0.37	0.13	2.81	0.96	2.26
8	12.53	0.04	0.17	0.82	0.45	0.20	2.90	1.70	2.03
9	14.98	0.06	0.18	0.61	0.36	0.20	2.41	1.60	1.53
10 - most deprived	19.65	0.24	0.31	1.00	0.45	0.40	3.79	2.46	2.03

Source: Census data supplied by ONS and GROS.

Pearson's correlations: When correlations between death rates and Carstairs were assessed among constituencies of all levels of deprivation, a strong, statistically significant, correlation of 0.727 was found (Table 39.2). However, this relationship was not statistically significant among any of the decile subgroups, and for the most deprived decile, the correlation was close to zero.

There were significant positive correlations for all constituencies combined between the Carstairs component deprivation indicators of unemployment, no car, low social class and overcrowding of 0.723, 0.709, 0.465 and 0.283, respectively. Among the deprivation decile subgroups, a statistically significant positive relationship was found only for unemployment and no car for the most deprived decile and low social class among the seventh and eighth most deprived deciles. A statistically significant negative association was found between overcrowding and death rates among the 7th–10th most deprived deciles of –0.327, –0.516, –0.263 and –0.368, respectively.

Analysis of correlations between death rates and population density found that for constituencies of all levels of deprivation, there was a positive association of 0.233, but among the 7th–10th most deprived deciles, there was a statistically significant negative association of –0.429, –0.399, –0.379 and –0.478, respectively. A similar pattern was found when BME population was considered with a positive association of 0.105 among all constituencies but a statistically significant *negative* association among the 7th–10th most deprived deciles of –0.436, –0.548, –0.500 and –0.490, respectively. A statistically significant negative correlation was found between change in population

Table 39.2: Correlations between age- and sex-standardized death rates and socio-demographic variables for all areas and by deprivation decile, Westminster parliamentary constituencies, Britain, 2001.

Carstairs decile	Carstairs score	Male unemployment (%)	No car (%)	Social classes IV and V (%)	Overcrowding (%)	Population density (per hectare)	Black and minority ethnic group (%)	Population change (%)
All deciles	0.727**	0.723*	0.709**	0.465**	0.283**	0.233**	0.105**	-0.483**
1 - least deprived	0.070	0.003	-0.059	0.062	0.136	0.018	0.150	-0.167
2	0.057	0.245	0.136	-0.144	0.005	.095	0.007	-0.245
3	0.065	0.211	-0.024	-0.085	0.042	0.074	0.018	0.047
4	0.182	0.167	0.240	-0.074	-0.079	0.130	-0.157	-0.337**
5	0.059	0.022	0.166	-0.036	-0.085	0.026	-0.126	-0.022
6	0.104	-0.057	0.350**	-0.151	-0.017	0.192	-0.068	-0.185
7	0.040	-0.067	-0.121	0.329**	-0.327**	-0.429**	-0.436**	0.171
8	-0.149	0.162	0.016	0.315*	-0.516**	-0.399**	-0.548**	-0.115
9	0.076	0.123	0.218	0.145	-0.263*	-0.379**	-0.500**	-0.475**
10 - most deprived	0.007	0.375**	0.360**	0.109	-0.368**	-0.478**	-0.490**	-0.717**

*0.05 significance level

**0.01 significance level

Note: Average all-cause death rates were calculated for the time period 1996–2001 using denominators based on straight-line (linear interpolation) estimates from Census data for 1991 and 2001. 2001 Census data were obtained from ONS and GROS and 1991 Census data, 'corrected' for undercount, from LCT. Age- and sex-standardized death rates were calculated using age groups 0–4, 5–9, 10–14, 15–19, 20–24, 25–29, 30–44, 45–59, 60–64, 65–74, 75–84 and 85 and over years.

Source: Death rates for constituencies were based upon death registrations from ONS and GROS. These two bodies also supplied the census data used here.

1971–2001 and death rates of −0.483 among all constituencies combined and −0.337, −0.475 and −0.717 among the 4th, 9th and 10th most deprived deciles, respectively.

Regression models: In the first linear regression model, examining the relationship between the dependent variable death rates and Carstairs score, when all constituencies were considered, there was a statistically significant coefficient of 0.727 (Table 39.3). However, when similar models were considered for separate deprivation deciles, the coefficients were low and not significant.

In Model 2, testing the association between death rates and the Carstairs component indicators, when all constituencies were considered, the coefficients for unemployment, no car and low social class were significant, positive figures of 0.218, 0.551 and 0.254, respectively, but the coefficient for overcrowding was a negative, significant figure of −0.242. In models for separate deciles, few or none of the deprivation indicator coefficients were statistically significant. In the most deprived decile, the coefficients for no car and overcrowding were statistically significant figures of 0.505 and −0.395, respectively.

In Model 3 of the association between death rates, Carstairs, population density, BME and change, when all constituencies were considered, there was a statistically significant positive coefficient of 0.849 for Carstairs. Population density, BME and change had negative coefficients of −0.083, −0.311 and −0.166, respectively. In

Table 39.3: Linear regression models for dependent variable age- and sex- standardized death rates, for all areas and by deprivation decile, Westminster parliamentary constituencies, Britain, 2001.

Model	Carstairs' decile										
	All decile	1- least deprived	2	3	4	5	6	7	8	9	10 - most deprived
Model 1											
Carstairs	0.727**	0.070	0.057	0.065	0.182	0.059	0.104	0.040	-0.149	0.076	0.007
Constant	1081.133	968.402	1002.363	1036.051	1087.001	1072.058	1092.784	1104.925	1243.160	1145.625	1264.303
Adjusted R^2	0.527	-0.011	-0.013	-0.012	0.017	-0.012	-0.005	-0.015	0.006	-0.010	-0.016
Model 2											
Male unemployment	0.218**	0.348	0.209	0.249	0.191	0.052	-0.147	0.127	-0.069	-0.041	0.135
No car	0.551**	-0.332	0.073	-0.070	0.477*	0.358	0.457	0.523	-0.046	0.377*	0.505**
Social classes IV and V	0.254**	0.176	-0.104	0.040	0.393	0.240	0.008	0.876	-0.165	0.299	0.188
Overcrowding	-0.142**	0.321*	-0.163	0.084	-0.022	-0.031	-0.221	0.138	-0.647*	-0.049	-0.396**
Constant	713.780	821.921	942.019	912.466	644.203	788.573	1016.388	236.677	1386.560	699.252	655.517
Adjusted R^2	0.624	0.013	0.013	-0.010	0.059	-0.009	0.115	0.115	0.221	0.075	0.358
Model 3											
Carstairs	0.849**	0.099	0.080	0.066	0.156	0.083	0.009	0.169	-0.071	0.051	0.281**
Population density	-0.083*	-0.256	0.212	0.144	0.162	0.144	0.422*	-0.236	-0.093	-0.280	-0.265**
Black and minority ethnic group	-0.311**	0.243	-0.288	-0.072	-0.424**	-0.214	-0.414*	-0.322*	-0.469**	-0.171	-0.259*
Population change	-0.166**	-0.153	-0.297*	0.085	-0.406**	-0.008	-0.114	0.035	-0.108	-0.431**	-0.532**
Constant	1127.711	982.287	1052.738	1030.739	110.336	1077.794	1098.223	1090.779	1240.205	1192.887	1172.489
Adjusted R^2	0.643	0.001	0.034	-0.049	0.643	-0.028	0.072	0.204	0.271	0.359	0.613
Model 4											
Male unemployment	0.156**	0.124	0.185	0.272	0.124	0.067	-0.201	0.065	-0.079	-0.124	-0.099
No car	0.675**	-0.332	0.057	-0.109	0.206	0.353	0.279	0.756	-0.069	0.133	0.462**
Social classes IV and V	0.155**	0.518*	0.004	0.056	0.479	0.206	-0.244	0.633	-0.309	-0.098	-0.092
Overcrowding	0.183**	-0.112*	0.028	0.165	0.277	0.144	0.192	0.410	-0.231	0.487*	0.266
Population density	-0.300**	-0.045	0.139	0.199	0.176	-0.018	0.071	-0.596	-0.185	-0.374	-0.728**
Black and minority ethnic group	-0.206**	0.633*	-0.312	-0.190	-0.426	-0.197	-0.674	-0.172	-0.428	-0.597**	-0.182
Population change	-0.095**	-0.304	-0.229	0.120	-0.436*	0.043	-0.129	0.105	-0.059	-0.437**	-0.369**
Constant	753.118	820.382	917.063	897.336	745.616	781.608	1175.818	290.489	1453.667	1226.705	1075.495
Adjusted R^2	0.666	0.079	0.010	-0.036	0.162	-0.051	0.129	0.243	0.239	0.459	0.688

*0.05 significance level **0.01 significance level

Note: Average all-cause death rates were calculated for the time period 1996–2001 using denominators based on straight-line (linear interpolation) estimates from Census data for 1991 and 2001. 2001 Census data were obtained from ONS and GROS and 1991 Census data, 'corrected' for undercount, from LCT. Age- and sex-standardized death rates were calculated using age groups 0–4, 5–9, 10–14, 15–19, 20–24, 25–29, 30–44, 45–59, 60–64, 65–74, 75–84 and 85 and over years.

Source: Death rates for constituencies were based upon death registrations from ONS and GROS. These two bodies also supplied the census data used here.

analysis of separate deprivation deciles, most coefficients in the models were not significant with the exception of the most deprived decile for which all variables were significant, a positive 0.281 figure for Carstairs and negative figures of −0.265, −0.259 and −0.532 for population density, BME and change, respectively.

In the fourth model, the relationship between death rates, the Carstairs indicators and the other socio-demographic variables were assessed. In analysis of all constituencies, all Carstairs' indicators, including overcrowding, had significant positive coefficients, the greatest being for no car at 0.675, and the other socio-demographic variables all had significant negative coefficients, the greatest being of −0.300 for population density. In models for separate deciles, few coefficients were significant except in the 9th and 10th deciles. In the model for the most deprived decile, the coefficient for overcrowding was also positive and coefficients were significant for no car, population density and change of 0.462, −0.728 and −0.369, respectively.

The R^2 for Models 1–4 for all constituencies combined was similar, at 0.527, 0.624, 0.643 and 0.666, respectively. Most of the R^2 for separate deciles were little above zero with the exception of the most deprived deciles. For the most deprived decile, the R^2 varied significantly with figures of −0.016, 0.358, 0.613 and 0.688 for Models 1–4, respectively.

Discussion

Main findings: This study finds a greater variation in death rates, Carstairs deprivation scores and indicators, population density and BME population among the most deprived decile of constituencies in Britain compared with less deprived deciles. This study also finds that the socio-demographic factors that are correlated with death rates vary between constituencies of all levels of deprivation and the most deprived decile of areas. When the most deprived decile is assessed separately, death rates were not always associated with socio-demographic variables in the 'expected' ways. In particular, this analysis finds that Carstairs, a deprivation index developed through analysis of death rates,[18] is not correlated with death rates among deprived constituencies.

The analysis indicates that the lack of correlation between death rates and Carstairs scores among the most deprived decile results, in part, from the negative association between death rates and one of the component indicators of the index, overcrowding. This study does not suggest that overcrowded housing is beneficial to health in deprived areas, but instead indicates that the negative correlation between death rates and overcrowding reflects the relationship between overcrowding and population density, BME population and population change.

Overcrowding, population density and BME are all positively correlated with death rates when all constituencies are compared but negatively correlated among the most deprived decile. In multivariate regression analysis, however, the direction of the associations between death rates and overcrowding, population density and BME are the same in models for all constituencies and the most deprived decile.

Among the most deprived decile, population density, BME and change were more strongly correlated with death rates than the deprivation indicators. The significance of population density, BME and change to death rates in the most deprived areas is also indicated by the multivariate model's R^2. Models for the most deprived decile which contained these variables had substantially greater R^2 than those containing only Carstairs' deprivation indicators.

What is already known: A number of previous studies have demonstrated that there is a significant variation in death rates between deprived areas of Britain.[4–16] Studies comparing countries and regions have found that areas in London have relatively better health, and North West England and Scotland worse health than would be expected from their levels of deprivation.[5,8–12,14,19] Analysis of ONS local authority classifications in England has also found that local authorities in 'mining, manufacturing and industry' and 'urban fringe' areas had lower life expectancies than their deprivation would predict,[11] while comparison of rural and urban wards in England and Wales have suggested that deprived rural areas have relatively low mortality.[20–22] The substantial diversity in deprivation indicators among the most deprived areas has also previously been demonstrated in England and Wales at a ward scale.[17] This analysis found much greater variation in Carstairs' 2001 deprivation scores and indicators among the most deprived fifth of areas in comparison to less deprived quintiles. Deprived areas' diverse experiences of deprivation have, however, not commonly been focused upon as a cause of variations in their death rates; instead, these differences have often been presented primarily as a methodological problem.

Analysis in Britain has commonly defined deprivation using census-based deprivation indices, such as the Carstairs index, the Townsend index and, more recently, the Government's Index of Multiple Deprivation, based on census and administrative data.[17,23,24] It has been suggested that variables that comprise these indices may misrepresent deprivation in some types of areas. In particular, the proportion of households without a car may 'overestimate' deprivation in cities, especially inner London.[5,20]

Some researchers have also stressed that it's not '*just deprivation*' that is important to understanding death rates in deprived areas in Britain.[16] Several studies investigating factors beyond the current degree of deprivation that may underlie health variations between deprived areas have considered population change[25–29] and ethnicity.[30,31] Other factors proposed include historical deprivation, spatial patterning of deprivation, selective migration, employment structure, education, social capital, drink and drug cultures and local social policies.[4–16,19,20,32–34]

What this study adds: This analysis builds on previous studies by demonstrating that there is a greater variation not only in death rates and deprivation indicators but also in population density and BME among the most deprived parliamentary constituencies in Britain compared with less deprived areas. The greater diversity in socio-demographic characteristics found among the most deprived areas is likely to be an important part of the explanation for their greater variation in death rates.

This study also demonstrates that the correlations between death rates and socio-demographic characteristics differ markedly between the most deprived decile of constituencies and those with all levels of deprivation. The opposite direction of association is found for overcrowding, population density and BME. The negative relationship between death rates and overcrowding among the most deprived areas is a significant limitation of Carstairs, Townsend and other indices that use overcrowding as a measure of deprivation in analysis of health.[17,23,24]

Previous studies have found that population change in local authorities in Britain and small areas in Scotland was associated with death rates,[25–29] but some analysis has suggested this association is an artefact of deprivation effects.[27,28] This studies' multivariate analysis provides further evidence of an independent association between population loss and high mortality separate from area's contemporary socio-economic status.[25,29] The results also support previous research, suggesting that population change has a greater impact upon death rates in deprived areas.[29] Notably, this analysis finds a stronger correlation between death rates and population change than any other socio-demographic variable in the most deprived decile.

The results indicating that BME population is associated with lower death rates in deprived areas, in bivariate and multivariate analysis, also support earlier research in London that found wards with higher proportions of New Commonwealth and Pakistan households have lower death rates after controlling for areas' socio-economic status.[30] However, the results contrast with research from the Netherlands that found deprived areas with lower death rates had fewer 'non-western immigrants'.[31]

The finding that low population density is also strongly associated with high death rates in deprived areas is novel. This contrasts with previous studies' findings of relatively better health in deprived rural areas.[20–22] Low population density may be related to risk of death directly because of its strong association with motor vehicle traffic injury fatalities,[35] or could be an indicator of long-term economic decline and population loss.

The strong associations among deprived constituencies between death rates and population density, BME and change demonstrated in this analysis could be perceived as evidence that factors other than deprivation are more important to health in deprived places. Alternatively, this could be interpreted as indicating that traditional deprivation indices like the Carstairs index have limitations in describing the diversity of disadvantage in deprived places.

Paradoxically, two weaknesses of traditional deprivation indices may be their limitations in describing continuity and change. There is evidence that the historical geography of deprivation in Britain over time periods as long as a century affects contemporary death rates.[36,37] BME and population change may be indicators of prolonged deprivation as deprived areas that have failed to attract international immigrants and had significant population loss in the period 1971–2001 are likely to have experienced long-term socio-economic disadvantage. Conversely, deprivation indices such as Carstairs, first developed with 1981 Census data,[17] may struggle to capture the diverse patterns of population mobility, affluence and ethnicity now found in deprived areas resulting from counter-urbanization, gentrification and international migration in recent decades. In this analysis, social class, traditionally central to the measurement of socio-economic status in Britain, was only weakly associated with death rates in the deprived areas. Moreover, the deprivation indicator overcrowding now interacts with some of these population characteristics to obscure relationships with health.

While this analysis does not directly address the causes of unexplained variation in death rates between regions of Britain, the results suggest some possible explanations. Deprivation indices such as Carstairs may not capture the experience of long-term economic decline in ex-industrial cities such as Glasgow or the growth of multi-ethnic and gentrifying populations in London. Deprived areas in Glasgow may have relatively high death rates, in part, because of their high proportions of residents of white ethnicity, low population density and population loss. Analysis comparing Censuses 1981–2001 indicates that over this period, Scotland, relative to England, experienced much larger falls in Carstairs' overcrowding while its mortality disadvantage, standardized for Carstairs score, increased substantially.[10] The decline in overcrowding, however, may have led to increasing 'underestimation' of the impacts of deprivation on health in Scotland. Longitudinal data that can describe both prolonged deprivation and how deprived areas have changed may be an important part of understanding variations in death rates across Britain.

Limitations of this study: The results will be dependent upon the scale of units and reflect the degree of internal variability within the areas.[8,38,39] The regression models should be interpreted with considerable caution because of the significant co-linearity between variables. Previous research has found greater heterogeneity in causes of death among deprived areas in England and Wales.[40] Further analysis should assess death rates by cause and age.

Conclusions

There is much greater variation in death rates and sociodemographic characteristics among the most deprived group of constituencies in Britain than among less deprived areas. Understanding of unexplained variation in death rates between deprived areas may be supported by detailed assessment of their diverse populations and histories of deprivation.

References[1]

[1] Shaw M, Dorling D, Gordon D *et al. The Widening Gap*. Bristol: The Policy Press, 1999.

[2] Woods LM, Rachet B, Riga M *et al*. Geographical variation in life expectancy at birth in England and Wales is largely explained by deprivation. *Journal of Epidemiology and Community Health* 2005;59:115–20.

[3] Thomas B, Dorling D, Davey Smith G. Inequalities in premature mortality in Britain: observational study from 1921 to 2001. *BMJ* 2010;341:291.

---

[1] Note that, in this chapter and in Chapter 42 below, to save space, references are formatted in medical journal style.

[4] Barker DJ, Osmond C. Inequalities in health in Britain, specific explanations in three Lancashire towns. *BMJ* 1987;294:749–52.

[5] Mays N, Chinn S. Relation between all cause standardised mortality ratios and two indices of deprivation at regional and district level in England. *Journal of Epidemiology andCommunity Health* 1989;43:191–9.

[6] Phillimore PR, Morris D. Discrepant legacies: premature mortality in two industrial towns. *Social Science and Medicine* 1991;33:139–52.

[7] Eames M, Ben-Shlomo Y, Marmot MG. Social deprivation and premature mortality: regional comparisons across England. *BMJ* 1993;307(6912):1097–102.

[8] Haynes R, Gale S. Mortality, long-term illness and deprivation in rural and metropolitan wards of England and Wales. *Health & Place* 1999;5:301–12.

[9] Doran T, Whitehead M. Do social policies and political context matter in the United Kingdom? *International Journal of Health Services Research* 2003;33:495–522.

[10] Hanlon P, Lawdor RS, Buchanan D *et al.* Why is mortality higher in Scotland than in England and Wales? Decreasing influence of socioeconomic deprivation between 1981 and 2001 supports the existence of a 'Scottish Effect'. *Journal of Public Health* 2005;27:199–204.

[11] Doran T, Drever F, Whitehead M. Health underachievement and overachievement in English local authorities. *Journal of Epidemiology and Community Health* 2006;60:686–93.

[12] Tunstall H, Mitchell R, Gibbs J *et al.* Is economic adversity always a killer? Searching for disadvantaged areas with relatively low mortality rates. *Journal of Epidemiology and Community Health* 2007;61:337–43.

[13] Reid JM. *Excess mortality in the Glasgow conurbation: exploring the existence of the Glasgow effect*. PhD thesis. University of Glasgow 2009.

[14] Whynes DK. Deprivation and self-reported health: are there 'Scottish effects' in England and Wales? *Journal of Public Health* 2009;31:147–53.

[15] Walsh D, Bendel N, Jones R *et al. Investigating a 'Glasgow Effect': why do deprived UK cities experience different health outcomes?* Glasgow Centre for Population Health, 2010.

[16] Walsh D, Bendel N, Jones R *et al.* It's not 'just deprivation': why do equally deprived cities experience different health outcomes? *Public Health* 2010;124:487–95.

[17] Morgan O, Baker A. Measuring deprivation in England and Wales using 2001 Carstairs scores. *Health Statistics Quarterly* 2006;31:28–33.

[18] Carstairs V, Morris R. Deprivation and mortality: an alternative to social class? *Community Medicine* 1989;11:210–9.

[19] Boyle PJ, Gatrell AC, Duke-Williams O. The effect on morbidity of variability in deprivation and population stability in England and Wales: an investigation at small-area level. *Social Science and Medicine* 1999;49:791–9.

[20] Charlton JR. Which areas are healthiest? *Population Trends* 1996;83:17–24.

[21] Phillimore P, Reading RA. Rural advantage? Urban rural-health differences in Northern England. *Journal of Public Health Medicine* 1992;14:290–9.

[22] Senior M, Williams H, Higgs G. Urban-rural mortality differentials: controlling for material deprivation. *Social Science and Medicine* 2000;51:289–305.

[23] Gordon D. Area-based deprivation measures—a UK perspective. In: Kawachi K, Berkman LF (eds). *Neighbourhoods and Health*. Oxford: Oxford University Press, 2003,179–210.

[24] Tunstall R, Lupton R. *Is targeting deprived areas an effective means to reach poor people? An assessment of one rationale for area based funding programmes.* CASEpaper 70, June 2003.

[25] Davey Smith G, Shaw M, Dorling D. 'Shrinking areas and mortality'. *Lancet* 1998;352:1439–40.

[26] Davey Smith G, Shaw M, Dorling D. Population change and mortality in men and women. *Journal of Epidemiology and Community Health* 2001;55:9.

[27] Exeter DJ, Feng Z, Flowerdew R *et al.* Shrinking area and mortality: an artefact of deprivation effects? *Journal of Epidemiology and Community Health* 2005;59:924–6.

[28] Exeter DJ, Boyle PJ, Feng Z *et al.* Shrinking areas and mortality: an artefact of derivation effects in the West of Scotland? *Health & Place* 2009;15:339–401.

[29] Brown D, Leyland AH. Scottish mortality rates 2000–2002 by deprivation and small area population and small area mobility. *Social Science and Medicine* 2010;71:1951–7.

[30] Congdon P. Deprivation in London wards: mortality and unemployment trends in the 1980's. The *Statistician* 1988;27:451–71.

[31] van Hooijdonk C, Droomers M, van Loon JA *et al.* Exceptions to the rule: Healthy deprived areas and unhealthy wealthy areas. *Social Science and Medicine* 2007;64:1326–42.

[32] Sridharan S, Tunstall H, Lawdor R *et al.* An exploratory spatial data analysis approach to understanding the relationship between deprivation and mortality in Scotland. *Social Science and Medicine* 2007;65:1942–52.

[33] Mitchell R, Gibbs J, Tunstall H *et al.* Factors which nurture geographical resilience in Britain: a mixed methods study. *Journal of Epidemiology and Community Health* 2009;63:18–23.

[34] Barnes J, Belsky J, Broomfield KA *et al.* Disadvantaged but different: variation among deprived communities in relation to family well-being. *Journal of Child Psychology and Psychiatry* 2005;46: 352–962.

[35] Eksler V, Lassarre S, Thomas I. Regional analysis of road mortality in Europe. *Public Health* 2008;122:826–37.

[36] Dorling D, Mitchell R, Shaw M *et al.* The Ghost of Christmas Past: health effects of poverty in London in 1896 and 1991. *BMJ* 2000;321:1547–51 [reproduced as Chapter 3 of this volume].

[37] Gregory IN. Comparison between geographies of mortality and deprivation from the 1900s and 2001: spatial analysis of census and mortality statistics. *BMJ* 2009;339:3454.

[38] Reijneveld S, Verheij R, de Bakker DH. The impact of area deprivation on differences in health: does the choice of the geographical classification matter? *Journal of Epidemiology and Community Health* 2000;54:306–13.

[39] Crayford T, Shanks J, Bajekal M *et al.* Analysis from inner London of deprivation payments based on enumeration districts rather than wards. *BMJ* 1995;311:787–8.

[40] Shelton NJ, Birkin MH, Dorling D. Where not to live: a geodemographic classification of mortality for England and Wales, 1981–2000. *Health and Place* 2006;12:557–69.

40

What if it were not the custard cream that did for them?

Dorling, D. (2012) 'What if it were not the custard cream that did for them? Review of *Disease maps: epidemics on the ground* by Tom Koch', *International Journal of Epidemiology*, vol 41, no 2, pp 572-3.

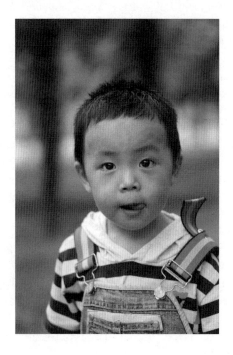

Disease Maps: Epidemics on the Ground. Tom Koch. Chicago: University of Chicago Press, 2011, pp. 344, $45.00, ISBN: 9780226449357. (Cover shown in Figure 40.1)

Tom Koch's book is a work of art that lovingly brings together hundreds of contemporary computer-generated and historical line-drawn maps to tell a tale of disease. Beginning by outlining the parallels between the developments of analytical cartography of the city and scientific anatomy of the body,[1] *Disease Maps* is an attempt to link Geography and Medicine, playing up the importance of images: 'For centuries the map has been a mechanism by which the rolls of the dead and the dying became shared realities whose relation to local environmental conditions could be assessed' (p. 2).

---

[1] Editorial Note: See Chapter 31, this volume: 'Anamorphosis, the geography of physicians, and mortality'.

The author himself says that his central argument is that we need to think about visualization, about 'seeing' at every scale (p. 4). To do this he tells numerous stories with maps and stories about maps. Most of these stories have a common format. They concern the cartographic search for the source of a particular disease. Early on in the book the disease is an outbreak of *Salmonella enteritidus* in British Columbia in the year 2000 and the source is traced back to a cream custard:

Figure 40.1: Cover image of *Disease Maps: Epidemics on the Ground,* by Tom Koch, 2011.

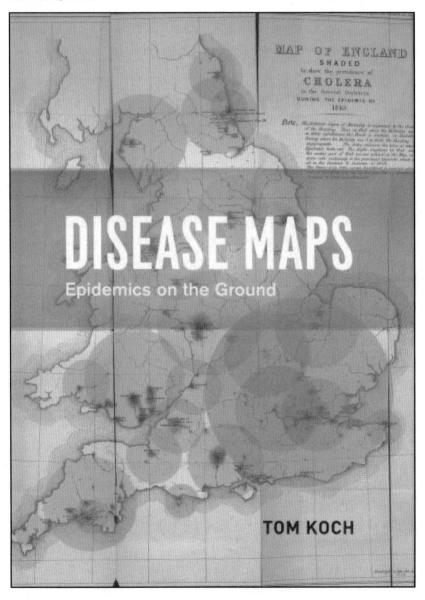

Source: Chicago: University of Chicago Press.

> *In the Vancouver example the patients were blameless and responsibility assignable in part to the local bakery whose cream custards were the apparent source of the outbreak. But the local baker brought supplies from wholesalers and they carried a predicate responsibility. Ultimately, the final responsibility rested with the hospitals that treated the patients and the health agencies that in theory but not always in practice assure restaurants and food producer practices are safe.* (p. 29)

I have no quibbles with the arguments against blaming the victims, or against seeing us all, through the agencies we fund and the hospitals we support, as being responsible, I have great admiration for the amount of work that has gone into documenting the stories behind so many maps and outbreaks in this book, I find Koch's arguments that there are no real heroes of great use, but I have a concern. What I am concerned about are the custard creams (which may have been vanilla slices—it is a little lost in translation). The problem is, for all the beauty of these maps, in almost every case there is very little evidence that the map was used to identify the causes of each outbreak.

In the case of the custard creams the health officials only 'tentatively identified that bakery as the origin of the outbreak' (p. 25). Why did they even do this? They did it because they were presented with a crude dot map, with a little spatial smoothing applied to the dots to suggest the bakery was near the place of greatest disease density. Officials then look in that place and, given their knowledge of the transmission at the time, finger a possible source. A few centuries ago it might have been a witch rather than a vanilla slice. Unless the cream custards are tested and found to be carrying the vector, all is pure speculation.

Disease Mapping does provide a wonderfully lucid history of graphical anatomy and human cartography developing side by side, of germ-theory spreading and of people learning, but it perpetuates the myth of map as microscope. A very large part of the book concerns the most celebrated case of all, John Snow's removal of the pump handle in Broad Street, Soho, England. Only at one point does Koch report that 'England's first great authority on microscopy, Arthur Hill Hassall, who examined the water from the Broad Street pump for the Board of Health inquiry, declared it "relatively bereft of microscopic animal life" that might be identified as a contaminant . . .' (p. 209). Labouring this point would not help the book's overall argument, so it is not laboured. Similarly, although the author does look in a little more detail at Snow's data with more modern techniques using rates, he concludes: 'Because these techniques were not in wide use in Snow's day they are not used here, with the exception of risk ratios, whose utility is so great it seemed wise to present them without dwelling on their significance' (p. 303, note 9).

The author makes what I think are mistakes when suggesting that Snow worked out an average rate of 3.83 incorrectly (p. 153). Snow in this case was right and Koch wrong. Snow might have added up some numbers incorrectly at this point, but, had he not made that mistake, the rate would have been 3.84. It is not an issue. Koch does find that his hero maps different numbers of deaths on two of his maps, in different places (see Figure 40.2 for the most famous map). This is far more serious a discovery than his reported rate of 3.83 possibly being 3.84 but is relegated to footnote 3 on p. 301.

Figure 40.2: Original map of Soho made by John Snow in 1854 showing cholera cases highlighted in black.

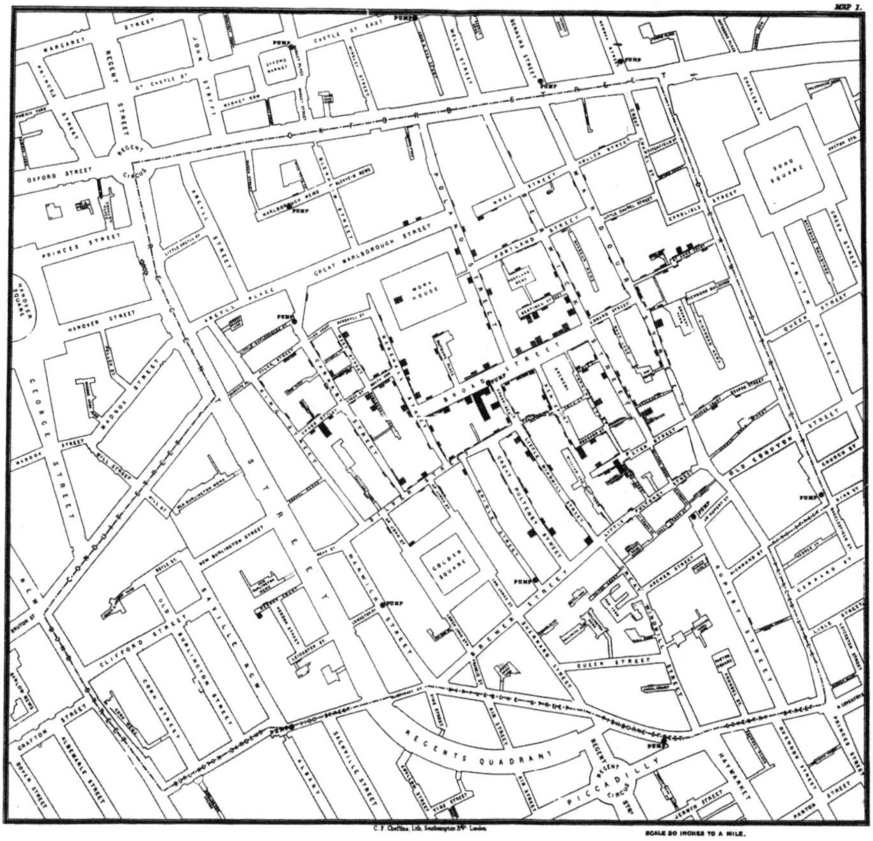

Source: This copy is publicly available at: http://en.wikipedia.org/wiki/File:Snow-cholera-map-1.jpg It was originally published by in Snow, J. (1855) *On the Mode of Communication of Cholera*, 2nd edn, John Churchill, New Burlington Street, London.

Just as in Monty Python's *The Meaning of Life* (part 7), only Death himself could identify the Salmon Mousse as the culprit. It remains an error to suggest that these disease maps did point the finger well enough to identify the source. There has been disease mapping that has sought to do a better job of cluster identification, including for Salmonella and Cholera. The maps from 1910 on p. 227, those of Hunter and Young from the 1970s referred to on p. 228, or Howe's of the 1960s were all redrawn at their various times using cartograms, on an equal population basis, to try to not make the custard cream errors, but this aspect of the history of disease mapping is ignored in this book. It does not fit the story.

It would be wonderful if, in a future edition some of the early disease mapping cartograms of Iowa, of Salmonella and cancers, of cholera and flu, Hunter and Young's projections and Howe's were mentioned. There also remain a number of less important errors that are most probably the publisher's fault and which could also be rectified. Publishers tend to write the blurb on book jackets. The last sentence on the inside cover of the book jacket ends '... only in maps do patterns emerge that allow disease theories to be proposed, hypotheses tested, and treatments advanced'. That is the way to raise a wry smile from knowledgeable epidemiologists, the majority of whom never use a map, but it does not add to the credibility of the book.

There are other irritants that I suspect are also more about the production than the writing. Sometimes a detail in a colour plate is enlarged (p. 44 of part of p. 43, p. 178 of part of an image on p. 177), but when this is first done the publisher forgot to enlarge the inset (p. 33 is drawn to the same size as p. 32). The English is, of course, American, but this does result in words about old London streets such as 'mews' being altered to 'news' (p. 204). It may be over-enthusiastic copy-editing, but copy-editing which did not spot that both the blue and red shades in the key of one of the first figures in the book (p. 17) are labelled with the same dates, or that % in the map on p. 236 should be ‰. Or that the last sentence of the book on p. 279 is simply not clear English.

Despite my complaints and concern over the propagation of possible myths, this remains a great work of scholarship, albeit one that also reveals fallibilities although often reporting them. But it is extremely well presented. You know that feeling when you pick up a book and it feels right, weighs right and smells right! Well, Chicago Press have certainly printed it beautifully and, regardless of my quibbles, there is nothing else that competes as well out there. It is also of interest to a wide readership, which is why I was asked to review the book for both an Epidemiology journal and one concerning Cultural Geography! This is the best book on disease mapping in print today. Its next edition could be even better[2].

---

[2] Editorial Note: Figure 40.3 shows the original map used as a backdrop for Figure 40.1, the book's cover. It is added here as there was not space in the original review to include it. Figure 40.2, included above, was also not in the original.version of this review but has been added here.

Figure 40.3: Map of England shaded to show the prevalence of cholera in several districts during the epidemic of 1849.

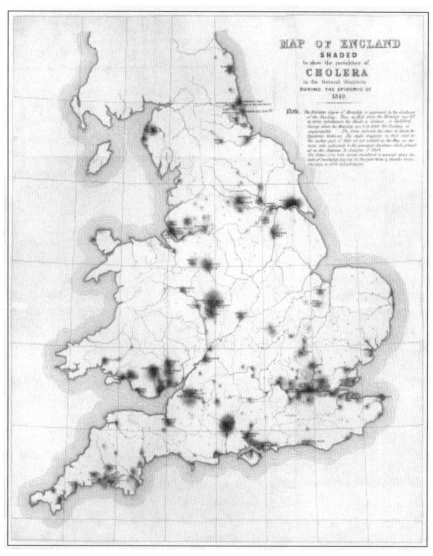

Note: Prevalance of the disease is indicated by dark shading and dates on the map suggest the time at which each epidemic broke out in each place.

Source: *Report on the mortality of cholera in England, 1848-49* (General Register Office. Printed by W. Clowes ... for HMSO, London, 1852. See: http://catalogue.wellcome.ac.uk/record=b1048030.

Following publication of the review I received the following email, April 2012:

Dear Danny,[3]

Just a note to let you know I've received, read, and appreciated your review (*Int. J. of Epidemiology*) of my book, *Disease Maps: Epidemics on the Ground*.

I was of course irritated by some of the errors that I either did not see when reading proofs ('news' for 'mews') or were introduced in production. The failure to see the blue and red shades in the map set on page 17 is an example. I think what happened was that, in reducing my maps to the page, some helpful production person changed the font size on the legends and in doing so ... destroyed them. This was, of course, the first page several friends turned to when they saw the book. It's been corrected, of course, for future editions.

Let me say I do think you miss the point, somewhat, in your reading of my treatment of Snow's work. I agree ... the addition error he made was trivial and certainly understandable when doing sums at night (after a day of surgery, probably) by candlelight. But the real point I tried to make, and one I think important, is that Snow's critics asked questions of what he did which could have been answered within the science of the day. This was especially true of the pump study—Rev. Whitehead's simple calculations in his brief monograph exemplify the type of work Snow might had done with his map and its data.

He had the skill—we know that—but did not take the time because he thought it unnecessary. He thought the point was made and refused to consider otherwise.

I'm sure there were cases that were missed in some of the maps. We know this in part from Snow's work and the case analytics of physicians who shared their casebooks with him. And his map has cases outside the designated study district; cases not included in Whitehead's, the Public Health, or Cooper's maps. But I think these outliers do little to change the ratio of deaths per population, per pump. Today, of course, we'd be a little more rigorous (I hope) in finding outliers and mapping the statistics. That said, Snow's ability to do as much as he did was ... impressive.

So, too, were, Whitehead's calculations in his short monograph. They were the work of an extremely gifted amateur and his use of statistics and his careful study of cases (for example, why older people were less affected than experience suggested) exemplary. And, too, he demonstrated the degree to which a simple statistical analysis—one Snow might have engaged but did not—was considered a basic of the study of localized outbreaks. We know Snow relied on Whitehead's materials, an example (if another is needed) that sciences of health and disease have always been communal and not individual pursuits.

---

[3] Editorial Note: This letter is reproduced with Tom's permission.

So while I admire Snow ... he stands for me as a cautionary example of one whose passionate belief in his correctness got in the way of the science he presented. According to other reviews, some have read it this way but obviously, you didn't; my fault as the author, not yours as a reader.

And too, I'd say the Vancouver case is a good example of how an intelligent use of mapping—of 'putting disease in place'—can offer insight into one kind of emerging public health event. It would not identify the egg-based pastries but would draw strong attention to the wholesaler whose materials were both geographically central as a restaurant and as a provider to area restaurants. That said, I wholly agree that the maps of Hunter and Young,[4] for example, provide an enormous insight into other types of public health events and do so clearly and with strong statistical backing. In my previous book, *Cartographies of Disease*, for example, I used their work on influenza to make this point.

I was aiming for a book that would serve the undergraduate as well as the professional, a public as well as a privileged audience. The Vancouver case served as an introduction to a simple kind of event and to the way its mapping may serve. But even there I might have been clearer (more strident?) in insisting this was only one 'simple' case and that others (for example, those of viral diffusion) call on a different approach.

But nobody can ask for more than a careful and honest review of another's work, one informed and based on a careful reading. And may I say I appreciated your praise of the general thrust of the book, its map collection, its history, and its presentation.

To me, it is the whole idea of science that is most important, here, our rectification of W.H. Frost's myth of Snow.

So, my regards, and my thanks for a clear and thoughtful review.

Sincerely,

Tom Koch

---

[4] Editorial Note: Hunter, J.M. and Young, J.C. (1971) 'Diffusion of influenza in England and Wales', *Annals of the Association of American Geographers*, vol 61, no 4, pp 637–53, www.jstor.org/stable/2562387, and for their innovative use of cartograms in medical mapping, see: Hunter, J.M. and Young, J.C. (1968) 'A technique for the construction of quantitative cartograms by physical accretion models', *Professional Geographer*, vol 20, no 6, pp 402–7, with images reproduced in Figures 4c and 4d on p 18 of: qmrg. org.uk.files/2008/11/59-area-cartograms-pdf

SECTION VII
Changing demographics and ageing populations

41

Growing old gracefully

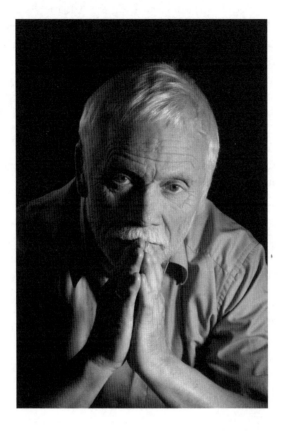

Lives curtailed are usually shortened by a series of insults rather than a single tragic event. Whether you get to grow old gracefully or die young depends, today, as much on where you grow up in Britain as it did a century ago.

Just over a century ago (some time shortly before 1920) was the last time when life expectancy gaps between areas were as large as they are today. Back then almost everyone lived shorter lives, but by 1936 they had also learned from the First World War, from the revolution in Russia, from the 1929 economic crash and during the 1930s depression, that they really could be 'all in it together'. In 1920, although hardly anyone realised it then, improvements had already begun. But a long human lifetime later, during 2012, life expectancy gaps had again grown to be greater than in 1920, but maybe not as great as in 1912.[1]

---

[1] Data on health inequalities were not collated between the 1890s (see Chapter 43, this volume) and the 1920s (see Table 38.1, Chapter 38, page 350, this volume). They were higher in the 1890s and slightly lower in the 1920s than now. A fair assumption might be that inequalities between geographical areas could have been greater in 1912 than today.

When today's centenarians were born

A single event, such as the sinking of RMS Titanic, brought into sharp focus the distinctions between social classes in 1912, and the need for all three social classes to be properly accommodated on a ship crossing the Atlantic. As contemplated by the Singaporean children shown in Figure 41.1, lists of the survivors and the deceased reveal that the passengers' segregation on board ship and their unequal access to lifeboats meant that while two thirds of first-class passengers survived, only half of second-class and a minority of third-class passengers (and crew) were rescued. Up close, the first names of the survivors and dead will have revealed the gender balance, but it was not all 'women and children first' – a third of the first-class men also survived (see Table 41.1).

Table 41.1: Casualties and numbers saved by age, sex and class on RMS Titanic, estimates produced by the British Board of Trade report.

Passenger category	Number aboard	Number saved	Number lost	% saved	% lost
Children, First Class	6	5	1	83	17
Children, Second Class	24	24	0	100	0
Children, Third Class	79	27	52	34	66
Women, First Class	144	140	4	97	3
Women, Second Class	93	80	13	86	14
Women, Third Class	165	76	89	46	54
Women, Crew	23	20	3	87	13
Men, First Class	175	57	118	33	67
Men, Second Class	168	14	154	8	92
Men, Third Class	462	75	387	16	84
Men, Crew	885	192	693	22	78
Total	2,224	710	1,514	32	68

Source: The Wikipedia page (http://en.wikipedia.org/wiki/RMS_Titanic#CITEREFMersey1912) relying in turn, it is said, on Mersey, Lord (1999) [1912] *The loss of the Titanic, 1912*, London: The Stationery Office, pp 110-11.

Some 80 years after the Titanic sank, social divisions in British society were clearly seen to have been growing again. In the 1992 General Election John Major's Conservatives won a majority despite (the then) 13 years of Conservative misrule. It was the people who lived in the places that enjoyed better health who supported the Conservatives most strongly in that fateful election (see Figure 41.2). The outcome of the 1992 General Election arguably resulted in the rise of New Labour, a party that then failed during its 13 years of rule (1997–2010) to prevent health inequalities growing even greater. We are currently waiting for the population data that will allow us to assess the last couple of years of New Labour's reign. It is not impossible that there was an improvement in inequalities towards the end, but it is impossible that that will have done anything other than to slightly curtail the rise in inequalities since 1997, itself a continuation of the social segregation that began in earnest in 1979.

Figure 41.1: The survivors and deceased lists by social class, RMS Titanic, 1912, viewed in Singapore in 2012.

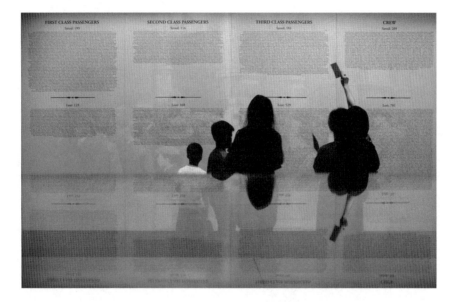

see colour version in plate section

Source: Image included in *The Guardian* newspaper, 11 April 2012, of people at an exhibition in Singapore (the world's most unequal rich country) looking at the RMS Titanic survivor lists.

It is worth comparing Figure 41.2 with Figure 39.1 on page 354 in Chapter 39, which shows how recently the correlation between deprivation and mortality has become a little weaker than that between voting and mortality (for very similar parliamentary constituencies). Voting patterns can reflect past traumas as well as current circumstances. The pattern of voting that occurred in 2010 saw the country become even more politically divided than before, as the greatest swings to the Conservatives occurred where health had been least damaged and the Conservative vote had been highest to begin with. Those parts of Britain that had suffered the most from growing division actually saw the share of the electorate voting Labour rise. It was similar in 1992 although then, because the country was less polarised, the Conservatives won an outright majority of seats (see Dorling and Thomas, 2011, p 50).

Figure 41.2: Scatterplots of Conservative and Labour voting in 1992 against all age-standardised mortality ratios, 1990–92.

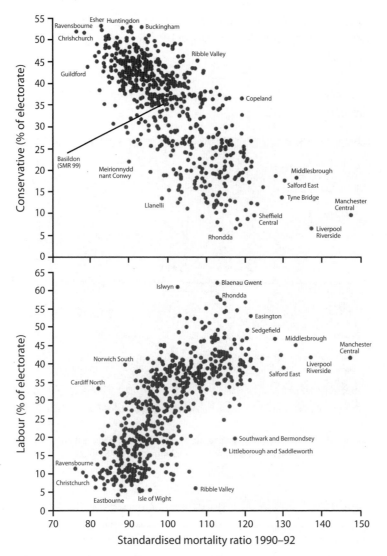

Source: Davey Smith, G. and Dorling, D. (1996) *British Medical Journal*. An open access copy is available at: www.ncbi.nlm.nih.gov/pmc/articles/PMC2359093/?page=3

What's worse, they don't care, either

Twenty years on from the 1992 General Election, and as numerous commemorations of the Titanic's sinking were taking place worldwide, under the surface of these commemorations was the uncomfortable recollection that the tragedy may have been as great as it was because there were only enough lifeboats for a fraction of the passengers. It was not just that the ship was thought unsinkable; it was that many of its passengers and crew were not considered a priority in planning for such an event. This has echoes in our present. The journalist John Harris has tried to explain how similar class prejudice and 'stupidity' remain in Britain:

> *Note also the words of backbencher Nadine Dorries, whose Liverpudlian dad was a bus driver: "The problem is that policy is being run by two public schoolboys who don't know what it's like to go to the supermarket and have to put things back on the shelves because they can't afford it for their children's lunchboxes. What's worse, they don't care, either." A saga is being played out, bound up with the enduring qualities of the English ruling class, and a mixture of gentry and parvenus (and, in Osborne's case, people stuck somewhere in between) who are failing power's most basic tests.*
>
> *It has all reminded me of the words of brilliant Old Etonian George Orwell, in 1941: "It is important not to misunderstand their motives, or one cannot predict their actions. What is to be expected of them is not treachery, or physical cowardice, but stupidity, unconscious sabotage, an infallible instinct for doing the wrong thing. They are not wicked, or not altogether wicked; they are merely unteachable. Only when their money and power are gone will the younger among them begin to grasp what century they are living in." (Harris, 2012)*

John Harris was writing in the immediate aftermath of the March 2012 Budget, what came to be called the 'Omnishambles' Budget. A conspiracy theorist might imagine that it deliberately contained so many policies that quickly had to be abandoned so as to avert attention from how it reduced tax-takes on the incomes of the rich, and reduced corporation taxes on the profit-take of the companies they owned and on their wealth (when the 'charity giving' proposals to reduce tax-dodging were abandoned). But no one could have had the foresight to have so carefully engineered such a spectacular cock-up. And it was not just the Chancellor's cock-up.

The Chancellor at least had taken a slightly different degree at university than almost everyone else involved in the public discussions – a reader of the same newspaper had commented just two days earlier, that:

> *As I watched the BBC coverage of the budget I was struck by the rich educational diversity of our politicians and pundits. Coalition: Osborne (history, Oxford), Cameron (PPE [Philosophy, Politics and Economics], Oxford), Hague (PPE, Oxford), Alexander (PPE, Oxford), Clegg (anthropology, Cambridge). Labour: Miliband (PPE, Oxford), Balls (PPE, Oxford). Pundits: Flanders (PPE, Oxford), Robinson (PPE, Oxford), Peston (PPE, Oxford). Strength in diversity? (Greenhaigh, 2012)*

In Britain health inequalities are so high not simply because 'policy is being run by two public schoolboys'. They were high and rising before that. They rose under Kesteven and Grantham Grammar School girl Margaret Thatcher's reign in office, stalled slightly under Rutlish Grammar School boy John Major's period of tenure, climbed during public school boy Tony Blair's years of office and perhaps stalled again during Kirkcaldy High School boy Gordon Brown's brief reign. Trends since 1998 are shown in Figure 41.3. It was not so much these leaders' segregated schooling[2] that is to blame, but the segregated schooling of so many they meet and work with in politics. This segregation is amplified by selection to university and then to courses and colleges within just a few universities. Just a few days later in the same newspaper it was explained that:

> The PPE clones often mate with lawyers in their attempt at world domination. They reaffirm each other's intellectual capacity by rarely deviating from the path. That path usually means a deference to the institutions which produced them and thus, at the top of the system, we have mind-numbing uniformity.... Education policy is made by those who loved it, and this is a fundamental mistake. People who never regarded school as a moronic prison full of inane rules should not be in charge of them. This is why, instead of looking to the future, the current fashion in education is to look only backwards. (Moore, 2012)

Were a small bunch of educationally segregated or otherwise socially segregated rich men steering the economy (as much as it was being steered) and reserving the lifeboats mostly for themselves? Is it because so many of them see it as in their personal self-interest to try to ensure that up to 49 per cent of beds in NHS hospitals are privately run that they push through policies such as the Health and Social Care Bill? Do they not want to mix on wards with poor people when they are old or ill just as they did not mix when they were young and well? Coalition government Ministers, MPs and supporters in the House of Lords appear to prefer to see parts of the NHS face bankruptcy and become available for rapid privatisation.

On Tuesday, 26 June 2012 it was announced that South London NHS Trust was being taken into administration. It was the first part of the NHS to go bankrupt in this way. The trust had brought mortality rates down from above the national average to below average in many poorer parts of London. It had done this within just a dozen years, but the lives that were prolonged were not the lives of the affluent.[3]

There are alternatives to NHS privatisation if a Minister wishes to avoid sharing a ward with the poor when they are old and fall ill. This is because Ministers have the power to redistribute wealth and opportunity. They could choose a fairer future for all, where fewer people are either very rich or very poor. This occurs in all other Western European countries. Ministers are able to reduce poverty. During early 2012

---

[2] In Gordon Brown's case his school was a comprehensive, but he was segregated within his school into an experimental fast-track scheme. He was sent to secondary school two years early and kept apart from other children, and is said to have loathed and resented this. The scheme was abandoned in 1967 (Macintyre, 2007).

[3] Radio 4, Today Programme, 8.52 am, 26 June 2012. On the same day the *British Medical Journal* announced that 900 stillbirths a year could be prevented in England if health inequalities were reduced rather than increased. Twice as many babies are stillborn in the most deprived part of the country as compared to the wealthiest: '*The UK had the highest stillbirth rate among 13 countries, including the US, Canada, Australia and European nations....*' (Boseley, 2012).

Figure 41.3: A measure of social integration between geographical areas: life expectancy estimates diverging in the UK, 1999–2010.

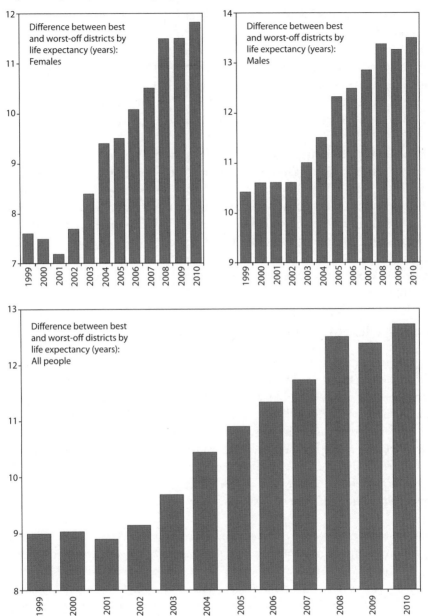

Note: The top two graphs show the trends of men and women separately. The bottom graph combines those trends. All show a similar picture, although the gap for men is greatest. The gap shown is simply the greatest range in officially reported life expectancies between local authorities across the whole of the UK.

Source: Local authority life expectancy estimates as published annually by ONS (three-year moving average to the year shown), and GRO (Scotland), 19 October 2011 release.

it was reported that just £20 million a year would have been enough to have ended the very worst child poverty in Britain. The mechanism to do this would simply be for a Minister to sign an order that would result in pressing a switch on the benefits computer. Currently some 10,000 children whose families are seeking asylum in Britain have to live on a daily family income of £17.86. That works out at £66 a week below the UK's official 'severe poverty line' (Ramesh, 2012). If you do not want to share an NHS ward with someone who is so poor, it is far cheaper to ensure they are not poor than to finance private healthcare for the rich. Health spending in the US demonstrates just how expensive a segregated healthcare system can become.

The argument that is made for not improving the living conditions of the poorest children in Britain up to the minimum, up to the level of living in severe (but survivable) poverty, is that this may, apparently, only encourage more families to seek asylum. However, no evidence has ever been provided to show that people seeking asylum in Britain have the detailed knowledge of welfare benefit levels and rights required for this argument to hold. Instead, there is a great deal of evidence that suggests that it is only through the immigration of poorer groups that the NHS has managed to keep wards staffed in recent decades, and that care homes were even able to operate.

Choosing who gets to grow old gracefully

Today we still ration the lifeboats to save a fraction of the money of those who already have the most. Worldwide, half of all children live below the US$2 a day international poverty line; 22,000 die a day, mostly of preventable illness. The majority of the remainder of the world's poor are adult women, and most poor adult women die of preventable diseases. The reason why it is worth differentiating children from adults, recognising that women bear the brunt of poverty among adults, is clearly spelt out by UNICEF in one of their recent reports (see Ortiz et al, 2012). There are good arguments as to why it is worth thinking of putting children on lifeboats before adults, although Table 41.1 shows when we didn't:

> The consequences of poverty and inequality are very significant for children. Children experience poverty differently from adults; they have specific and different needs. While an adult may fall into poverty temporarily, falling into poverty in childhood can last a lifetime – rarely does a child get a second chance at an education or a healthy start in life. Even short periods of food deprivation can impact children's long-term development. If children do not receive adequate nutrition, they grow smaller in size and intellectual capacity, are more vulnerable to life-threatening diseases, perform worse in school, and ultimately, are less likely to be productive adults. Child poverty threatens not only the individual child, but is likely to be passed on to future generations, exacerbating inequalities in society. (Ortiz et al, 2012, p 1)

Look back at Figure 41.1. Then try to imagine a future world when, in a hundred years' time, children in the area that is then the world's richest but most *unequal* country look at an exhibition of events in 2012. What might be singled out? Could it be reports produced in 2012 that showed that we knew that medical '... *interventions that improve childhood health directly improve the quality of life and, in addition, have multiplier effects, producing sustained population and economic gains in poor countries*' (Bhalotra and Pogge, 2012, p 2), in particular interventions concerning vaccines, but that we chose not to act? All this despite knowing that it was poor children within poor countries who bore the brunt of the entire global burden of disease in 2012, and despite knowing that '... *the current global economic order may contribute to perpetuating poverty and poor health in less-developed countries*' (Bhalotra and Pogge, 2012, abstract). In other words, we already know that there are too few lifeboats. We know we could easily build more. But we choose not to.

The chapters in the remainder of this section are brought together because each tries to look at one facet of the body of reasons as to why we – those of us mostly mostly housed in first-class, in rich nations – choose not to act. First, in Chapter 42, a study is reproduced that attempts to list what it is that most concerns us – on average, the end of our most personal relationships (divorce and separation) ranks just above the deaths of our parents in importance. Deaths of children create the most distress, exceeded only by the deaths of grandchildren.

Conversely, we tend to express most contentment in the years in which we report starting personal romantic relationships with other people, next when we get a job, and next when we buy a home; strangely, just below these events in apparent (self-reported) importance is our average expressed happiness when first expecting a child (Chapter 42, Table 42.3, page 394), with mothers much more likely to report the birth of a child as a significant event in the past year than fathers! Such high average self-absorption, including different members of one family having such varying recollections, is perhaps a significant part of any explanation for such widespread general apathy.

Grandparents recalled the births of grandchildren as even more important than the parents. Perhaps they have, on average, a better sense of perspective? They certainly have a different perspective given that they are no longer the primary carers and can step back. But maybe by older age many of us better value what should matter most in life – health more than wealth. What appears most important as we rush around in mid-life, quickly driving from meeting to meeting, may look misguided and possibly dangerous in hindsight.

Chapter 43 is a transcript and slideshow from a lecture on what will soon replace AIDS as one of the biggest premature killers of people worldwide: road crashes. Our roads should be seen as the equivalent in the 21st century to the problem of open sewers in the 19th century. This issue is connected to Chapter 44, a review of the World Health Organization's Commission on the Social Determinants of Health report of 2008, in which it is repeated yet again that '... *addressing health inequalities will require a radical shift in policy priorities away from a focus on individual responsibility, to a more potent upstream strategy'*. And, in that light, Chapter 45 considers who might provide healthcare for all the centenarians predicted to be living in affluent countries in the future. Again, the conclusion is that a radical shift in policy priorities is needed, in this case, welcoming the immigration of young people from countries where more people are young, and not trying to discourage young people from emigrating to countries with rapidly ageing populations.

Chapter 46 provides estimates of just how many young people there might be in the almost foreseeable future, which may reassure any reader who thinks that there are billions upon billions more humans to come, and that the barricades need building up now around their affluent ageing nations. These projections cover a period forward in time of almost 100 years, and there is a discussion of how the United Nations (UN) makes guesses as to whether there will be nine, ten or many more (or many less) billion of us around at that early 22nd-century point of 2100. This is followed by Chapter 47, which complements the discussion by looking more precisely at which places we know have been losing and gaining the most people since 1990, again worldwide, and again looking forward, but only to 2015.

Finally, Chapter 48 returns to the UK and asks how we can better confront the tendency of those with power to behave unethically, to ignore the evidence and to follow policies that will reduce all of our collective chances of all growing old gracefully together. The following sums up the direction in which we in Britain, and those in similarly divided states, are currently heading. It is through the continuing scandal of unequal health that the harm caused by tolerating our current course will become most clearly measured in the immediate years to come:

Titanic Inequality,

Nigel Jones (Review, 14 April) says of the author of a book on the Titanic, 'with great sensitivity, [he] dissects the apartheid-like social distinctions on board – with the rich paying 10 times as much as the steerage class for their passage, and the poor forbidden to enter the liner's lounges and libraries reserved for their betters', as if things were better now.

One doesn't need 'great sensitivity' to see all manner of similar 'apartheid-like social distinctions' of class in our contemporary society. Anybody sitting in a coach-class carriage of a train who has tried to walk through a first-class carriage to step off on to the platform, or has tried to use a business-class bathroom on any airline when they're sitting in 'steerage', will have come up against similar barriers. Today, the lowest-paid have incomes less than one-third of one per cent of the highest-paid, and the research evidence shows that a wide range of health and social problems become worse with greater inequality. Our society is now rapidly heading towards being as unequal as it was in the Titanic era, and the iceberg we'll crash into will do far more damage. (Pickett, 2012)

References

Bhalotra, S. and Pogge, T. (2012) *Ethical and economic perspectives on global health interventions*, IZA Policy Paper No 38, Bonn: Forschungsinstitut zur Zukunft der Arbeit (Institute for the Study of Labor, IZA) (http://ftp.iza.org/pp38.pdf).

Boseley, S. (2012) 'How 900 stillbirths could be prevented', *The Guardian*, 25 June (www.guardian.co.uk/uk/2012/jun/25/stillbirths-900-preventable-england).

Davey Smith, G. and Dorling, D. (1996) '"I'm all right, John": voting patterns and mortality in England and Wales, 1981–92', *British Medical Journal*, vol 313, no 7072, December, pp 1573-7.

Dorling, D. and Thomas, B. (2011) *Bankrupt Britain: An atlas of social change*, Bristol: The Policy Press.

Greenhaigh, P. (2012) 'Rich diversity', Letter, *The Guardian*, 23 March (www.guardian. co.uk/theguardian/2012/mar/23/toll-roads-budget-mad-men).

Harris, J. (2012) 'The Tories are no closer to shaking the taint of privilege issue', *The Guardian*, 25 March (www.guardian.co.uk/commentisfree/2012/mar/25/cruddas-tories-privilege-arrogance).

Macintyre, B. (2007) '"Cruel" experiment that left its mark on a very precocious boy', *The Times*, 19 May (http://journalisted.com/article/2p3).

Moore, S. (2012) 'Gove is so busy trying to recreate the narrow education of the past that he's blind to the future', *The Guardian*, 4 April (www.guardian.co.uk/commentisfree/2012/apr/04/gove-is-blind-to-future).

Ortiz, I., Daniels, L.M. and Engilbertsdóttir, S. (2012) *Child poverty and inequality: New perspectives*, New York: UNICEF (www.unicef.org/socialpolicy/index_62108.html and www.unicef.org/socialpolicy/files/Child_Poverty_Inequality_FINAL_web. pdf).

Pickett, K. (2012) 'Titanic inequality', Letter, *The Guardian*, 16 April (www.guardian. co.uk/society/2012/apr/16/titanic-inequality-poverty-society).

Ramesh, R. (2012) 'Young migrants living "far below poverty line"', *The Guardian*, 9 April (www.guardian.co.uk/uk/2012/apr/09/young-migrants-below-poverty-line?newsfeed=true).

WHO (World Health Organization) Commission on Social Determinants of Health (2008) *Closing the gap in a generation: Health equity through action on the social determinants of health*, Final Report of the Commission on Social Determinants of Health, Geneva: WHO.

42

Measuring the impact of major life events upon happiness

Ballas, D. and Dorling, D. (2007) 'Measuring the impact of major life events upon happiness', *International Journal of Epidemiology*, vol 36, no 6, pp 1244-52.

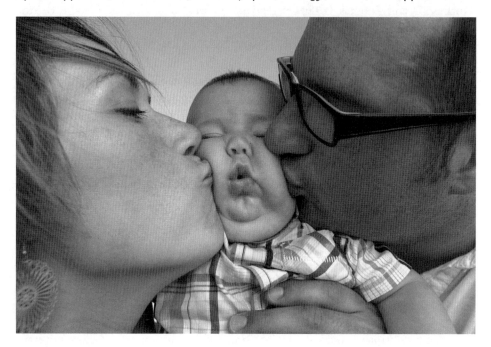

Key messages

1. Secondary data analysis of self-reported happiness and major life event data can provide an initial suggestion, of which dynamic events appear to matter most in people's lives and some measure of to whom and where those events are most likely to occur.
2. Our analysis suggests that in British society at the end of the 20th century personal relationships were extremely important in terms of happiness, just surpassing the importance of relationships at work on individual well-being.
3. Births and deaths as well as health and employment-related events, also appear to have a considerable effect on happiness. In contrast, events such as 'going on holiday' or 'buying a pet' do not seem to have any significant consistent impact on happiness.

Abstract

Background: In recent years there have been numerous attempts to define and measure happiness in various contexts and pertaining to a wide range of disciplines, ranging from neuroscience and psychology to philosophy, economics and social policy. This chapter builds on recent work by economists who attempt to estimate happiness regressions using large random samples of individuals in order to calculate monetary 'compensating amounts' for different life 'events'.

Methods: We estimate happiness regressions using the 'major life event' and 'happiness' data from the British Household Panel Survey.

Results: The data and methods used in this article suggest that in contrast to living states such as 'being married', it is more events such as 'starting a new relationship' that have the highest positive effect on happiness. This is closely followed by 'employment-related gains' (in contrast to employment status). Also, women who become pregnant on average report higher than average levels of subjective happiness (in contrast to 'being a parent'). Other events that appear to be associated with happiness according to our analysis include 'personal education related events' (e.g. starting a new course, graduating from university, passing exams) and 'finance/house related events' (e.g. buying a new house). On the other hand, the event that has the highest negative impact upon happiness according to our analysis is 'the end of my relationship', closely followed by 'death of a parent'. Adverse health events pertaining to the parents of the respondents also have a high negative coefficient and so does an employment-related loss.

Conclusion: The analysis presented in this chapter suggests that what matters the most in people's lives in Britain is to have good dynamic interpersonal relationships and to be respected at work with that respect being constantly renewed. These 'goods' are as much reflected through dynamic events as static situations. Relationships at work appear to be of a similar order of importance to those at home. Other factors that contribute to higher than average levels of subjective happiness, at least at a superficial level, include delaying death and keeping illness at bay, having babies, buying homes and cars, and passing exams. The analysis presented here also suggests that people should not expect too much from their holidays and wider families. The findings presented in this article may help us to understand a little better the propensity for groups to be more or less happy and may help us to begin to better understand the importance of the dynamics of social context—the context in which we come to terms with reward and loss.

Keywords: Happiness, well-being, major life events, British Household Panel Survey

[Note – all references in this chapter are numbered and are listed at the end.]

Introduction

Human perceptions of happiness vary and depend on a wide range of factors. Efforts to define and understand happiness date back long ago to include, for instance, Buddhist traditions and practices. However, the origins of western thought in this area can be found only a few decades later than Buddhist scripts in the work of Socrates, Plato and Aristotle. In particular, Aristotle, in his work *Nicomachean Ethics,* attempted to give an answer to the question: what is the good life for man?[1,2]

For Aristotle (born almost exactly a century after Gautama Buddha died), happiness is the highest good achieved by human action. Aristotle suggested that the attainment of happiness involves the satisfaction of the human desires that are necessary to live a full and rich life.[1] However, Aristotle believed that the question of what is a full and rich life cannot be answered for an individual in abstraction from the society in which they live, in contrast to some Buddhist traditions.

The meaning of happiness varies through space and time and there have been numerous attempts to understand and define happiness since the work of Aristotle. Attempting to determine the factors that make individuals happy has long been represented as a research challenge that spans many academic disciplines. There have been numerous recent studies of happiness and well-being issues, often from very different perspectives. On the one hand there are critiques of the idea that happiness can be measured such as by Sumner[3] who argues that happiness is subjective and that no objective theory about the ordinary concept of happiness has the slightest plausibility. Nevertheless, there have been several researchers who suggested that happiness can be measured[4–7] and should be measured,[8] and there has been an ongoing debate over how to measure it.[9–11]

In an epidemiological context, it would be of practical use to have good measurements of happiness and well-being and to be able to also determine what the key psychosocial and environmental factors affecting well-being are. Among these factors are major events and experiences that occur throughout the life course. Such events have often been classified on the basis of their association with depression and ill-health and of how stressful they are in various contexts.[12–17] Cumulative exposure to 'negative' major life events throughout the life course may be linked to increased risks of chronic unhappiness, mental illness and premature mortality.[18] In contrast, cumulative lifetime exposure to 'positive' major life events may be associated with increased probabilities of sustained happiness, good health and well-being.[19]

Recent research has been[20] aimed at measuring the importance of different life events expressed in the form of money, in determining personal happiness, using data from the British Household Panel Survey (BHPS), a representative sample of some 10 000 individuals living in Britain in the 1990s (see Taylor *et al.*[21] for more details). This survey includes a question that asks whether the respondents have been recently unhappy or depressed, and a number of the straightforward questions that seek to measure individual contentment such as whether respondents feel 'able to enjoy normal day-to-day activities'; whether they 'have been losing self-confidence'; and whether 'they are losing sleep over worry'.

Clark and Oswald[20] fitted regression models of happiness that measured the impact of different life events upon human well-being. In particular, using pooled data from the first seven waves of the BHPS (1991–97), they defined an occurrence of a 'life event' as a change between different states such as 'single' to 'married', 'employed' to 'unemployed' and 'health excellent' to 'health good'. They then estimated ordered probit regression equations, with measures of subjective well-being as their dependent variables and 'life event' (state change) dummy variables as well as monthly income as their independent variables and they used these equations to estimate the 'compensating amounts' for various changes of states. For instance, they estimated that a change between a state of having 'Excellent Health' to having 'Good Health' was equivalent to losing, on average, £12,000 a month[*] in income.

This chapter builds on the work of Clark and Oswald[20] and complements the work of Oswald and Powdthavee[22] by investigating further the potential of the BHPS to measure the impact of life events on happiness. However, we do not attempt to attach monetary values to life states. Instead, this chapter focuses on BHPS variables that explicitly pertain to 'life events' for a similar time period to that examined by Clark and Oswald. In particular, the so-called 'Major Life Event' BHPS data (see the appendix to this chapter, pp 401–2, and Taylor *et al.*[21] for a detailed description of all event categories) were utilized in order to investigate the degree to which these events affect subjective well-being by using simple cross-tabulations of 'Major Life Events' and 'Subjective Happiness'. A multiple regression equation was also fitted on the 'Major Life Event' data in order to measure the relative importance of different events in relation to subjective happiness.

Data and method

Examining happiness and major life events in the BHPS

Between September 1992 and December 1995, members of the BHPS were asked to: 'state in your own words what in the last year has happened to you (or your family) which stood out as important'. Up to four events were recorded on up to four occasions in four consecutive years (1992, 1993, 1994 and 1995). [This question was discontinued in 1996 but was then asked again in 1999, 2001 and 2004. In the context of this chapter, we focused on the years when the question was asked consecutively (1992–95), which also represent a relatively similar period to that examined by Clark and Oswald (1991–97).] These were coded as 80 types of event that were placed by us into the following categories:

[*] Editorial Note: This may appear a very high amount and it is. Average monthly income in Britain as reported by the study authors at the time of their study was £2,000. They estimated the value of not losing your job as equivalent to an additional £23,000 a month in income! These sums are partly so high because, despite our everyday suspicions, additional income above average is not associated with great increases in happiness, whereas losing your job or experiencing a decline in health is associated with greater declines in expressed well-being.

- Health-related events
- Education
- Employment
- Leisure

- Births and Deaths
- Relationships
- Finance and Other

In addition, each of these events related to 21 possible subjects (see the appendix to this chapter, pp 401-2). For instance, one of the events was coded as: 'my mother' (subject 8) 'passed her driving test' (event 32).

In the context of this chapter, different combinations of 'major life events' and 'event subjects' have been explored in order to define a smaller number of more 'statistically manageable' events. It should be noted that in practice, of the 1680 possible events only 34 combinations accounted each for more than 1% of all recorded events and so an aggregation of major life events to these 34 combinations is used here. Table 42.1 lists these 34 combinations of 'major life events' and 'subjects'.

In order to explore the possible relationship between different events and subjective well-being, we used the following GHQ (General Health Questionnaire): 'General Happiness' BHPS question: 'Have you recently been feeling reasonably happy, all things considered?' with the responses: 'More so than usual', 'Same as usual', 'Less so' and 'Much less'. For the purposes of exploring the impact of different variables upon happiness, it was more meaningful to aggregate the third and fourth responses, so we recoded these into one category entitled 'Less so than usual'. We also reversed the scores, so that higher values indicate 'higher happiness'. We then used the data from the years in which the event data discussed above were also collected (1992–95) in order to explore the impact of our 34 'Major Life Events' (Table 42.1) upon subjective happiness. Table 42.2 gives an indication of what these relationships might be. In particular, it shows how average happiness levels, measured on the 1–3 scale varies across different events.

Results

As can be seen in Table 42.1, according to the data most survey respondents are likely to report that there were no major life events in the previous year: 'nothing important happened' makes up 66.12% of all 'events'. Next most commonly occurring are events that can be labelled: 'Finance and other'; and then 'Relationships' events that make up 6.49 and 6.02% of the total number of recorded events, respectively.

It should be noted that the frequency of the various 'major life events' described in Table 42.1 vary considerably across different age groups. Figure 42.1 shows this variation by single year of age group for events in each of the seven categories described in Table 42.1. There are many notable patterns in Figure 42.1, for instance, the tendency of younger people to report 'education'-related events as major, whereas older people tend to report 'health'-related events. People of an age likely to be parents of school age children also have a higher than average interest in education. Many events that matter to folk are not those that immediately affect them but those that affect people they care about and/or for (or who care for them).

Table 42.1: 'Major life event' and 'subject' combinations, BHPS waves 1992–95 (pooled), Britain.

Description of event combination	Frequency	Frequency (%)	Description of event combination	Frequency	Frequency (%)
Nothing important happened	94911	66.12	**Births and deaths**		
Health related events			Pregnancy/birth (other)	97	0.07
Health 1-9[a] (other[b])	991	0.69	Pregnancy/birth (mine)	1284	0.89
Health 1-9 (mine)	2678	1.86	Pregnancy/birth (child's)	1309	0.91
Health 1-9 (partner)	755	0.52	Pregnancy/birth (family)	1264	0.88
Health 1-9 (child)	620	0.43	Death (other)	384	0.27
Health 1-9 (parent)	648	0.45	Death (parent)	708	0.49
Subtotal	5692	3.96	Death (family[c])	1674	1.16
Education			Subtotal	6720	4.67
Education (other)	903	0.63	**Relationships**		
Education (mine)	2185	1.52	Relationships (family 35, 41-42)	988	0.69
Education (child)	1828	1.27	Relationships (mine starting 35, 42)	1597	1.11
Subtotal	4916	3.42	Relationships (child's starting 35, 42)	830	0.58
Employment			Relationships (mine ending 36, 43)	637	0.44
Employment (other)	1808	1.26	Relationships (family 46-53, 55-59)	3728	2.59
Employment (job change)	2615	1.82	Relationships (pet ownership/ companionship 54)	560	0.39
Employment (job gain)	1143	0.79	Subtotal	8661	6.02
Employment (job loss)	1370	0.95	**Finance and other**		
Subtotal	6936	4.82	Finance (other 60-69, 73-79)	2563	1.78
Leisure			Finance (car 70)	973	0.68
Leisure (other)	1824	1.27	Finance (house 71)	772	0.54
Leisure (our holiday)	1223	0.85	Moving home (44, 80-81)	2810	1.95
Leisure (my holiday)	3635	2.53	Other event (10-11, 32-34, 37-39, 90-95)	2224	1.55
Subtotal	6682	4.64	Subtotal	9342	6.49
			Total number of recorded events*	143860	

Notes: * The total number of recorded events include all reported 1st, 2nd, 3rd and 4th important life events. Respondents were asked to list all events in order of importance. In the cases when respondents only reported at least one important event but not all four, we assumed that the rest of the events were equivalent to the 'nothing important happened' category (e.g. if an individual reported 'employment, job change' as the 1st important life event, but did not report any other events, we recorded the rest of the event responses as 'nothing important happened').
[a] '1–9' and all other numbering in this table refers to the major life event categories, as coded by the BHPS, see http://ije.oxfordjournals.org/content/36/6/1244.full.pdf Appendix.
[b] 'Other' refers to any person or subject other than 'mine', 'partner', 'child' (e.g. it could be 'friend/ colleague/neighbour/employer' or 'grandparents', etc, see http://ije.oxfordjournals.org/content/36 /6/1244.full.pdf Appendix).
[c] Note that thankfully too few children in the BHPS died in these years for enough of their parents to record the event for us to include it in this analysis. Results not reported here, however, do suggest that death of a child or grandchild is extremely traumatic and future research using more years of life histories should examine this further.

Source: British Household Panel Study questions asked between September 1992 and December 1992 on what happened to respendents or their family.

Table 42.2 shows how subjective happiness levels vary across different events and which events are characterized by higher than average levels of 'happiness' or 'unhappiness'. For instance, 32% of the observations that recorded 'relationship mine ending' as a major life event also record subjective happiness, which is 'less so than usual' (relationships ending are generally a source of unhappiness; however, for a smal but quantifiable group the end of the relationship is reason for celebration). The respective figure for average unhappiness of those that recorded 'death of a parent' as a major life event is 25% (perhaps most of these deaths occurred at a time that was more predictable than are the demise of most partnerships). On the other hand, 33% of the people that recorded the start of a personal relationship as a major

Table 42.2: Major life events and happiness, BHPS waves 1992–95 (pooled), Britain.

Event	Subjective general happiness (%)			
	Less so than usual	As usual	More so than usual	Total
Nothing important happened	13	74	13	100
Health (other[a] 1-9[b])	18	70	12	100
Health (mine 1-9)	22	68	10	100
Health (partner 1-9)	17	75	8	100
Health (child 1-9)	18	73	9	100
Health (parent 1-9)	25	61	14	100
Education (other 12-19)	11	74	15	100
Education (mine 12-19)	13	62	25	100
Education (child 12-19)	15	73	12	100
Employment (other 23, 26-29)	18	64	18	100
Employment (job change 20-21)	12	68	20	100
Employment (job gain 22)	10	67	23	100
Employment (job loss 24)	24	64	12	100
Leisure (other 30-31)	10	73	17	100
Leisure (our holiday 30)	11	76	13	100
Leisure (my holiday 30)	11	74	15	100
Pregnancy/birth (other 40)	17	64	19	100
Pregnancy/birth (mine 40)	12	64	24	100
Pregnancy/birth (child's 40)	10	78	12	100
Pregnancy/birth (family 40)	11	71	18	100
Death (other 45)	23	66	11	100
Death (parent 45)	26	66	8	100
Death (family 45)	20	69	11	100
Relationships (family 35, 41-42)	12	70	18	100
Relationships (mine starting 35, 42)	11	56	33	100
Relationships (child's starting 35, 42)	11	76	13	100
Relationships (mine ending 36, 43)	32	48	20	100
Relationships (family 46-53, 55-59)	14	73	13	100
Relationships (pet ownership/companionship 54)	17	68	15	100
Finance (other 60-69, 73-79)	15	70	15	100
Finance (car 70)	10	72	18	100
Finance (house 71)	9	66	25	100
Moving home (44, 80-81)	14	68	18	100
Other event (10-11, 32-34, 37-39, 90-95)	16	68	16	100
Population mean levels	13	73	14	100

Note: For all [a]subject codes and [b]numbered category codes see http://ije.oxfordjournals.org/content/36/6/1244.full.pdf Appendix.

Source: British Household Panel Study questions asked between September 1992 and December 1992 on what happened to study members or their family.

life event also record 'more than usual' levels of subjective happiness (in this case, it is interesting how many are sanguine). In addition, 25% of the people that record 'education, mine' as a major life event also report 'more than usual' levels of happiness. It is also interesting to note that 'pregnancy/birth, other' is associated with relatively high rates of both 'happiness' (19% of 'more than usual') and 'unhappiness' (17% of 'less than usual', possibly expressing unwanted pregnancies or post-natal depression, and often of people's grown-up children being pregnant, perhaps cementing a relationship with an offspring's partner that the parents had hoped would end).

In order to evaluate the effect of the events described in Tables 42.1 and 42.2 upon happiness, we employed the statistical tool of ordinary least squares (OLS) multivariate regression, building on the work of Clark and Oswald briefly reviewed in the previous section. It should be noted though that, unlike Clark and Oswald, we fitted an OLS model (instead of ordered probits) on data pertaining to changes of state—events—that respondents themselves declare as important (instead of differences in state) and we did not attempt to assign a monetary value upon different events (and hence we did not include an income variable in the analysis).

Table 42.3 summarizes the results of the OLS regression analysis (listing the life event regression coefficients in ascending order). High negative values imply an association of the event with 'unhappiness', whereas high positive values indicate that an event has an association with 'happiness'. As can be seen in Table 42.3, the event 'the end of my relationship' has the highest negative coefficient and therefore according to the BHPS data and the method used here, it has the highest positive association with 'unhappiness'. This is followed by 'death of a parent' and the effect upon the individual of health events pertaining to the parents of the respondents. A 'death of some other person' (not family member) also has a high negative coefficient and so does an employment-related loss (e.g. being made redundant or

Figure 42.1: Major life themes by age in Britain (aged 15–97), frequency of reporting events in the last year concerning subject.

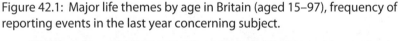

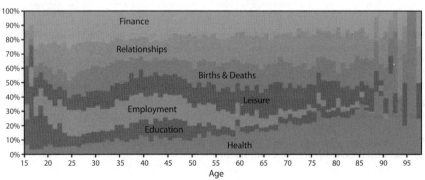

Source: British Household Panel Study questions asked between September 1992 and December 1992 on what happened of significance to all study members or to a member of their family.

see colour version in plate section

Table 42.3: Subjective happiness and major life events, BHPS waves 1992–95 (pooled and weighted), Britain.

Life Event	Coefficient	P-value[a]	Frequency (%) x Regression coefficient	Original regression rank	Prevalence-based regression rank
Relationships (mine[b] ending 36, 43[c])	-0.178	0.00	-0.08	1	6
Death (parent 45)	-0.166	0.00	-0.08	2	5
Health[d] (parent 1-9)	-0.139	0.00	-0.06	3	7
Death (other 45)	-0.137	0.00	-0.04	4	11
Employment (job loss 24)	-0.129	0.00	-0.12	5	3
Health (mine 1-9)	-0.117	0.00	-0.22	6	2
Death (family 45)	-0.098	0.00	-0.11	7	4
Health (partner 1-9)	-0.092	0.00	-0.05	8	9
Health (child 1-9)	-0.084	0.00	-0.04	9	13
Health (other 1-9)	-0.073	0.00	-0.05	10	8
Education (child 12-19)	-0.029	0.12	-0.04	11	12
Employment (other 23, 26-29)	-0.028	0.13	-0.04	12	15
Other event (10-11, 32-34, 37-39, 90-95)	-0.026	0.14	-0.04	13	10
Nothing important happened	-0.022	0.11	-1.47	14	1
Relationships (pet ownership/companionship 54)	-0.020	0.44	-0.01	15	17
Finance (other 60-69, 73-79)	-0.019	0.27	-0.03	16	16
Relationships (family 46-53, 55-59)	-0.014	0.39	-0.04	17	14
Relationships (family 35, 41-42)	0.002	0.91	0.00	18	18
Leisure (our holiday 30)	0.010	0.61	0.01	19	20
Moving home (44, 80-81)	0.013	0.46	0.02	20	24
Education (other 12-19)	0.024	0.27	0.02	21	21
Finance (car 70)	0.027	0.22	0.02	22	22
Leisure (my holiday 30)	0.029	0.07	0.07	23	30
Pregnancy/birth (other 40)	0.031	0.56	0.00	24	19
Pregnancy/birth (family 40)	0.034	0.09	0.03	25	25
Relationships (child's starting 35, 42)	0.037	0.10	0.02	26	23
Employment (job change 20-21)	0.040	0.02	0.07	27	29
Leisure (other 30-31)	0.043	0.02	0.05	28	28
Education (mine 12-19)	0.052	0.00	0.08	29	33
Pregnancy/birth (child's 40)	0.053	0.01	0.05	30	26
Pregnancy/birth (mine 40)	0.084	0.00	0.08	31	31
Finance (house 71)	0.097	0.00	0.05	32	27
Employment (job gain 22)	0.097	0.00	0.08	33	32
Relationships (mine starting 35, 42)	0.160	0.00	0.18	34	34

Notes: OLS regression equation of subject happiness adjusted for gender, age, age squared and education, weighted on the basis of the 1995 cross-sectional weights; note that the value of the constant is 2.25. For all [a]subject codes and [b]numbered category codes see http://ije.oxfordjournals.org/content/36/6/1244.full.pdf Appendix.
[c] See chapter appendix for a detailed description of all event category codes.
[d] Health-related events include 'negative' (e.g. injury) as well as 'positive' events (e.g. recovery, positive test results); the same applies to many of the other variables listed here; see above appendix for more details.

Source: British Household Panel Study questions asked between September 1992 and December 1992 on what happened to them or their family.

experiencing a pay cut). Note that, as stated earlier, we only considered events that when aggregated, accounted for more than 1% of all recorded events. By using this aggregation, major events such as 'death of a child'—which accounted for <1% of all events—were subsumed in the 'death in family' overall category.

The events listed at the bottom of Table 42.3 have the highest positive coefficients and therefore can be considered to have a relatively high association with 'happiness'. 'Starting a new relationship' has the highest positive coefficient and this is closely followed by 'employment-related gain' (e.g. a new job, or a promotion or pay rise) and 'financial, house related events' (e.g. buying a new house). Other events that appear to be associated with happiness according to our analysis include pregnancies and 'personal education-related events' (e.g. starting a new course, graduating from university, passing exams).

The regression model takes into account the frequency of the different events and this is expressed to a degree through the '*P-values*' (second column in Table 42.3)—infrequent life events with unpredictable consequences are less likely to show effects with small, and hence more significant, *P-values*. However, it is useful at this stage to combine the frequency data presented in Table 42.1 with the regression results of the rough importance of an event in order to give prominence to events that both matter (have a not insignificant effect), and which are more likely to happen in people's lives (and also more likely to be reported as 'major life events'). For example, it is interesting to note that there were 1597 events (1.11% of total events) described as 'relationship, mine, starting' which, as seen in Table 42.3, has the highest regression coefficient and can therefore be considered to be the (aggregate) life event type that is most associated with happiness. In addition, the event with the second highest positive coefficient ('employment, job gain') was reported 1143 times (0.79% of all major life events). It is noteworthy that the top 10 events in terms of positive regression coefficients were reported 14,283 times in the survey (10.32% of all events). On the other hand, the event with the highest negative coefficient ('end of my relationship') was reported 637 times in the survey (0.44% of the total). The event with the second highest negative coefficient ('death of a parent') was reported 708 times (0.49% of the total). The top 10 events with the highest negative coefficient were reported 10,465 times (7.29% of all major life events). People may thus, presumably, be a little averse to reporting bad news in social surveys. As many relationships have to end as start, albeit some that last long will end only through death.

It is interesting to see how the life events would be ranked if their prevalence were taken into account. The fifth column of Table 42.3 shows how the life events would be ranked if the overall impact on population happiness is taken into account by multiplying the frequency of events (second column in Table 42.1) by the regression coefficient (first column in Table 42.3). When ranked in this way, the event category 'nothing important happened' is on top (compared with 14th place in the regression coefficient-based rank). This 'event' category has a very low regression coefficient but also has the highest frequency. Thus, it can be argued that the slow, mundane aspects of most of everyday existence, when nothing of interest happens, have some of the highest negative impacts on our happiness. Comparing columns 4 and 5 in Table 42.3, it is also interesting to note that there is a considerable shift in the order of the events associated with unhappiness. Events pertaining to personal health problems ('health, mine') are, when ordered by magnitude in this way, on top of the list, followed by 'employment, job loss' and 'death of a family member'. 'End of my relationship', which has the highest negative regression coefficient is the 6th event when ordered by magnitude. Looking at the events in the bottom of the alternative prevalence-based regression rank, it is also interesting to note that events pertaining to a new personal relationship ('relationships, mine starting') still have the highest positive position even when measured as the product of frequency and regression coefficient (life is not as simple as the song lyric '*all you need is love*', but love gets you most happiness in the short term). New social/emotional relationships are followed in happiness rankings by new school/collegiate friends and challenges: 'education, mine starting', and then the same for the slightly less best-days-of-your-life world of new work: 'employment, job gain'.

Discussion

The results presented in this chapter can be used to paint a picture of the life events that superficially matter the most in people's lives. Our analysis suggests that in British society by the end of the 20th century personal relationships were extremely important in terms of happiness. In short, the analysis presented in this chapter suggests that what matters the most in British people's lives is to have good interpersonal relationships (to be respected and cared for at home) and to be respected at work. Respect at the workplace is shown best by promotion and events related to that which we have similarly coded.

Over love—it is easy to recognize that interpersonal relationships are good when they are new. Many in happy relationships may well adapt to seeing that state as normal. However, our methods will not effectively measure long-lasting happiness when relationships do not change other than very obliquely through the general negative reporting of 'nothing changing'. What the research presented in this chapter has hopefully provided is, instead, an initial suggestion of which dynamic events appear to matter most in people's lives and some idea of to whom and where those events are most likely to occur. It can be argued that the findings presented here may help us to understand the propensity for groups to be more or less happy, better or worse-off, made more or less ill through sustained worry or cumulative good fortune.

The findings appear to be consistent with much recent research on happiness, but they hopefully add some more concrete examples to that work and further clues as to the proximal mechanisms involved. For instance, the importance of interpersonal relationships is consistent with relevant research findings highlighting the importance of social wellbeing [23] as well as social trust and local community networks to our quality of life[24] and suggesting that friendship is one of the biggest sources of happiness and well-being.[25,26] The strength of the importance of employment is unexpected but is consistent with new theories of the importance of respect and self-esteem in societies in general.[27] It can also be argued that the negative impact of the 'nothing happened' event category is consistent with arguments made by Bauman,[28] according to which in modern materialistic societies being bored, in addition to making one feel uncomfortable, is also turning into a shameful stigma and a testimony of negligence or defeat, which may lead to a state of acute depression.

Instead of the GHQ, there are a number of alternative measures of happiness and subjective well-being in the BHPS that could be used as a dependent variable in the regression model described above. In the context of this research, we explored these measures and re-fitted the regression equations in order to examine whether there were any differences in the results.

It is also interesting to compare the relative importance of the 34 life event variables with that of the variables examined by Clark and Oswald.[20] In order to do so, we added the following variables to the regression model described in Table 42.3: 'health status', 'educational qualifications' and 'employment status'. According to this alternative model, if included, 'health status' has a much higher impact on happiness when compared with other life events. In particular, the coefficient of the dummy variable 'Health Excellent' (with having 'poor' or 'very poor' health as a reference category) has a value which is more than double that of the 'start of my relationship' life event. This is perhaps to be expected given that good health and happiness are often interchangeable concepts. [For instance, in many languages the expression 'good health' is commonly used (instead of 'cheers') upon having a drink.] Apart from the health-state variable, the inclusion of the other 'state' variables analysed by Clark and Oswald did not change the relative magnitude of the top-ten positive and top-six negative coefficients of the original equation described in Table 42.3. Nevertheless, it is interesting that being 'separated' and being 'unemployed' are in the top-ten list of negative coefficients (eighth and ninth in the list, respectively). It is also noteworthy that the state of being unemployed has a smaller (in absolute terms) coefficient than the life event of job loss (which includes 'becoming unemployed'). It can be argued that this adds quantitative evidence supporting the idea that people adjust to new circumstances through adaptation and habituation processes.[29–31]

It should be noted that one of the limitations of the analysis presented here is that the data and methods that were used would not allow us to consider possible 'memory recall bias' effects and in particular the degree, to which the psychological state of subjective happiness might influence which life events are retrospectively retrieved from memory and which are nominated as 'major'. It may be the case, for instance, that an 'unhappy' survey respondent may be less likely to remember or report as important a desirable life event★ and, in contrast, happy respondents may recall more desirable events.[32]

Conclusion

The findings presented in this chapter build upon an existing and rapidly growing body of interdisciplinary research on the determinants of well-being adding to the debate on whether increasing happiness should be a key public health policy goal.

★ Editorial Note: It may even be possible to predict which people are more likely to see the same glass as half empty and which as half full, but further research would be required.

Among the aims of such policies could be to raise the occurrence of lifetime exposure to 'positive' major life events and to minimize the exposure to and/or outcome of 'negative' events (or 'non-events' in the case of 'nothing important happening'). Our results could be used to inform more humane versions of cost–benefit analysis. For instance, at the national level, it could be argued that there is a need for policies that would increase leisure and social time (possibly via taxation change).[25] It is also possible to enhance the chances of events such as 'job gains' to occur in people's life and to increase educational opportunities. To give just one example, employers could be encouraged (through taxation) to adopt a policy of small pay rises spread across many employees over many years rather than larger rises for the few.

It should be noted that there might be a considerable degree of interdependencies between life events and other factors. For instance, the ability to make and maintain friends may be affected to a certain degree by factors such as income and occupational status. Thus, the probability and severity of major life events can be influenced by life course and socioeconomic position and further research is needed to study such influences that would have major policy implications. Furthermore, it has long been argued that there is a strong relationship between inequalities and health, although that relationship is more about one's place in a society than about a locality.[27,33] It can similarly be argued that there is a relationship between subjective happiness and inequalities[34] and in this context the degree, to which there are inequalities in the probabilities of major life events to occur to different social groups would mirror a similar inequality in the distribution of happiness.

The degree to which people compare themselves most with their 'near equals' in a society[35] or 'peer groups'[36–39] will affect the relative impact of different life events upon happiness (if everyone else is getting a promotion or boyfriend/girlfriend, why not you?). Finally, the ability of people to adjust to new circumstances through adaptation processes[40,41] may also affect their responsiveness to different life events. Whatever else may be true, it is hard to argue that we should not be looking a little more closely at what folks themselves say most matters to them in their lives.[42]

References[*]

[1] Lear J. Aristotle: *The Desire to Understand*. Cambridge: Cambridge University Press, 1988.

[2] Ross WD. *Aristotle*. London: Methuen & Co., 1923.

[3] Sumner LW. *Welfare, Happiness and Ethics*. Oxford: Clarendon Press, 1996.

[4] Griffin J. *Well-being: Its Meaning, Measurement and Moral Importance*. Oxford: Clarendon, 1986.

[5] Broome J. *Ethics Out of Economics*. Cambridge: Cambridge University Press, 1999.

[6] Frey B, Stutzer A. *Happiness and Economics*. Princeton: Princeton University Press, 2002.

---

[*] Note that in this chapter and in Chapter 39 above, to save space, references are formatted in medical journal style.

[7] Blanchflower DG, Oswald AJ. *Hypertension and Happiness Across Nations.* Working Paper, University of Warwick, 2007.

[8] Shah S, Marcs N. *A Well-being Manifesto for a Flourishing Society.* London: New Economics Foundation. Available at: http://www.neweconomics.org/gen/z_sys_publicationdetail.aspx?pid193, 2004.

[9] Little IMD. *A Critique of Welfare Economics.* Oxford: Clarendon Press, Oxford, 1957.

[10] Sen A. *Choice, Welfare and Measurement.* Oxford: Blackwell, 1982.

[11] Sen A. *On Ethics and Economics.* Oxford: Blackwell, 1987.

[12] Holmes TH, Rahe RH. The social readjustment rating scale. *Journal of Psychomatic Research* 1967;11:213–8.

[13] Kessing LV, Agerbo E, Mortensen PB. Does the impact of major stressful life events on the risk of developing depression change throughout life? *Psychological Medicine* 2003;33:1177–84.

[14] Voss E, Stegmann A, Schro¨der J. Stressful life events, protective factors and depressive disorders in middle adulthood In: Wahl H-W, Hermann B, Heidrun M, Dietrich R, Christoph R (eds). *The Many Faces of Health, Competence and Well-Being in Old Age.* New York: Springer, 2006, pp. 99–113.

[15] Brilman EI, Ormel J. Life events, difficulties and onset of depressive episodes in later life. *Psychological Medicine* 2001;31:859–69.

[16] Brown GW, Harris T. *Social Origins of Depression: A Study of Psychiatric Disorder in Women.* London: Tavistock Press, 1978.

[17] Brown GW, Harris T. *Life Events and Illness.* London: Unwin Hyman, Guilford Press, 1989.

[18] Davey Smith G. Socio-economic differentials In: Kuh D, Ben-Sholmo Y (eds). *A Life Course Approach to Chronic Disease Epidemiology: Tracing the origins of ill-health from early to adult life,* Oxford: Oxford Medical Publications, 1997, pp. 242–73.

[19] Hatch S, Huppert FA, Abbot R *et al.* A life course approach to wellbeing In: Haworth J, Hart G (eds). *Well-Being: Individual, Community, and Social Perspectives.* Basingstoke: Palgrave, 2007, pp. 187–205.

[20] Clark AE, Oswald AJ. A simple statistical method for measuring how life events affect happiness. *International Journal of Epidemiology* 2002;31:1139–44.

[21] Taylor MF, Brice J, Buck N, Prentice-Lane E. *British Household Panel Survey User Manual Volume A: Introduction, Technical Report and Appendices.* Colchester: University of Essex, 2001.

[22] Oswald A, Powdthavee N. *Death and the calculation of hedonic damages.* Preliminary draft of paper for June 1–2 2007 workshop at the University of Chicago, 7 May 2007. Available at http:// www2.warwick.ac.uk/fac/soc/economics/staff/faculty/oswald/ jlschicagojune2007.pdf

[23] Keyes C. Social well-being. *Social Psychology Quarterly* 1998;61:121–40.

[24] Putnam R. *Bowling Alone: The Collapse and Revival of American Community.* New York: Simon and Schuster, 2000.

[25] Layard R. *Happiness: Lessons from a New Science.* London: Allen Lane, 2005.

[26] Diener E, Selingman ME. Very happy people. *Psychological Science* 2002;13:81–84.

27 Wilkinson R. *The Impact of Inequality: How to Make Sick Societies Healthier*. New York: The New Press, 2005.

28 Bauman Z. *Ill being in the world of consumers*. Paper presented at the Joseph Rowntree Foundation workshop 'Social ill-being real or imagined?', London, 22 November 2006.

29 Brickman P, Coates D, Janoff-Bulman R. Lottery winners and accident victims: is happiness relative? *Journal of Personality and Social Psychology* 1978;36:917–27.

30 Frederick S, Lowewnstein G. Hedonic adaptation In: Daniel K, Ed D, Norbert S (eds). *Well-being: The Foundations of Hedonic Psychology*. New York: Russell Sage Foundation, 1999, pp. 302–29.

31 Clark AE. Are wages habit-forming? Evidence from micro data. *Journal of Economic Behaviour and Organization* 1999;39:179–200.

32 Seidlitz L, Diener E. Memory for positive versus negative events: theories for the differences between happy and unhappy persons. *Journal of Personality and Social Psychology* 1993;64:654–64.

33 Wilkinson RG, Pickett KE. Income inequality and population health: a review and explanation of the evidence. *Social Science Medicine* 2006;62:1768–84.

34 Ballas D, Dorling D, Shaw M. Social inequality, health, and wellbeing In: Haworth J, Hart G (eds). *Well-Being: Individual, Community, and Social Perspectives*. Basingstoke: Palgrave, 2007, pp. 163–86.

35 Runciman W. *Relative Deprivation and Social Justice*. London: Routledge and Kegan Paul, 1966.

36 Clark AE, Oswald AJ. Satisfaction and comparison income. *Journal of Public Economics* 1996;61:359–81.

37 Bolton A. *Status Anxiety*. UK: Pantheon, 2004.

38 Diener E, Horwitz J, Emmons RA. Happiness of the very wealthy. *Social Indicators Research* 1985;16:263–74.

39 Marmot M. *Status Syndrome*. London: Bloomsbury, 2004.

40 Dolan P, White M. Dynamic well-being: connecting indicators of what people anticipate with indicators of what they experience. *Social Indicators Research* 2006;75:303–33.

41 Easterlin R. Explaining happiness. *Proceedings of the National Academy of Sciences of the United States of America*, 100,19, pp. 11176–11183. Available at: http://www.pnas.org/cgi/reprint/100/19/11176, 2003.

42 Dorling D, Gunnell D. Suicide: the spatial and social components of despair in Britain 1980–2000. *Transactions of the Institute of British Geographers* 2003;28:442–60 [reproduced as Chapter 20, this volume].

Appendix

This appendix provides more information on the ways in which the responses to the open-ended BHPS question asking people to state in their own words 'what has happened to you (or your family), which has stood out as important?' were coded in the BHPS (for a more detailed discussion see Taylor *et al.*[21]). Answers were recorded verbatim, but verbatim responses were not made available for public release, because of confidentiality concerns. However, the following numeric codes were developed to capture the full range of events:

Health: '01 Ill Health/Concern about Health', '02 Hospitalization/Operation', '03 Accident (Involving Injury)', '04 Health Tests (Positive & Negative)', '05 Loss of Mobility/ House-Bound', '06 Recovery/Continuing Good Health', '09 Health (not elsewhere classified—nec)'

Caring: '10 Caring Responsibilities—Not Childcare (ascertained by asking: Who is Cared For?)'; '11 Babysitting (made clear by asking: Who is the Sitter?)'.

Education: '12 Starting/In School', '13 Leaving School', '14 Starting/In Further Education (inc. Sixth Form)', '15 Leaving Further Education', '16 Studying For/ Passing Educational/Vocational Qualifications/Acquiring Skills/Training (nec)', '17 Travel Related to Study', '19 Education (nec)'.

Employment: '20 Change of Job (inc. Hours, Status)/Starting Own Business'; '21 Planned/Possible Change of Job', '22 Getting Job (Following Economic Inactivity)', '23 Work-related Training (inc. Apprenticeship/HGV Licence/Work Experience)', '24 Redundancy/Unemployment (Threat of or Actual)', '25 Retirement', '26 Travel Related to Work (Who Travels?)', '27 Work-related Problems', '29 Jobs/Careers (nec)'.

Leisure/Political: '30 Vacation/Travel (nec)', '31 Leisure Activities', '32 Learning to Drive/Passing Test (not HGV)', '33 Political Participation/ Voluntary Work (inc. Committee Work)', '34 Reference to National/World Events (subject is determined by asking: Who is Concerned by Event?)'.

Non-familial relationships: '35 Began Friendship (including Girl/ Boyfriend)', '36 End Friendship (including Girl/Boyfriend)', '37 Spending Time with/Visiting Friends (Coded as Holiday as Appropriate)', '38 Problems with Neighbours (Who has the Problem?)', '39 Non-Family Relationship (nec)'.

Family events: '40 Pregnancy/Birth (Identity of Parent?)', '41 Cohabitation', '42 Engagements/Weddings', '43 Separation/ Divorce/End of Cohabitation', '44 Leaving Parental Home', '45 Death (Who Died?)', '46 Wedding Anniversaries', '47 Birthday Celebrations', '48 Becoming Godparent', '50 Spending Time/Visits with Relatives (Not Within Household)', '51 Day-to-day Family Life', '52 Family Problems (Person Causing Problems?)', '53 Domestic Incident (e.g. Fire/Burst Pipes, etc)', '54 Pets/ Animals (Pet Coded)', '59 Family Event/Family Reference (nec)'.

Financial matters: '60 Money Problems/Drop in Income/Debt', '61 Forced Move (Repossession/Eviction) (Residential Move Not Included)', '62 Improved Financial Situation', '63 Received Money (Inheritance/Compensation/Pools)', '69 Financial Other (nec)'.

Consumption: '70 Bought/Buying Vehicle (Car, Caravan, etc)', '71 Bought/ Buying/Building House', '72 Household Repairs/ Improvements/Appliances', '73 Won Prize (Not Cash)/Award', '74 Received Present (from whom?)', '79 Other Purchases (nec)'.

Residential move: '80 Moved in Past Year', '81 Future Intention to Move', '82 Move into Residential Home (Nursing/ Retirement, etc)', '83 Move into Respondent's Household (Who is Moving In?)'.

Crime: '90 Victim of Crime (Burglary, etc)', '91 Committed Crime/In Trouble with Police'.

Religion: '92 Joined/Changed Religion', '93 Other Religious Reference (Not Confirmation/Baptism of Children)'.

Other: '94 Plan Not Fulfilled/Something That Didn't Happen (e.g. Didn't Have a Holiday)', '95 Civil Court Action/Battles with Bureaucracy', '96 Other Occurrence (nec) given low priority', '97 Nothing Happened'.

People's answers to the BHPS event question included not only events that happened to them personally but also events that happened to other family members or friends. Each event has, therefore, been assigned a *subject code* as follows:

'00 Not Mentioned', '01 We/Household', '02 Self (Explicit or Inferred or No Pronoun)', '03 Spouse/Partner', '04 Daughter(s)', '05 Son(s)', '06 Child(ren) (nec)', '07 Son/Daughter in-law', '08 Mother', '09 Father', '10 Parents (both or not specified)', '11 Parent(s) in-law', '12 Siblings (sister/brother)', '13 Sister-in-law/Brother-in-law', '14 Grandparent(s)', '15 Grandchild(ren)', '16 Other Family Members/Family Members Unspecified', '17 Friend/Colleague/Neighbour/Employer', '18 Other', '19 Pet', '20 Not Specified'.

43

Roads, casualties and public health: the open sewers of the 21st century

Condensed version of: Dorling, D. (2011) 'Roads, casualties and public health: the open sewers of the 21st century', Publication of PACTS 21st Westminster Lecture, London: Parliamentary Advisory Council for Transport Safety (PACTS).

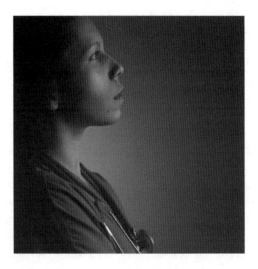

...

I am going to start by reading out part of a letter that appeared this morning in a newspaper. The letter is by Michael O'Hare and appears on page 7 of *The Independent*, today. In part of the letter, he says:

> *... there is no doubt that the number of road deaths worldwide per annum is astonishingly high. In the worst-case scenarios (which include pollution and extrapolated deaths in nations which don't record specific car-related incidents) the estimate is 2.4 million people killed due to motor vehicles every year. This exceeds easily the annual military death toll from the First World War. Even the most conservative estimates, which include only road deaths reported in developed nations and only down to direct motor-vehicle accident, put the current annual road-death toll at 100,000 per year.*
>
> *Within six months of the September 11th attacks on New York and elsewhere, it is estimated that the number of people subsequently killed on the roads because they chose not to fly because of the chance of a repeat atrocity had well exceeded the death toll caused by the terrorists on that day, an unintended and gruesome consequence of their actions.*
>
> *It is clear that humans have a blind spot when it comes to road deaths ...*[1]

---

[1] Michael O'Hare, Northwood, Middlesex, Letters, *The Independent*, 23/11/2010, http://www.independent.co.uk/opinion/letters/letters-how-animals-are-killed-2141067.html

I read that and I thought that – if anything – I am being a bit weak in what I am about to tell you, not forceful enough in the argument I am going to try to make.

My argument

Every century comes with a major public health warning about the harm that we inflict on ourselves. In Britain in the nineteenth century it was the diseases we spread by tolerating open sewers. In the twentieth century it was tobacco that we slowly learnt to love then fear. In the twenty-first century it is the way we tolerate how cars are allowed to travel on our roads.

My basic argument is quite simple. The argument comes not from being a road safety campaigner: it comes from being somebody who has spent a large part of his career looking at what it is that kills people at different times in our history. Every century has had a major killer. In the nineteenth century it was open sewers and poor public health which led to all kinds of diseases being widespread. In the twentieth century the major killer, not just through lung cancer but also through heart disease and other routes, was tobacco – what is called the 'tobacco epidemic' – and we are seeing the end of the worst period of that now so that in the twenty-first century the public health epidemic is and will be: road crashes. This is the argument. The question is: how long will it take us to recognise this and how slow will we be to treat crashes as an epidemic? Obviously we have a long and proud history of campaigning but as yet road safety has not been put on the same kind of pedestal as public health once was, and as tobacco still is.

The map [in Figure 43.1] was drawn by a young German man whose father had sent him to Manchester in 1842 to help run his mill. The young German was shocked at what he saw. He was quite industrious. The book it is taken from is called *The Condition of the Working Class of England* and the young man was Friedrich Engels. Little Ireland was a district in the middle of Manchester (area 8 on the map in Figure 43.1). I want to show you one quote taken from that book that Friedrich Engels wrote of his experiences, and especially his experiences in Little Ireland, in 1842:

> *As I passed through the dwellings of the mill-hands in Irish Town, Ancoats, and Little Ireland … found a whole street following the course of a ditch, because in this way deeper cellars could be secured without the cost of digging, cellars not for storing wares or rubbish, but for dwellings for human beings.* Not one house of this street escaped the cholera. (emphasis as in original)

Engels said that a remarkable thing about this particular street was that the entrepreneurs had chosen this ditch to build in because they did not have to dig the lower cellars out because the ditch had already excavated the land so they could save money when they jerry-built. As a result people were literally living in sewage. Although it took about 100 years, and hundreds of thousands of premature deaths, agitation such as this meant that we now have decent sewer systems; although still not decent enough worldwide. It took a long time for us to realise that speculative building spread disease.

... Sewage is still the biggest killer of children worldwide today. There are 82 million cases at any one time of diarrhoea amongst children in the world. Figure 43.2 shows a stretched map (a 'cartogram') where the area is proportional to the number of cases. Eighty-two million is the whole area. You can just make out Western Europe there – small, but still with cases. At any one time, the map makes clear that there are far more cases of diarrhoea among children in Nigeria than are found across the whole of Western and Eastern Europe.

I am not saying that the problems of public health infection and issues of sewerage haven't gone away. At its height in Britain poor sanitation was key in maintaining high infant mortality and, as a result Manchester's life expectancy, from 1801 to 1850, was the lowest ever recorded (bar pandemic), calculated at 25.3 years, affecting a population of 235,000 people in 1841[2]. In Liverpool registration district itself life

Figure 43.1: Nineteenth-century Manchester.

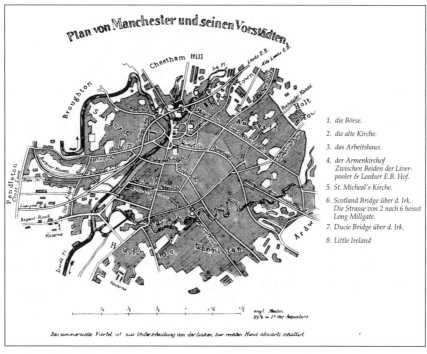

Source: http://www.marxists.org/svenska/marx/1845/02-d030.htm
Illustration from page 515 of the collected work of Marx and Engels Volume 4, printed by Progress Publishers of the Soviet Union in collaboration with Lawrence & Wishart (London) and International Publishers (New York).

---

[2] Szreter, S. and Mooney, G., 1998, Urbanization, mortality, and the standard of living debate: new estimates of the expectation of life at birth in nineteenth-century British cities, *Economic History Review*, 51, 1, 84–112 (table 3).

Figure 43.2: Childhood cases of diarrhoea in the world today.

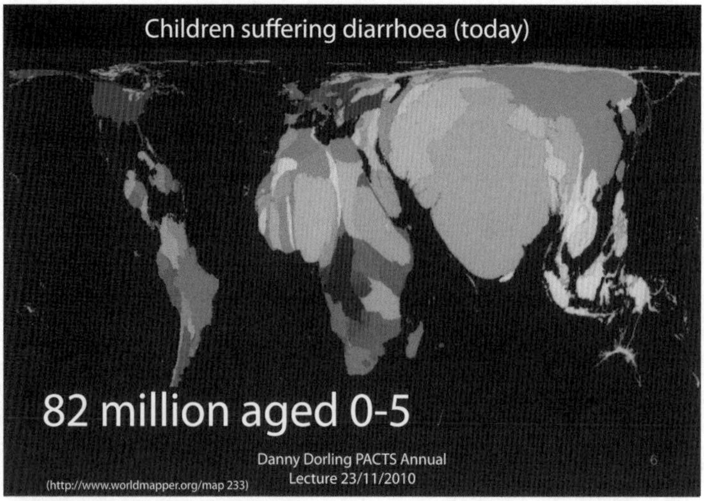

Note: Area of each country proportional to numbers suffering (total area is equal to 82 million children aged under six).

Source: World Bank's 2005 World Development Indicators, from the series named Diarrhoea prevalence (% of children under 5) (SH.STA.DIRH.ZS). The underlying source that the World Bank cites is the United Nations Fund for Children's (UNICEF) publication, *The State of the World's Children*.

expectancy in the 1880s was only 29 years of life, some 19 years lower than the 48 years recorded then in the affluent Clifton district of Bristol[3]. In Glasgow, in earlier years, similarly low rates as in Liverpool were recorded, as low as age 27 around 1840[4].

We led the world with public health and sewers because we had to[5]. Because we industrialised first, we brought together so many people in such cramped conditions that we created the circumstances that were first this bad. For about fifty years the life expectancy for Manchester was round about 25 years due to infant deaths. The only time I have seen reported an equivalent large-whole-city-population life expectancy as low as that is in Madras, in India, during the 1918–19 flu pandemic.[6] If you go to a Victorian graveyard (the one I know best is Undercliffe in Bradford), there you will see the whole of Victorian society laid out in the gravestones. The industrial titans such as Sir Titus Salt had the biggest gravestones; smaller gravestones were reserved for the vast bulk of lesser people. Almost all of the 80,000 infants buried there have no gravestones because you couldn't fit them in and because so many who died were born to the poor or very poor.

---

[3] *Ibid* (table 2).

[4] *Ibid* (table 5).

[5] Editorial Note: See Chapter 2 of this volume.

[6] Editorial Note: Those Victorian years were an exceptional period in Britain. In the 1880s you still had a life expectancy of 29 years in Liverpool and great health inequality: that average of 29 was 19 years lower than in Clifton (now in Bristol). Earlier, in Glasgow, people were dying at age 27 on average which means almost unimaginable numbers of infant deaths.

Figure 43.3 shows the current worldwide distribution of part of the poor sanitation death toll, largely of children and very small children still dying incredibly preventable early deaths from diarrhoea: 1.87 million a year[7]. And falling. Getting better, and getting interventions, getting drips. Fewer dying.

Figure 43.3: Deaths due to diarrhoea in the world today.

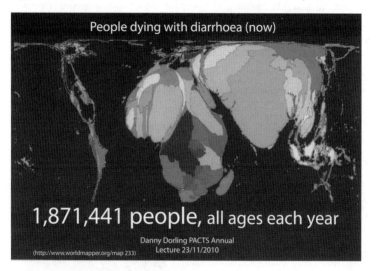

People dying with diarrhoea (now)

1,871,441 people, all ages each year

Danny Dorling PACTS Annual
Lecture 23/11/2010
(http://www.worldmapper.org/map 233)

see colour version in plate section

Note: Area proportional to number of deaths.

Source: The data used here are from the World Health Organization's (WHO) Global Burden of Disease (GBD) statistics on death and disability worldwide as measured in 2002. Diarrhoeal diseases, ICD U010, (causing 17% of deaths worldwide included in the category: Infectious and parasitic diseases).

Even in the global recession this figure is finally beginning to go down[8]. Western Europe has disappeared from this map of deaths in contrast to its size in terms of cases shown in Figure 43.2, on p 406. Near where Europe has shrunk to near-invisibility you can see Turkey, still reporting too many deaths, and you will see that Africa has a much larger share of world deaths than it has cases, and that the Congo (the largest dark red area[9]) in particular is very significant, as is India (although the overall child population there is far higher). People are still dying as a result of poor public health, but not many in rich countries any more.

---

[7] Figures are derived from the World Health Organisation's estimates, which are due to be updated after the end of 2012. For all the detail on these numbers and our assumptions see: http://www.worldmapper.org/extraindex/text_causedeath.html

[8] Along with the slight fall reported in infant deaths overall worldwide by WHO in their latest 2010 annual report, and continuing trends first widely reported to be becoming established a decade earlier: *Bulletin of the World Health Organization*, 2000, 78 (10): http://www.who.int/healthinfo/statistics/mortbulletinchildmortalitydecline/en/index.html [The falls in infant mortality reported for 2011 may be even faster.]

[9] See colour version in plate section.

Public health in Britain today

The reason why I told you earlier the figures for Liverpool in the 1880s, and Clifton in Bristol in the 1880s, is that we have to go back to the 1880s to find a gap in life expectancy as wide as we have currently have in Britain (Figure 43.4). The gaps between north and south in Britain (in life expectancy) are the widest gaps in Western Europe. The next widest gap was found in Germany shortly after the Wall fell but it was narrower, and the gap in Germany, despite the population of the East being added, has narrowed since 1990 whereas our gap has widened[10]. This is the gap in years between the area where people live the longest, which is Kensington and Chelsea now, and the shortest, which is Glasgow; a gap of about 12.4 years, and it has been rising in recent years. In the very last year it actually stabilised if not narrowed (by just a week) but nobody noticed that. It remains a source of great shame to the last government that this gap widened. And the reason for showing

Figure 43.4: The life expectancy gap between the extreme districts of Britain.

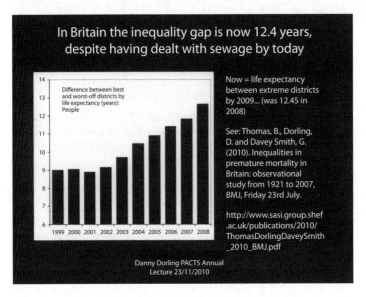

Source: Office for National Statistics and General Registrar Office (Scotland) estimates of life expectancy by local authority authority, three-year moving averages.
By 2008–10 the gap had grown to 12.65 years: http://www.guardian.co.uk/news/datablog/interactive/2011/oct/20/life-expectancy-map-local-authority-uk.

---

[10] Recent statistics are easier to locate given so many sources now on the web. For the 1990s figures and analysis of the early trends found then see: Shaw M., Orford S., Brimblecombe, N. and Dorling, D. (2000) Widening inequality in mortality between 160 regions of 15 countries of the European Union, *Social Science and Medicine* 30, 1047-1058.

you the gap today is that a large contribution to the gap is the inequality between areas in your chances of being killed on the roads between poor areas and rich areas.

I realise that the damage done from road crashes that don't involve deaths is widespread but I am going to concentrate on mortality because that is the way in which we end up recognising that road safety is vehemently important.

Back again to sewage. In 1950 my mum was playing on the beach in Filey[11]. Luckily she was not playing near the sewage outlet on the beach so she was not one of those children who contracted polio and died or were maimed (Figure 43.5 includes for Britain some adults of a similar age to my mother dying prematurely today due to catching polio as a child).

Figure 43.5: Deaths in the world today with polio as underlying cause.

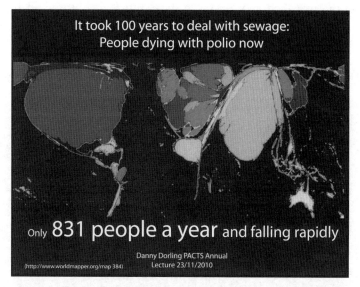

It took 100 years to deal with sewage:
People dying with polio now

Only **831 people a year** and falling rapidly

Danny Dorling PACTS Annual
Lecture 23/11/2010
(http://www.worldmapper.org/map 384)

Source: World Health Organization's (WHO) statistics for 2002, as reported in Worldmapper. Most of the polio deaths that year were of people who had been severely disabled by polio years before who eventually died because of polio's long-term effects. Poliomyelitis caused 0.0015% of all deaths worldwide in 2002 with an average of 1 death per 10 million people.

It took us a long time to learn to deal with sewage. We got it out of the back streets, we got it down the pipes, but to get it off the beaches took over 100 years from when Friedrich Engels was writing about these English people who were building their homes on top of open drains. The number shown in Figure 43.5 above is not a typo. It is only 831 people worldwide who die due to having originally contracted polio and most of these contracted the disease as a child. Polio has almost been eradicated. These few die today having had polio as the 'underlying condition'. It

---

[11] Just below Filey Brigg on the Yorkshire coast.

takes a long time to deal with a public health disaster and the longer you take over it the more pain and unnecessary suffering are caused.

Road traffic today

…

If you look at the wards around where I live, the three nearest wards, you find that not a single child has been killed over several years, or in fact has even been involved in an accident under the age of twelve. And the reason is because for almost all the day there are no unaccompanied children under the age of twelve on the streets. Not one. You don't see them, because they are imprisoned in their homes. They will of course live and not be damaged, but this leads to an acceleration in the inequality between areas. [Across the parliamentary constituencies of Sheffield children in the worst-off area are seven times more likely to be hit by a car than in the best-off area. While, worldwide, people driving cars and other vehicles and crashing is accelerating in importance as a global killer.]

Figure 43.6: Deaths in the world today due to road traffic collisions.

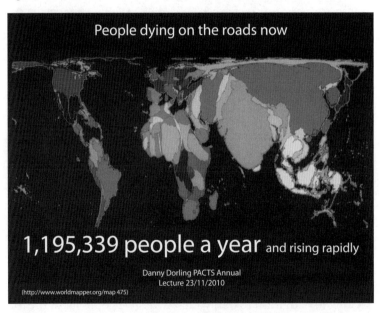

Note: In 2002 road traffic accidents (now more commonly labelled 'crashes') caused 2.1% of all deaths worldwide, an average of 191 deaths per million people per year. This number is rising rapidly.

Source: World Health Organization's (WHO) Global Burden of Disease (GBD) statistics on death and disability worldwide in 2002.

WHO estimates from a few years ago now suggest that the number of people dying directly as a result of being hit (mostly) by cars was approaching 1.2 million, and rising rapidly as the car spreads around the world (Figure 43.6). Europe is not negligible in size on the map above, but India, China, Nigeria and Brazil suffer far more deaths in absolute terms. Worldwide and in Britain the car is our new major public health problem. It is the problem that is on the rise as our old public health problems are diminishing in importance.

Figure 43.7 lists the birth and death dates of a few characters I am going to tell you about. The lists start off with a communist or, more accurately, one of the men who invented communism but who also highlighted just how poor British public health was (Friedrich Engels). He is followed historically over at the other end of the political spectrum by Charles Booth. You may know Charles from his maps (one of which I will show you in a minute). Charles was a liberal philanthropist who joined the Conservative party in old age and was very concerned with poverty. His research assistant (who helped in drawing up the maps of poverty about 100 years ago) was a young lady called Beatrice Potter, who married someone called Sidney Webb and they were among the forces that created the modern British Labour party. Another young man who was involved in this tale was Seebohm Rowntree, whose Quaker family fortune still funds the office of the Liberal Democrat leader. Politics and health have always been interlinked. Next, on smoking, I am going to tell you a little bit about Richard Doll, an epidemiologist, and finally, on poverty

Figure 43.7: Some pioneers who most helped to improve our public health.

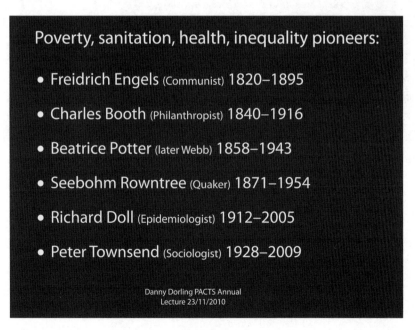

Poverty, sanitation, health, inequality pioneers:

- Freidrich Engels (Communist) 1820–1895
- Charles Booth (Philanthropist) 1840–1916
- Beatrice Potter (later Webb) 1858–1943
- Seebohm Rowntree (Quaker) 1871–1954
- Richard Doll (Epidemiologist) 1912–2005
- Peter Townsend (Sociologist) 1928–2009

Danny Dorling PACTS Annual
Lecture 23/11/2010

Source: Davey Smith, G., Dorling, D. and Shaw, M. (eds) (2001) *Poverty, inequality and health: 1800–2000 – a reader.* The Policy Press: Bristol.
http://en.wikipedia.org/wiki/Peter_Townsend_(sociologist) and
http://www.guardian.co.uk/society/2009/jun/11/obituary-letters-peter-townsend.

and inequality, something of Peter Townsend (who died last year [2009] and who was a sociologist).

Top right in Figure 43.8[12] is the famous map of London from the 1880s that Charles Booth commissioned and that people like Beatrice Potter as she was (not the Beatrix Potter who drew pictures of hedgehogs, the other one) went out and surveyed. It shows some parts of London having servant-keeping classes and living in luxury up by the British Museum, and other parts being '*rookeries of the vicious semi-criminal poor*', as they were called. Bottom right is a map of York drawn by Seebohm Rowntree, Joseph Rowntree's son. And, on that, the dark green areas[13] are the districts inhabited by the '*servant-keeping classes*'.

Figure 43.8: Some early maps of social divisions which influenced public health.

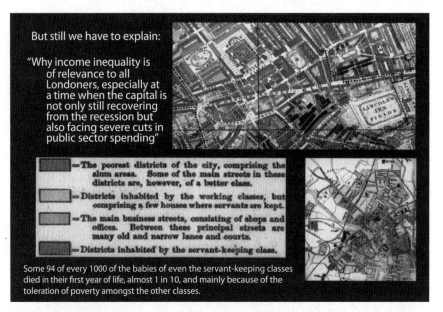

Source: Dorling, D. (2012) *Fair play: A Daniel Dorling reader on social justice*, Bristol: The Policy Press, reproducing figures in turn produced under the direction of Charles Booth and Benjamin Seebohm Rowntree, but drafted by others with data collected by yet others that they employed.

The key statistic of the time, all the way through the 1880s to at least 1905, was that almost one in ten of the children of the servant-keeping classes, just a hundred years ago, were dying in their first year of life. [The rates for other social classes were even higher.]

As affluent people began to realise that these deaths were caused by infection and disease, not acts of God, they learnt that they could not leave the poor suffering in

---

[12] From figures also reproduced in turn and original sources given in Dorling, D. and Pritchard, J. (2010) The Geography of Poverty, Inequality and Wealth in the UK and abroad: because enough is never enough, *Applied Spatial Analysis and Policy*, 3, 2-3, pp 81-106.

[13] See colour version in plate section.

such bad conditions if they wanted their own children to have a better chance of survival. I think we can learn from these lessons and use what we know about past public health movements to do a better job of how we organise ourselves today.

Figure 43.9[14] is the only slide I show on smoking, I will explain it in a little bit of detail. The X axis shows the passage of time from 1850 to around about now. The Y axis represents age, from the first year of life all the way up to people who make it to 100. People who just make it to 10, but die at that age, contribute to the colour shown along the horizontal line of cells within the figure by the number 10 to the left[15]. The colour scale is the difference between how many men and boys died out of all those then alive at that age, the rate of male deaths at those ages, and the rate of female deaths. It is based on a billion people, people living in the richest countries of the world (all added up together) so you get more reliable estimates.

What you see in the past, in the colour version of Figure 43.9 at least, are lots of red areas: men and women being equally likely to die. Then we have an event where, for a few years, men between the ages of eighteen and their early thirties were

Figure 43.9: Two world wars, the smoking cloud, emancipation and repeated recessions.

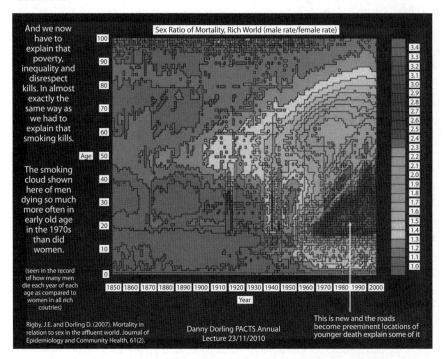

Source: The data used here were drawn from the Human Mortality Database collated by John R. Wilmoth (Director, University of California, Berkeley) and Vladimir Shkolnikov (Co-Director Max Planck Institute for Demographic Research). Access is free and may be found here: http://www.mortality.org/

[14] From a figure first published in Rigby, J.E. and Dorling, D. (2007). Mortality in relation to sex in the affluent world. *Journal of Epidemiology and Community Health*, 61(2).
[15] See colour version in plate section.

much more likely to die than women. That's the First World War. You can see it as a short vertical band of blues and green around 1914–19. And, in the early 1940s, the second distinct vertical band of differently coloured cells is the Second World War. Later, great green contours can be seen centred around people dying in their early 60s in the late 1970s – this is the smoking cloud, a smoking epidemic. It is men being twice as likely (or even 2.4 times and 2.3 times more likely) as women to die in their 50s or 60s because they had started smoking during the First World War, and/or for those who grew up in countries which saw the first boats arriving carrying mass machine-rolled cigarettes. When you see it like this you can see how effective cigarettes were as a killer. We can only see the lighter green smoking cloud in Figure 43.9 because it was not socially acceptable for women to smoke back then and we have a controlled experiment worldwide.

You, however, when studying Figure 43.9 are probably looking at the more recent triangle of dark blues and purples [the triangular area in the bottom right of the figure]. This is a three-to-one ratio now for young men. Obviously chances for everyone in these countries have got much better over time, but we are seeing something new: for young adults recently, far fewer deaths than involved at older ages, but far more dramatic inequalities between young men and young women than seen before (outside wartime). There are a whole lot of reasons: it is overdoses on drugs, it's suicide, it's fights, it's risky behaviour, but we don't help with how we allow our roads to be places where speeds (that humans never faced during our evolution) kill so often.

Twenty-first century health threats

I am going to show you a whole series of pie charts next. The pie charts are described in more detail in a publication that comes out in a few months' time in which Bethan Thomas (who drew the pie charts) and I wrote this about the cuts that are going to occur. I am going to talk a bit about the cuts in the road safety budget, but the statement was one Bethan and I made about the cuts in general in writing on the changing situation in 2010:

> *In June 2010 the Department for Communities and Local Government published what is likely to become one of the most infamous documents of the economic depression/ recession. It was titled: 'Local government contribution to efficiencies in 2010/11.... the cuts this document specified will result in more people, and especially young children, being killed. That is because road safety funding is to be cut by £37 million: £20.592m is proposed to be removed from the road safety revenue grant (paid out via area based grant) in the last four months of 2010/11 and a further £17.205m from the road safety capital grant originally due to be paid in May. This represents a reduction of 27 per cent in the revenue grant and all of the capital grant.*[16]

---

[16] Dorling, D. and Thomas, B. (2011) *Bankrupt Britain: An atlas of social change*, Bristol: The Policy Press, which is the source for all of the charts which now follow – based in turn on mortality data for 2006-2007 by cause for all deaths recorded in Britain.

An argument that I want to make today, which many of you have heard before, and which I think needs making more widely, is that the way that we currently allow our roads to be used doesn't just harm those most likely to be hit by a cars, it actually reduces the freedom of almost everybody. It reduces the freedom of our children enormously, particularly posh middle-class children who no longer get to play in the way that I got to play: I was out on my trike at the age of six to go and explore my estate and went under the subway under what was (at that point) a six-carriageway road at the age of six on my own. We don't allow children to do that any more. Perhaps rightly, but I don't think we should live in that way.

Roads trap affluent children in their homes and are the main site of killing of poorer children. What is key is how large this contribution to death has become. Figure 43.10 shows the first of the series of pie charts. I have scaled this one to be very small because the numbers of deaths involved at these ages are very small, partly because we are cosseting children at these ages. These are just the external causes of death. And this is the latest data, the 2006 and 2007 mortality rates by cause. As I give this lecture, data for 2008 still has not been published, let alone 2009[17]. Figure 43.10 is

Figure 43.10: Deaths of children aged 5 to 10 in Britain not attributed to disease (2006–07).

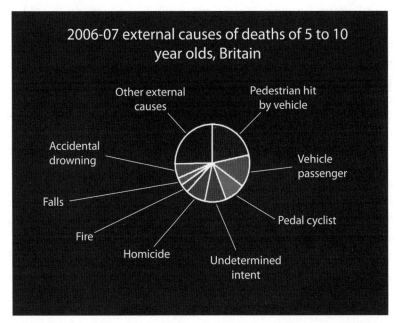

see colour version in plate section

Source: Shaw, M., Davey Smith, G., Thomas, B., and Dorling, D. (2008) *The Grim Reaper's road map: an atlas of mortality in Britain*, Bristol: The Policy Press, relying in turn on data supplied by the Office for National Statistics and General Registrar Office (Scotland).

---

[17] Editorial Note: Data for all deaths in England and Wales for both years arrived at our offices a few days after I gave this lecture. We already held data for Scotland, which are processed more speedily and for which different regulations apply. Updated images based on more recent data are included here: http://sasi.group.shef.ac.uk/bankruptbritain/Material.html

showing you the relative importance of all the external non-disease causes of death amongst children aged five to ten. The area of each slice of the pie is proportional to the number of deaths in Britain attributed to that underlying cause and also to the areas in the pie charts below. [The overall areas for older age groups are larger as far more children of older ages and young adults die than those in the 5–10 age group.]

When you worry about people murdering children aged five to ten and when you hear about them dying in a house fire, or tragedies of drowning, you have to weigh those events against what you see in Figure 43.10. When you look at the figure and think of the deaths of children being hit by vehicles, those who are in cars and die, and young child pedal cyclists – think of me aged six on my trike – think of actual potential victims to accompany each label on that chart. If you have children think of them, or think of yourself when at these ages. If we are worried about our children aged five to ten then we need to be much more worried about cars than pedal cycling. It is the collisions with cars that mostly kill.

Cutting road safety spending

As to the government's cuts to the road safety budget, £37m is nothing. Or to put it more precisely, it is about three quarters of the annual salary of Bob Diamond, the boss of Barclays Capital[18]. It is a tiny amount of money. You would only cut this money from the road safety funding budget if you didn't think road safety was a good idea, I think; although I am happy to argue this with you. I am shocked at the cuts. Especially as to how many people are losing their extremely lowly paid and very part-time jobs. This includes those who man (but mostly woman) zebra- and other assisted school-crossings. If you know about Government budgeting and how everything adds up to billions, the savings these cuts make appear after the decimal point.

We should look at the cuts to road safety budgets and lollipop crossings in the context of Figure 43.11, which shows what most often kills all eleven- to sixteen-year-olds who die in Britain. I know it is a complicated diagram but I wanted to put in every cause of death from which those eleven- to sixteen-year-olds have died. Obviously, far fewer eleven- to sixteen-year-olds die now than used to die, but that doesn't stop how much we care, or how much we worry, or how important those deaths are, and all the illness, accidents and non-fatal suffering that is caused to the people of these ages who don't die.

Look closely at Figure 43.11. You will see that the biggest slice of the pie is vehicle passenger or driver deaths, obviously driving illegally in most cases. The figure also

---

[18] Editorial Note: Bob Diamond was, in effect, sacked in 2012, but continued to receive some income from Barclays due to the nature of his contract. However, in future the British will be wasting a little less of their monies on his salary. Some think it would be better to spend a higher proportion of such monies slowing cars down rather than trying to teach future generations of children and young adults to do something they were never designed to do, to stay constantly alert and to be able to spot heavy objects moving at great speed, passing so near them so often without those youngsters making a single mistake and not looking before they step into the road.

Figure 43.11: Underlying cause of deaths of children aged 11 to 16 in Britain (2006–07).

2006-07 all causes of death of 11 to 16 year olds, Britain

Pnuemonia
Other respiratory
Meningitus
Asthma
Other infections
Other cancer
Pedestrian hit by vehicle
Leukemia
Cancer of brain
Other diseases
Vehicle passenger or driver
Sudden death, cause unknown
Disease of blood
Pedal cyclist
Disease of digestive system
Deaths due to drugs
Epilepsy
Suicide & undetermined intent
Endocrine disorders
Cardiovascular
Homicides
Congenital defect
Falls
Accidental drowning
Disease of nervous system
Other external causes

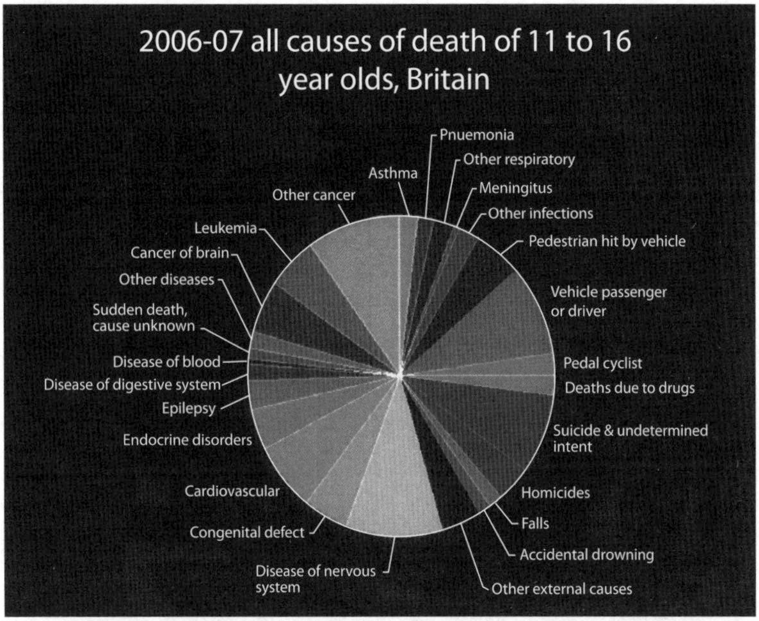

Source: Shaw, M., Davey Smith, G., Thomas, B., and Dorling, D. (2008) *The Grim Reaper's road map: an atlas of mortality in Britain*, Bristol: The Policy Press, relying in turn on data supplied by the Office for National Statistics and General Registrar Office (Scotland).

shows that at these ages pedal cyclists dying are a significant addition, but fewer in number. I want you to remember that as you read on because I am later going to show you pedal cyclist deaths as a proportion of all deaths at an older age and compare that to the numbers of pedestrians being hit and killed by vehicles. At these ages when considering road casualties you are considering about a fifth of all deaths, and the majority of those are resulting from the most preventable causes.

We pay millions of pounds worth of money for advanced medical research to try to prevent mortality at younger ages, to try to work out ways in which we could possibly further curtail mortality from causes such as childhood leukaemia, while we still treat road collision deaths as if they were largely unforeseeable accidents, as if they were an act of God.

Let me turn to the reason why cars are no longer the greatest threat to five- to ten-year-olds as they were for most of my career. I always used to say that cars are killing more five- to ten-year-olds than anything else. It is because we now do really incarcerate our five- to ten-year-olds so effectively that fewer under-elevens are killed on the roads today. And, if you live in a posh middle-class area, you can even start to see twelve-year-olds being walked to school, normally by mum (a larger number are now driven, ironically due to road safety fears).

The reason we closet our young teenagers now is because almost half of the deaths of those who die from non-disease causes are due to road traffic 'accidents'.

Compare the human road deaths shown in Figure 43.12 below to the prevalence of other 'external' causes that usually get the most press attention.

By age ten cars have become the greatest danger to children living in Britain, and that danger then increases substantially with each subsequent birthday for a child. Figure 43.12 shows the relative magnitude of risks by showing all the deaths due to external causes which have occurred among eleven- to sixteen-year-olds across Britain in the two most recent years for which I had access to data. Parents know about the reality that Figure 43.12 makes visible, but they don't know it directly, they kind of hear it on the grapevine and it is all so obvious as you walk down the pavement – you see the cars going past fast.

Figure 43.12: Deaths of children aged 11 to 16 in Britain not attributed to disease (2006–07).

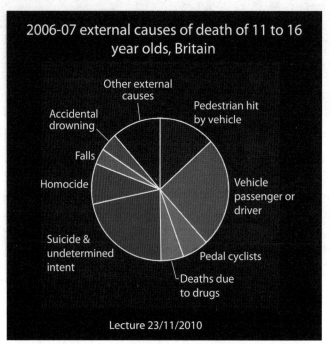

Source: Shaw, M., Davey Smith, G., Thomas, B., and Dorling, D. (2008) *The Grim Reaper's road map: an atlas of mortality in Britain*, Bristol: The Policy Press, relying in turn on data supplied by the Office for National Statistics and General Registrar Office (Scotland).

Freedom to walk

The threat of death by collision reduces our freedom to move as children, and we become more socially isolated. By the onset of adulthood the car and a small number of cases of suicide together account for half of all deaths at these young ages: nine deaths a week of 17-, 18- and 19-year-olds from these causes alone, almost all due to cars and their drivers (Figure 43.13). The numbers of deaths per week from such causes continue to rise throughout young adults' 20s, only falling relative to other risks when these young adults reach their late 30s.

Figure 43.13: Underlying cause of all deaths of people aged 17 to 19 in Britain (2006–07).

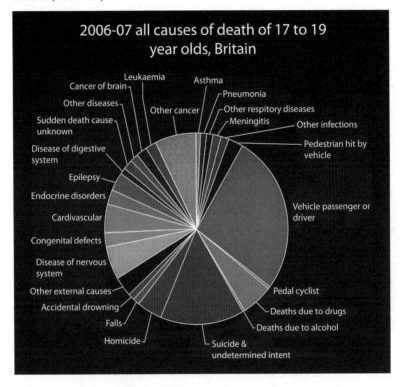

Source: Shaw, M., Davey Smith, G., Thomas, B., and Dorling, D. (2008) *The Grim Reaper's road map: An atlas of mortality in Britain*, Bristol: The Policy Press, relying in turn on data supplied by the Office for National Statistics and General Registrar Office (Scotland).

We always worry about our children. We are innately programmed to worry about our children. We are innately programmed as it is very sensible for us to worry about our children because our children had such a high chance in the past of being hurt, of getting diseases, dying of measles and other such things. The worry does not diminish because the world has become safer. The worry gets translated into more and more actions to try to make things safer, but only safer at an individual level. At an individual level we try to wrap our child, metaphorically, in cotton wool, but we fail to do this at an aggregate level.

Around 30,000 people of all ages are killed or seriously injured on roads in Britain every year. In 2008 some 27,855,000 cars were registered to be driven on the country's roads. That rose slightly to 27,868,000 during 2009 (partly with government encouragement for new car buying with a 'scrappage scheme'). Very young adults

see colour version in plate section

now cycle less. Figure 43.14 shows just how much less. It is not that they now still cycle but are surrounded by some kind of force-field that protects them. It is that they cycle less, walk less and they exercise less as a result.

Figure 43.14: Deaths of people aged 17 to 19 in Britain not attributed to disease (2006–07).

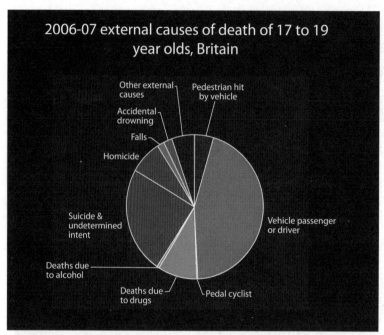

Source: Shaw, M., Davey Smith, G., Thomas, B., and Dorling, D. (2008) *The Grim Reaper's road map: An atlas of mortality in Britain*, Bristol: The Policy Press, relying in turn on data supplied by the Office for National Statistics and General Registrar Office (Scotland).

You will be grateful to know that I am not going to take us all through the age range up to our dotage. I will stop at our mid-20s. I particularly regret not having time to tell the whole story through the age ranges because I would have liked to have talked about so many pensioners being hurt as well. But I think that, for campaigning purposes, children have a certain *capital*. Things are not their fault. They didn't decide to be born into a world at a time and in a place when you so commonly have one tonne of steel moving at 40 miles per hour when you walk to school. [And they have had no time to change the world.]

Figure 43.13 showed 17- to 19-year-olds and all causes of death that most afflict them. Underlying how it differs from Figure 43.11 for younger ages, these older teenagers' bodies have become much stronger, and often the causes which would have been congenital are risks that by these ages have largely past. If you happen to be a parent and are worried about your 17- to 19-year-olds, for instance if you are sending them off to university, then the figures above suggest that there is one little thing above all other little things to tell them to be worried about: worry first about being a vehicle passenger or driver who may die in a car.

Freedom to cycle

Please look again at Figure 43.14 and at how slight is the risk of dying as a pedal cyclist at these ages. Teenagers hardly cycle any more. Fat, middle-aged men like me cycle, and some younger children cycle, but we don't any more have many of our children of these ages cycling. This often means that the first time that they are on the road is as a car driver, not when in control of a pedal bike, but as a new car driver (which is not a good way to be on the road for the first time).

In comparison to almost any other way in which our older children and younger adults are likely to die, traffic collisions are becoming more important as a cause of death. If you are a really mean-spirited neo-liberal economist, and you see the world through the lens of profit, then look at the threat of car collisions this way: you have just invested your maximum amount in the education and health of these people to get them to the point where they are going to be economically productive, then cars are the most likely thing that is going to damage your investment. Or think of how much interest you'll lose on each student loan that won't be repaid and future taxes not collected due to a road death today. With a little inflation (and the inclusion of multiplier effects) you are talking millions of future pounds.

As you can see I am trying to work out ways to talk to the new government, to think in their mind-set. Because one problem is that folk can be really callous, and some people are really callous. If you do a crude cost-benefit analysis you can decide that it is not worth spending on expensive intensive therapy unit beds (to treat crash victims who might otherwise die) and that a certain number of deaths on the road are worth the price we pay. But you have just got to get yourself out of that way of thinking and see the wider benefits of far fewer road deaths and of not being so narrow minded.

Reining in the motor industry

Today we prioritise what is good for the motor industry over what is good for human beings. We do this because the industry has become a force in its own right as there is so much profit to be made from selling the dreams that go with cars. Take the car 'scrappage scheme'. The car scrappage scheme actually resulted in more cars on our road than there were before. It was introduced because we felt we had to support the banks. And we had to support the car companies because what the car companies actually do is not so much make cars, as sell debt.

General Motors was going to go under a few years ago because it was having trouble raising money, to loan people the money, to get them to buy cars, often cars sold as devices for *protecting* people! Buy a huge American car and your children are less likely to be injured within it during a collision as long as the car or small lorry you hit is smaller than your huge car. Such selling encourages both selfishness and an inability to see the aggregate effect.

Imagine if cars had to be sold with health warnings such as having some of these pie charts painted on their bodywork (like warnings printed on cigarette packets). I am not advocating that, but I think information about how dangerous road traffic is, in comparison to almost every other threat, should be information that is given out in schools, and should be known.

Look again at the pie charts above and road casualties versus suicides (the second most greatest 'external' threat to 17- to 19-year-olds, in Figure 43.14). The road collision casualities are people who did not want to die. But sadly quite a few of those who died at their own hands are people who did want to die[19]: there is a lot you can do to reduce suicides, but almost everyone killed on the roads didn't want to die. It is only now, decades on, in fact for the first time since the 30mph speed limit was introduced, that we are just beginning to better recognise that that limit is too high. So now, finally:

> We want to encourage highway authorities to introduce, over time, 20 mph zones or limits into streets which are primarily residential in nature and into town or city streets where pedestrian and cyclist movements are high, such as around schools, shops, markets, playgrounds and other areas ... We want to draw attention to the initial evidence from the trial of wide area signed-only 20mph limits in Portsmouth, and want to make clear that 20 mph limits over a number of roads may be appropriate elsewhere. (Department for Transport circular, December 2009)

We are moving forward very slowly. In terms of the equivalent to how we dealt with sewage, we are in the 1840s, today – at the equivalent point as in the run-up to the famous 1848 Public Health Act. Above is a quote from a circular from the Department for Transport in 2009, giving (maybe) a bit more than lukewarm support for 20mph in both residential and other urban areas. But the policy is really about leaving 20mph zones as options to be devolved down to local government. When you go to local government and they tell you that with the cuts 'everything is terrible', and you say there is one thing you can do which would tackle the biggest killer of young people in your area very cheaply, they are still reticent[20]. I know there are problems about the funding and putting in the hard material (if you think speed bumps help, which

---

[19] It is particularly unfortunate that the label 'external cause' includes cases of suicide as if they were due entirely to outside influence. However, rates of suicide vary greatly between countries and even within countries so the majority of suicides are preventable, as they are due to the social context in which people are living. They are just not as easily and obviously preventable as are road traffic deaths. For an estimate of how many suicides could be prevented in Britain if everyone had the life chances of the best-off of their age and sex, see: Dorling, D. and Gunnell, D. (2003) Suicide: the spatial and social components of despair in Britain 1980–2000, *Transactions of the Institute of British Geographers*, 28, 442–60. [An extract of that paper is reproduced as Chapter 20 in this volume.]

[20] Editorial Note: Two years after giving this lecture, in Sheffield where I live, only seven 20mph zones are to be introduced into just a few parts of the city. The reason the council gives for doing so little is that the cuts mean they can only afford a few 20mph signs.

I don't), but we are beginning to finally move towards mass advocacy that 20mph is appropriate where roads are shared with nearby humans, especially human children. However, the greatest cull on the roads is of young adults:

The epidemiology of road death

Figure 43.15: Underlying cause of all deaths of people aged 20 to 24 in Britain (2006–07).

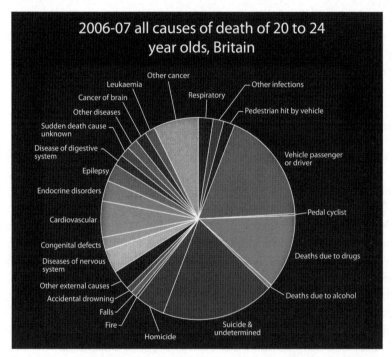

Source: Shaw, M., Davey Smith, G., Thomas, B., and Dorling, D. (2008) *The Grim Reaper's road map: An atlas of mortality in Britain*, Bristol: The Policy Press, relying in turn on data supplied by the Office for National Statistics and General Registrar Office (Scotland).

Figure 43.15 above shows what have recently been the most common causes of mortality among 20- to 24-year-olds in Britain. Deaths due to drugs are beginning to become an important cause, but road collision deaths are still far more common than drug overdoses. Death on the road is just as important (and far more preventable) as the other leading cause of mortality in young adulthood, which is suicide. We are beginning to get the medical evidence from epidemiological work on traffic accidents. If you think back to all those studies to try to understand cholera, to the advent of germ theory, to pioneering epidemiological work continuing today on smoking, and then to research on road crashes, you can trace a lineage. But now the context is very different:

The introduction of 20 mph zones was associated with a 41.9% (95% confidence interval 36.0% to 47.8%) reduction in road casualties, after adjustment for underlying time trends. The percentage reduction was greatest in younger children and greater for the category of killed or seriously injured casualties than for minor injuries. There was no evidence of casualty migration to areas adjacent to 20 mph zones, where casualties also fell slightly by an average of 8.0%.[21]

This quote is taken from the *British Medical Journal*, from a paper published in 2009. The 'slight difference' between this study and most epidemiological studies is that the 'effect' number isn't 0.041, or 4.1%. It is 41.9%! A 41.9% reduction in casualties from a single intervention! Now if you had a drug that gave you a 41.9% reduction in people suffering from an illness you would make a fortune, especially if that illness was something which affected quite a lot of people.

...

Conclusions

The deaths that I have been talking about are really only the tip of the problem. The problem really extends not just to the accidents, the major accidents, or minor accidents. It's the obesity that's caused and rises because people don't get out on their trikes at the age of six. It's the timidity that begins to result should you begin to realise how dangerous the environment is outside you. And it's this lack of freedom: taking away the freedom from children; the freedom from other adults; the freedom from older people; the freedom from people on their bikes to travel safely; the freedom for your bus to run on time because there are so many cars. And also the collective stupidity of ending up stuck in traffic jams so often because of the way we currently run things.

I find it very hard to think of anything else in the Western world which has as bad an effect on our health, and is as easy to begin to mitigate, as our current car transport system. I find it very hard to believe that we won't – in the very near future – change things quite dramatically. My concern is that we might be as slow as we were over the sewage, or have as many deaths as we had from tobacco, before we began to really target our current greatest public health disaster. Thank you very much for your attention.

---

[21] Grundy, C. *et al.* (2009) Effect of 20 mph traffic speed zones on road injuries in London, 1986–2006: controlled interrupted time series analysis, *British Medical Journal*, 2009;339:b4469

Further reading

Billington, J., Wilkie, M., Field, D.T. and Wann, J.P. (2010) Neural processing of imminent collision in humans, *Proceedings of the Royal Society B, Biological Sciences,* published online 27 October 2010, doi: 10.1098/rspb.2010.1895

Dean, J.S. (1947) *Murder most foul… a study of the road deaths problem,* London: George Allen & Unwin Ltd. Reprint 2007 by RoadPeace.

Roberts, I. with Edwards, P. (2010) *The energy glut: climate change and the politics of fatness,* London: Zed Books.

Wang, J. (2010) 'Traffic at 30 mph is too fast for children's visual abilities, scientists reveal', University Press Release, http://www.rhul.ac.uk/aboutus/newsandevents/news/newsarticles/speedchildren.aspx

WHO (2009) *Global status report on road safety,* Geneva: World Health Organisation.

Figure 43.16: How we might view roads had we more time to evolve with them.

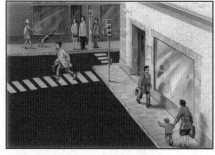
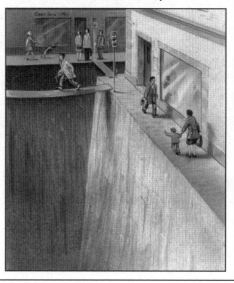

The wrong way to see a road

How to view the relative risk correctly

Note: We have learnt to be afraid of heights because those people who were not afraid of heights got to become parents a little less often than those who were afraid. Being hit by a car is a little like falling horizontally. Not something we have evolved to fear.

Source: Johansson, R., (2009) Presentation: Chief Strategist, Road Safety Division, Swedish Road Administration, Improving Road Safety in Scotland: Prevention and Best Practice. Edinburgh, Tuesday 3rd of February.

44

Tackling global health inequalities: closing the health gap in a generation

Pearce, J. and Dorling, D. (2009) 'Tackling global health inequalities: closing the health gap in a generation', *Environment and Planning A, Commentary*, vol 41, pp 1-6

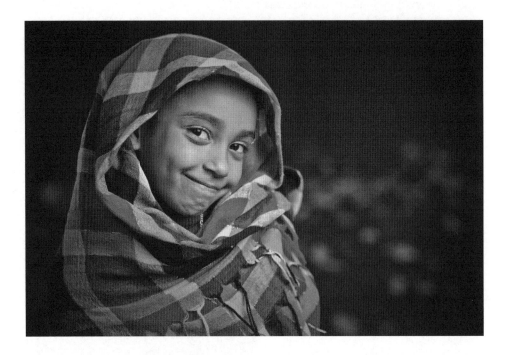

Social injustice is killing people on a grand scale. (WHO Commission on Social Determinants of Health, 2008, p 26)

It is well established that good health is not evenly shared. Both between and within most nation-states, inequalities in health outcomes, health care expenditure, and health care utilisation among various social and ethnic groups are profound. Socially and economically disadvantaged groups and areas, as well as ethnic minority and indigenous populations, commonly have relatively worse health than more advantaged groups. The recording and revealing of health inequalities have a long history, which in England extends as far back as the pioneering work of Edwin Chadwick, Friedrich Engels, and others during the mid-19th century (Davey Smith *et al*, 2001). Chadwick, for example, documented the marked health gap between social class groups in Victorian London. For males in the parish of Bethnal Green, life expectancy ranged from 16 in the 'lower class' group to 45 among the 'middle class' (Chadwick, 1843). A life expectancy of 16 was sustained through persistently high infant mortality rates, and the significant number of the rural poor migrating into London. In Britain infant mortality rates peaked in the hot summer of 1905. By age group, by far the largest numbers of bodies buried in (often unmarked) Victorian graveyards were of newly born infants (Dorling, 2006).

By the end of Queen Victoria's reign, as many as a quarter of the infants born in English working-classes towns were dying within the first year of life. In his 1899 survey of poverty in York, Benjamin Seebohm Rowntree documented that the lowest recorded mortality rates among the least deprived classes were still as high as one in ten of all young children (Rowntree, 1901). Importantly, Rowntree noted a clear *gradient* in infant mortality across three working-class districts of the city that were arranged by occupation type and income (Table 44.1). The rates incrementally decreased from the most deprived to least deprived district or group. For example, the infant mortality rate (under 12 months) of babies in the poorest area of the city was more than 2.5 times that of the 'servant-keeping' classes. For the first time, these studies began to reveal that health was causally related to social position, which itself was embedded in the social structures around which society was built.

Table 44.1: Mortality rates in York, England, in 1898, by social class, according to area of residence.

Working-class area	Overall[a,b]	Children aged 1-4 years[c]	Children under 12 months[d]	Persons over 5 years[a,b]
Area 1 (poorest)	22.78	13.96	247	13.8
Area 2 (middle)	20.71	10.50	184	10.2
Area 3 (Highest)	13.49	6.00	173	7.5
Servant-keeping class			94	
Whole of York	18.50	7.37	176	11.1

Notes: All figures exclude deaths in public institutions (e.g. workhouses).

[a] Deaths per annum per 1000 of the population.

[b] Figures not age adjusted.

[c] Deaths per annum per 1000 population of all living ages.

[d] Deaths per annum per 1000 children born.

Source: Davey Smith, G., Dorling, D. and Shaw, M. (2001) *Poverty, Inequality and Health in Britain, 1800-2000: A reader* (Bristol, The Policy Press), pp 102-104.

More than a century later, inequalities in health in England, and most other countries, persist. This 'health gap' remains unrestricted to simple dichotomies (e.g. rich/poor; black/white) but, instead, a social gradient in health remains across all groups. When individuals or geographical areas are stratified by measures of poverty or socioeconomic status (e.g. wealth, education, ethnicity, occupation, or social deprivation), average health status incrementally improves from the least to most advantaged groups. Importantly, it has been observed that since the 1970s relative inequalities in health status have tended to widen both between (Dorling *et al*, 2006) and within (Mackenbach *et al*, 2003) many countries. For example, since the early 1980s in nation-states such as the United Kingdom, the United States, and New Zealand, geographical inequalities in life expectancy have sharply increased by between 50% and 60% (Pearce and Dorling, 2006; Shaw *et al*, 2005; Singh and Siahpush, 2006).

There is a substantial literature seeking to explain the recent social and spatial polarisation in health. A range of structural, material, and sociocultural factors have been implicated. The premise of the argument is that access to resources and opportunities such as wealth, education, employment, and health care are themselves unevenly distributed, and this injustice underlies the social distribution in health status. Recently, market-oriented economic and social policies intended to deregulate the labour market and constrain social security have widened inequalities in social position. However, the story is not straightforward. Recent evidence suggests that the uneven allocation of resources in non-egalitarian societies is not only disadvantageous for more socially deprived groups, but is also harmful to more affluent groups. National-level income inequality, a marker of social stratification, is also a key driver of a nation's health and well-being (Dorling *et al*, 2007). For example, among richer nations, countries that have maintained high levels of income inequality in recent years have the highest prevalence of mental illness.

In the United States, the United Kingdom, Australia, and New Zealand, it takes the poorest fifth of society at least seven days to earn or be awarded what the richest fifth receive for a single day's labour (see www.worldmapper.org, maps 151 and 152). The rates of inequality in these countries are the highest of all affluent nations worldwide. It is unlikely to be a coincidence that of the twelve countries with comparable data, it is the same four countries that also have the highest rates of mental illness. In other affluent countries, where rates of inequality are 50% lower than in these four countries, the prevalence rates of mental illness are also halved (Wilkinson and Pickett, 2007, figure 1, page 1968). It is almost certain (but remains to be established) that the richest fifth of residents of more unequal countries do not fare as well as the richest fifth in more equitable affluent countries. Support for this notion is provided by recognising which cities in a variety of countries experience the lowest working-age mortality rates (Ross *et al*, 2005, figure 1). It is thought that inequalities create and nurture fear and anxiety in more unequal countries. They harm the mental health of all involved (in living in the more competitive and cut-throat societies they foster). They harm the health of the poor the most, but also of those who supposedly benefit from their poverty: the rich. However, whilst there is a plethora of evidence describing and explaining the rising inequalities in health, to date many high-level reports and public inquiries into health inequalities have been reluctant to fully acknowledge the underlying drivers of social inequalities in health, as well as policy remedies that are likely to succeed in addressing these disparities.

Given this inertia, the recent publication of the report by the World Health Organisation's Commission on Social Determinants of Health entitled *Closing the*

Gap in a Generation: Health Equity through Action on the Social Determinants of Health marks a welcome shift in emphasis (WHO Commission on Social Determinants of Health, 2008). The report questions, for example, how a child born in Japan can expect to live more than 80 years, whereas in many African countries less than 50. Stark inequalities in health are also evident at a local level including, for example, the 28-year difference in life expectancy between two Glaswegian children living only a few suburbs apart. The report, which was authored by a twenty-strong international commission from a range of academic, political, and advocacy backgrounds, is overt and sufficiently courageous to claim that *'social injustice is killing people on a grand scale'* (page 26). Given the breadth and the strength of the presented evidence, it is difficult not to be convinced by the authors' assertion that the social distribution in health is not a natural phenomenon but rather that the *'toxic combination of poor social policies and programmes, unfair economics, and bad politics is responsible for much of health inequity'* (page 35). Importantly, the report is unequivocal in elucidating the causal pathways between an array of social factors and various health and health-related outcomes. So what needs to be done? The Commission sets out a suite of policy priorities that provide an unambiguous agenda for action. The authors are appropriately ambitious, and challenge policy makers to close the health gap in a generation. The report is structured around three overarching recommendations (see Table 44.2 for an overview) that are prescribed to achieve this radical objective:

Table 44.2: Recommendations from the World Health Organisation Commission on Social Determinants of Health.

Overarching recommendations	Subthemes
1. Improve daily living conditions: enhance the social and physical environments in which people are born, grow, live, work, and age.	Equity from childhood; healthy places; employment and working conditions; social protection across the lifecourse; universal health care.
2. Tackle the inequitable distribution of power, money, and resources: address the deeper social structures and processes that shape inequalities in daily living conditions.	Health equity across all government policies and programmes; target public finances to addressing the social determinants of health; market responsibility; empowerment of women; political empowerment and fair representation in decision making.
3. Measure and understand the problem and assess the impact of action: ensure the basic data systems for collecting vital statistics as well as monitoring health inequalities and social determinants of health are in place.	The social determinants of health: monitoring, research and training.

Source: Adapted from Davey Smith, G. and Krieger, N., 2008, 'Tackling health inequities', *British Medical Journal* 337, 529-530.

1. The first recommendation highlights the need to address the conditions of daily life such as improving educational levels, employment status, and working conditions; eradicating poverty and providing sufficient income and welfare; addressing key urban design issues such as affordable housing, transport, and the provision of water and sanitation; and ensuring universal health care. Whilst the authors of the report recognise that these and other social and material circumstances are important throughout the lifecourse, the living conditions into which children are born are identified as a priority.

2. Second, the report recognises that it is the deeper social structures and processes that initially generate, and then perpetuate, the inequalities in the conditions required to lead a healthy life (the 'determinants of the determinants'). It is considered essential that the structural drivers of the inequities in social conditions are challenged, including the uneven distribution of power, money, and resources. The authors assert that responsibility for addressing health inequalities must be placed at the highest level of government, and a whole-of-government strategy that considers health inequalities in all aspects of policy making should be established. It is argued that coherent policy making is likely to strengthen governmental resolve to finance action on the social determinants of health, expand the commitment to global aid, as well as equitably allocate government resources for addressing the needs of marginalised populations including, for example, indigenous groups disadvantaged by the legacies of colonialism.

3. Finally, it is necessary that the magnitudes of health inequalities are precisely measured and continuously monitored. The authors call for local, national, and inter- national surveillance systems to be in place to improve the monitoring of both health inequalities and the social determinants of health. A consistent monitoring framework will better enable the evaluation of the impacts of various health and social policies.

The three principles are bold, and achieving these aims requires effective action from key players operating from the global to local level. Multilateral agencies, the World Health Organisation, national and local government, civil society, a chastened private sector, as well as the researcher community will all be integral. Importantly, successful policy initiatives will have to be underpinned by robust research findings. Research that describes and explains the current situation, which generates new understandings, as well as work identifying what works successfully in addressing health inequalities will all be required.

Geographers have made, and can continue to make, important contributions to the debates on health inequalities. Recent geographical work includes: monitoring spatial inequalities in health; evaluating macro-level health determinants including income inequality; considering the role of mobility and migration in establishing health disparities; as well as the voluminous literature on 'place effects' such as neighbourhood poverty, housing, social capital, and access to assorted community resources (Curtis, 2004; Smyth, 2008). This research agenda has been successful in identifying and understanding pertinent structural and place-based determinants, numerous underlying social processes such as globalisation, poverty, and social exclusion, as well as the spatial mechanisms that are often important in rendering these processes into measurable inequalities in health status. Many of these findings have been translated into policy recommendations. Area-based interventions (e.g. the Healthy Cities model, New Deal for Communities) have had traction. Whilst this brief overview of the geographical work that has contributed to the health inequalities debate barely scratches the surface, the growing body of literature emphasises that understanding the implications for health inequalities of the geographical context in which people are born, live, and age will continue to be important.

The report from the WHO Commission on Social Determinants of Health is timely. The report reveals that globally, nationally, and locally, health is becoming increasingly socially and spatially polarised. The findings provide a stirring reminder that for most people health is not a choice that can be readily modified by simply expanding options in health care provision and encouraging greater personal responsibility in disease prevention. This point remains important because the health strategies of many national governments remain firmly fixated on health campaigns that encourage us to amend our health-related behaviour (quit smoking, eat better, exercise more, etc). Key health policy documents continue to ignore the social determinants of health framework and many health policy makers remain wedded to largely discredited victim-blaming philosophies.

At the time of writing (October 2008) the New Zealand general election campaign is in full swing. It is notable that, in their manifestos for health, both of the major political parties (National and Labour), as well as most of the smaller parties, continue to promote individual responsibility, and advocate providing greater (often private sector) choice in health care services. There is little explicit or implicit recognition (with the notable exception of the Green Party) that health is socially embedded. Similarly, it is instructive that the United Kingdom government's White Paper on addressing the 'obesity epidemic' was entitled *Choosing Health: Making Healthier Choices Easier* (Department of Health, 2004), a title that would appear to downplay any recognition that obesity, like most health conditions, is strongly embedded in a range of social and economic issues. The tenet of these health policy statements is clearly at odds with the more holistic recommendations of the Commission.

Although increasing inequalities in health status over the past three decades are execrable, their rapid escalation also attests that health inequalities are amendable. Whilst an array of micro-level and macro-level social forces are driving the widening health divide, addressing the common structural, material, sociocultural antecedents – unequal power, colonial attitudes, business 'ethics', and the like – will have considerable and rapid benefits. If there is global support for the report's recommendations then it has the potential to become a landmark document. Coupled with a heightened worldwide awareness that the financial systems that exacerbate health inequalities may not necessarily be beneficial for everyone in the long run, it is an opportune moment to relay the report's key message that reducing inequalities in health is important. The long-term success of the report will depend on the response of the WHO and the national governments, and peoples of the member states. A sustained commitment and the political will to implement a progressive social and economic agenda will be required.

The conclusions of the WHO report are a salient reminder to the governments of member states that reducing health inequalities should be a political priority. Not only are health inequalities unfair and avoidable but, at the very least, the spill-over effects such as crime, violence, the spread of infectious disease, as well as alcohol and drug use, affect all of society. Further, determinants-oriented interventions to reduce inequalities in health are cost effective (Woodward and Kawachi, 2000). More probably, even the affluent in highly unequal Anglophone countries are not content with their circumstances. For many governments (including those of New Zealand and the United Kingdom), addressing health inequalities will require a radical shift in policy priorities away from a focus on individual responsibility, to a more potent

Figure 44.1: Infant mortality rates in England and Wales, 1996–2010.

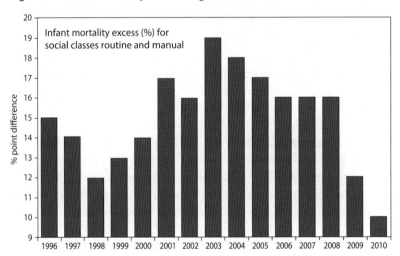

Note: Social class was NS-SE 90 classification prior to 2000, NS SEC in 2001 and after, and rates are three-year averages ending in the year shown. Only infants with a registered father were included.

Source: Department of Health (2005) *Tackling Health Inequalities: Status Report on the Programme for Action*, London: HMSO. Department of Health (2006) *Tackling Health Inequalities: 2003-05 data update for the National 2010 PSA Target*, London: HMSO. Department of Health (2008) *Tackling Health Inequalities: 2007 Status Report on the Programme for Action*, London: HMSO. Department of Health (2011) *Mortality Monitoring Bulletin: Infant Mortality, inequalities*, updated to include data for 2010, published 8 December 2011, table 16, page 6.

upstream strategy for confronting the numerous and multifaceted social determinants of health, and the social processes that determine their unequal distribution[1].

References

Chadwick, E. (1843) *Report on the Sanitary Condition of the Labouring Population of Great Britain. A Supplementary Report on the Results of a Special Inquiry into the Practice of Interment in Towns*, London: W. Clowes and Sons for HMSO.

Curtis, S. (2004) *Health and Inequality: Geographical Perspectives*, London: Sage.

Davey Smith, G. and Krieger, N., (2008) Tackling health inequities, *British Medical Journal*, 337, 529-530, Commentary 5.

Davey Smith, G., Dorling, D. and Shaw, M. (2001) *Poverty, Inequality and Health in Britain, 1800–2000: A Reader*, Bristol: The Policy Press.

Department of Health (2004) *Choosing Health: Making Healthy Choices Easier*, Cm 6374, London: Department of Health.

Dorling, D. (2006) Infant mortality and social progress in Britain, 1905–2005, in E. Garrett, C. Galley, N. Shelton, R. Woods (eds) *Infant Mortality: A Continuing Social Problem*, Aldershot: Ashgate, pp 213-228 [reproduced as Chapter 4, this volume].

Dorling, D., Shaw, M., Davey Smith, G. (2006) Global inequality of life expectancy due to AIDS, *British Medical Journal*, 332, 662-664 [see Chapter 28, this volume].

Dorling, D., Mitchell, R., Pearce, J. (2007) The global impact of income inequality on health by age: an observational study, *British Medical Journal*, 335, 873-875 [reproduced as Chapter 32, this volume].

Mackenbach, J.P., Bos, V., Andersen, O., Cardano, M., Costa, G., Harding, S., Reid, A., Hemstrom, O., Valkonen, T. and Kunst, A.E. (2003) Widening socioeconomic inequalities in mortality in six Western European countries, *International Journal of Epidemiology*, 32, 830-837.

Pearce, J. and Dorling, D. (2006) Increasing geographical inequalities in health in New Zealand, 1980-2001, *International Journal of Epidemiology*, 35, 597-603.

Ross, N., Dorling, D., Dunn, J., Henriksson, G., Glover, J., Lynch, J. and Weitoft, G. (2005) Metropolitan income inequality and working-age mortality: a cross-sectional analysis using comparable data from five countries, *Journal of Urban Health*, 82, 101-110.

Rowntree, B.S. (1901) *Poverty: A Study of Town Life*, London: Macmillan.

Shaw, M., Davey Smith, G. and Dorling, D. (2005) Health inequalities and New Labour: how the promises compare with real progress, *British Medical Journal*, 330, 1016-1021.

---

[1] Editorial Note: Figure 44.1 has been added to this chapter to illustrate what reduced health inequalities actually look like when shown on a graph. It has been so many years since health inequalities fell in Britain that this is a rare sight. However, we need to be careful that part of this is not a slowing down in the overall infant mortality progress in England and Wales in 2009 and 2010. It will take time and research to tell and discern this. A huge number of factors may be involved, from the introduction of free healthy food for pregnant women, to the large increase in the rate at which babies were being taken away from their parents following the death of Baby Peter in August 2007 and the conviction of his abusers in November 2008, see: http://en.wikipedia.org/wiki/Death_of_Baby_P

Singh, G.K. and Siahpush, M. (2006) Widening socioeconomic inequalities in US life expectancy 1980–2000, *International Journal of Epidemiology*, 35, 969-979.

Smyth, F. (2008) Medical geography: understanding health inequalities', *Progress in Human Geography,* 32, 119-127.

WHO Commission on Social Determinants of Health (2008) *Closing the Gap in a Generation: Health Equity through Action on the Social Determinants of Health*, Final Report of the Commission on Social Determinants of Health, Geneva: World Health Organisation.

Wilkinson, R.G. and Pickett, K.E. (2007) The problems of relative deprivation: why some societies do better than others, *Social Science and Medicine*, 65, 1965-1978.

Woodward, A. and Kawachi, I. (2000) Why reduce health inequalities?, *Journal of Epidemiology and Community Health*, 54, 923-929.

45

How will we care for the centenarians of the future?

Dorling, D. (2011) 'How will we care for the centenarians of the future?', *The Guardian*, 23 May.

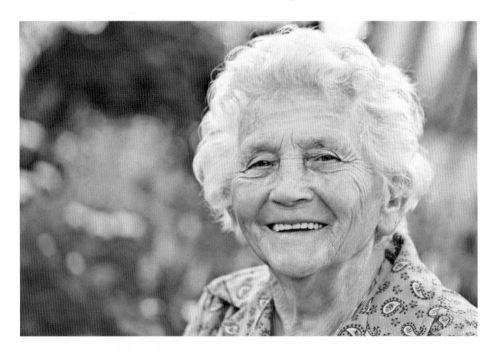

The future potential care bill for the elderly in Britain is so great that it could threaten family ties, according to a report released by the Organisation for Economic Co-operation and Development yesterday[1]. It suggests that, by 2050, the country will spend more than a fifth of its entire national output on services for the elderly.

In our new social atlas, *Bankrupt Britain*, I document with Bethan Thomas how the current economic woes have revealed a whole series of potential financial, residential and moral future bankruptcies[2]. The harsh truth is that by 2048, advances in medicine, a better-ordered society, and even huge amounts of care being provided by the young elderly, will not be enough to help us care for our rising population of

[1] Ross, T. (2011) OECD: huge elderly care bill threatens family ties, *The Telegraph*, 22 May, http://www.telegraph.co.uk/news/politics/8501333/OECD-huge-elderly-care-bill-threatens-family-ties.html
[2] Hill, A. (2011) It's grim in Kensington and Chelsea, claims author of social geography atlas; new atlas shows levels of crime, pollution and antisocial behaviour mean quality of life in affluent areas is declining, *The Guardian*, 20 May, http://www.guardian.co.uk/society/2011/may/20/britain-social-geography-atlas

the very old. Last year, the Department for Work and Pensions upped their estimates of future centenarians considerably, to suggest that there will be more than half a million aged over 100 by 2066[3].

To aggravate the situation, there is great uncertainty over how many young people there will actually be in the future in Britain, compared to how many we need. When the present Queen was just a couple of years on the throne, and then again a dozen years later, she was told wildly different stories about how many future subjects she should expect to reign over. Her advisers were uncertain, but such uncertainty matters when we try to prepare for our dotage.

In the 1955 and 1965 projections, published by the precursors of the Office for National Statistics for the UK, population around the time of the millennium differed by some 22 million people. The 1955 projection of 53 million by 1995 was far closer to the final outcome than was the 1965-based estimate of 75 million by 2001. We tend to overestimate future populations rather than underestimate them. The 1965-based projections, published around the Queen's 42nd birthday, projected that there would be more than 1.5 million babies born in the year 2000, a projection that turned out to be over twice the actual number.

When the 2011 census results are released in less than a couple of years' time, we will find out again if we have been over-estimating the population and perhaps then we will recognise that we do need censuses, we do need to plan and we could be much better organised than we are.

However, better organisation only gets you so far. No matter how well we organise ourselves in future, we do have a problem with how few youngsters there are projected to be in future in Britain. Even if (like almost every other nation state in Europe) we disband the households of servants that royalty and the super-rich have established to care for them, so that the cost of these servants can be redistributed to allow the rest of us to be cared for more efficiently, there may well not be enough younger people to go around in Britain. It is when people find that this is the case that the fear of an each-for-their-own attitude prevails most strongly.

Most of the world's population who are projected to be very elderly in 2050 are not living in those places where the vast majority of people currently being born are projected to live. Those born today are people who will, by 2050, be in the prime of their lives. But almost all of them won't be living in Britain, unless we change our attitude to immigration (in this country and across all of Europe) – the greatest fall in fertility in the world recently has been in eastern Europe, so we shouldn't expect help from Polish carers in future.

If our current population and household projections are allowed to run their course then, just as there was a 73% rise in single (mainly elderly) households between 1981 and 2008, with just a 12% rise in households containing more than one person, so too we should expect a similar rise over the course of the next 27 years.

---

[3] DWP (2010) Over ten million people to live to 100, Press release, 30 December, http://www.dwp. gov.uk/newsroom/press-releases/2010/dec-2010/dwp186-10-301210.shtml

However, as we can see, though, from the contradictory advice given to the Queen, there is nothing inevitable about projections. They have been out by millions before, mainly because what actually occurs is very much out of our hands. A higher proportion of single-occupancy households is what you get when you combine an ageing population with a curtailment of immigration.

Britain's full up, you might say, and – apart from when petrol prices rise suddenly and incomes fall – our roads are pretty full. But that has more to do with people taking more journeys in Britain than is usual in Europe, than with British population density being too high. Many of the more affluent British currently emigrate in great numbers to some of the most densely populated areas of Europe to enjoy their retirement in the sun: to Malta, to the Spanish Costas and other hotspots.

We have as many emigrants as immigrants; it's just that being a very unequal country the exchange has not always been that fair – more affluent Brits out (for at least the colder part of the year) and more poorer immigrants in.

This imbalance is a product of the inequalities we tolerate. Inequalities which, if they are allowed to increase unabated, result in a very unattractive image of a future society. Not the kind of place that will find it easy to care well for that first tally of half a million centenarians. I'm 'young' enough to be among that cohort (Table 45.1)[4]. If I should live that long I have a huge vested interest in Britain changing for the better beforehand.

---

[4] Editorial Note: The three footnotes above were included in the original piece as web-links. Understandably the *Guardian* could not include a table of data as well. Table 45.1 is shown here so you can work out for yourself, should you have been born after 1950, what your chances of living to 100 are thought to be. For me, born in 1968 and male, there is a 90% chance I'll make it to age 65, having lived to age 44; a 50% chance I'll live to 86 (and hence a 50% chance I will not) and a 13% chance I'll live to be a centenarian. My daughter's chance of living to 100 is estimated to be 32%, and my sons' chances are 24% and 26% (for the younger). The assumptions at play here include a presumption that future medical progress will be great. But these are the 'official' future projections. Thus the chance that any of my children reach age 100 is 62%, calculated as $1-(1-0.24)\times(1-0.32)\times(1-0.26)$. That is a better reason for me to worry about how we care for older people in the future than my own very selfish concerns, even if it is still quite personal. The 62% chance of at least one of the three seeing in the 22nd century assumes that their chances are independent of each other, and much else, which they clearly are not. Should they cooperate their chances improve. That is why this book is dedicated to all three of them ☺

Table 45.1: Office of National Statistics Projections of UK population future mortality rates, people born 1951–2013.

	Male cohort mortality rate by date of birth chance of living to age			Female cohort mortality rate by date of birth chance of living to age		
	90%	50%	% living to 100	90%	50%	% living to 100
1951	69	85	9	72	89	12
1952	69	85	9	72	89	13
1953	68	85	9	72	89	13
1954	68	85	9	71	89	13
1955	68	85	9	71	89	13
1956	67	85	10	71	89	14
1957	67	85	10	71	89	14
1958	67	86	10	70	89	14
1959	66	86	10	70	89	15
1960	66	86	10	70	89	15
1961	66	86	11	70	89	15
1962	66	86	11	70	89	16
1963	66	86	11	70	90	16
1964	66	86	11	70	90	16
1965	65	86	12	70	90	17
1966	65	86	12	70	90	17
1967	65	86	12	70	90	17
1968	65	86	13	70	90	18
1969	65	87	13	70	90	18
1970	65	87	13	70	90	18
1971	65	87	14	70	90	19
1972	65	87	14	70	90	19
1973	65	87	14	70	91	19
1974	65	87	14	70	91	20
1975	65	87	15	70	91	20
1976	65	87	15	70	91	20
1977	65	87	15	70	91	21
1978	65	88	16	70	91	21
1979	65	88	16	70	91	22
1980	65	88	16	70	91	22
1981	65	88	17	71	92	22
1982	65	88	17	71	92	23
1983	65	88	17	71	92	23
1984	65	88	18	71	92	24
1985	65	88	18	71	92	24
1986	65	89	19	71	92	24
1987	65	89	19	71	92	25
1988	65	89	19	71	92	25
1989	65	89	20	71	92	26
1990	65	89	20	71	93	26
1991	65	89	20	72	93	27
1992	66	89	21	72	93	27
1993	66	90	21	72	93	27
1994	66	90	22	72	93	28
1995	66	90	22	72	93	28
1996	66	90	22	72	93	29
1997	66	90	23	72	93	29
1998	66	90	23	73	94	29
1999	66	90	24	73	94	30
2000	67	91	24	73	94	30
2001	67	91	24	73	94	31
2002	67	91	25	73	94	31
2003	67	91	25	73	94	32
2004	67	91	26	74	94	32
2005	67	91	26	74	94	33
2006	67	91	26	74	95	33
2007	68	92	27	74	95	33
2008	68	92	27	74	95	34
2009	68	92	28	74	95	34
2010	68	92	28	74	95	35
2011	68	92	29	74	95	35
2012	68	92	29	75	95	36
2013	69	92	29	75	95	36

Note: These numbers are derived from those data and the rates shown assume that people have lived until at least 2012.

Source: Historic and projected mortality rates (qx) from 2010-based UK life tables – principal cohort projection.

46

We're all ... just little bits of history repeating[1]

Dorling, D. (2011) 'We're all ... just little bits of history repeating, Part 1: History, Part 2: Future', *Significance Magazine* website, 13 June.

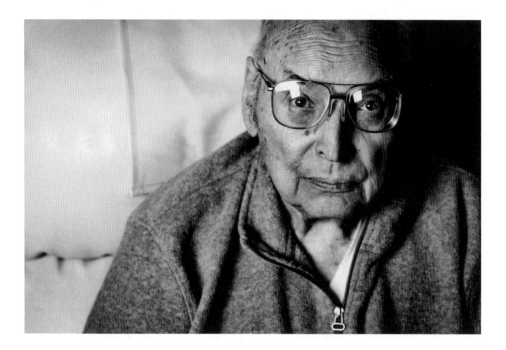

Part 1: History

In May 2011 the United Nations Population Division released 'The 2010 Revision' of its world population estimates and projections. The headline story was that the projection was up greatly on the previous medium variant estimate. We were now projected to number 10.1 billion within the next 90 years, 9.3 billion by 2050. The Division's press release came with a health warning *'Small variations in fertility can produce major differences in the size of populations over the long run. The high projection variant, whose fertility is just half a child above that in the medium variant, produces a world population of 10.6 billion in 2050 and 15.8 billion in 2100. The low variant, whose fertility*

---

[1] Online at: http://www.significancemagazine.org/details/webexclusive/1081285/Were-all___just-little-bits-of-history-repeating-Part-1---History.html and http://www.significancemagazine.org/details/webexclusive/1082185/Were-all___just-little-bits-of-history-repeating-Part-2---The-Future.html

remains half a child below that of the medium, produces a population that reaches 8.1 billion in 2050 and declines towards the second half of this century to reach 6.2 billion in 2100.[2]

Why had the medium variant projection gone up, and just how sensitive were the projections to small variations? Well, it turns out they had gone up because there had been a very small and very recent variation. Worldwide we had experienced a mini baby boom during the last decade. Take a look at Figure 46.1. On the left-hand axis, and as depicted by the thick line, are shown the new UN medium variant population projections in millions of people. On the right-hand axis, and by the thin line, is shown the first derivative of that trend – the change – births less deaths. I've put a black dot on the curve of change in case you miss it. The dot marks the end of a previously unexpected mini baby boom. It marks *now*.[3]

Figure 46.1: World population estimates and projections and annual population change.

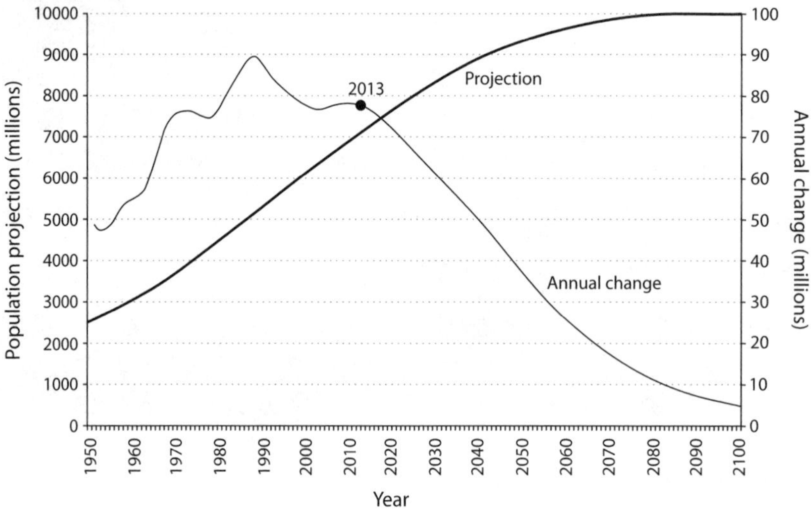

Source: UN median variant scenario, May 2011.

Demography is a complex science, but it is also an art. The correct way to look at projections is to calculate life tables and tables of fertility rates by age, to carefully project them forward year on year, to do this for each country, maybe even taking into account international migration trends and their impacts, add up the results

---

[2] United Nations Population Division (2011) World population to reach 10 billion by 2100 if fertility in all countries converges to replacement level, Press release embargoed until 3 May 2011, 11:00 a.m., New York time, see: http://esa.un.org/unpd/wpp/Other-Information/Press_Release_WPP2010.pdf
[3] 'Now' being 2013 for the version included here as that is when this book is published. You can get the data here: Rogers, S. (2011) World population by country: UN guesses the shape of the world by 2100, Guardian Datablog, 26 October, http://www.guardian.co.uk/news/datablog/2011/may/06/world-population-country-un

and publish your global projection. But there is another way to look at a projection. Just take the past trend and look at the change, and the change in the change, and see if there is a pattern.

Figure 46.2 shows the change in the change that the UN Division *both* estimates to have occurred and projects to occur in future, all in one thick line. It is the second derivative of population. It is births in one year less births the year before plus deaths the year before less the deaths this year. It is the degree to which population numbers are accelerating (change in change above zero) or decelerating (change in change below zero). The UN Division does not now estimate population change to decelerate as quickly in future as it did in its previous revision. Instead, based on the most recent evidence, it suggests the greatest deceleration will be by, at most, about one million people a year and that itself will flatten out towards almost no change in change by the century's end.

Figure 46.2: World population estimates and projections, annual change in population change.

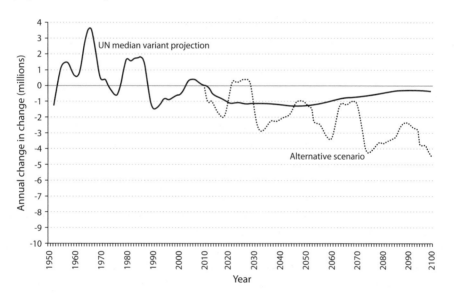

Source: UN median variant scenario, May 2011. Alternative scenario drawn as dotted line.

But what if the future is as spiky as the past? Look at the trend in Figure 46.2 of what we think occurred before 2011. Compare that to what is projected to come after (the solid line from 2011 onwards). The projection is very smooth as compared to its precedent. Perhaps change in change is just too hard to project and the UN demographers are sensible to suggest an asymptotic turn towards stability. However, we know something about what we are predicting here. These are people, but they are being treated as if they were drops of water flowing in and out of a bathtub.

The length of time between the most recent peak in Figure 46.2 (2006) and the one before it (1986) is 20 years, the one before that (1966) is 20 years. Do these lengths of time ring a bell? Remember, it's people we are talking about, not baboons or fruit-flies and not water running in and out of the tub. What is it that people tend to do every… 20 odd years? The answer: it's have more people, on average, worldwide. It is the current compressed length of a generation across most of the world.

So what if those peaks and troughs were to repeat? That is what the faint dotted line in Figure 46.2 illustrates. It is a projection based simply on repeating, from 2012 onwards, the last 32 years of peaks and troughs. It is just what you get with that little – generation and a half – bit of history repeating. Extending the pattern of change forward, as the faint dotted line does, suggests that what we have just experienced globally is a mini baby boom, many more babies born recently because many of the children of 1986 have recently become parents. They in turn, were more numerous because of the worldwide boom of 1966. And so we should expect a further smaller boom around 2026, 2046 and so on, perhaps becoming more spaced out, hopefully damping down as compared to the strict repletion shown by the dotted line in Figure 46.2.

Contraception has become more popular worldwide, especially where infant mortality has fallen most recently. Next, I'll show you what effect that tiny change in the future trajectory of the trend would have.

Part 2: The future

Estimating the past is hugely uncertain. Most people in the world are still born without being issued a well-recorded birth certificate and most die without their deaths being systematically counted. We estimate the past. The troughs and peaks of population from 1966 to 2011 that I showed above are all estimates and include estimates of better infant survival and estimates of prolonged lengths of life that will all have errors associated with them. What we can be most sure of is how uncertain the future is. That health warning the UN Division gave was very apposite because small fluctuations really do have huge effects, especially now that the second derivative of population shown in Figure 46.1 is hovering around the zero line.

To illustrate the uncertainty I had added that faint dotted line to the graph in Figure 46.2 which shows not the change, but the change in change projected forward if the peaks and troughs of the past were to continue into the future.[4] Introduction of this little bit of variation has a huge impact on how population could change in future. By altering the predicted change in change rates ever so slightly, to reflect the global baby booms of the recent past, the rate of population change itself is then projected to begin to fall rapidly shortly after 2030. The revised figures are shown

---

[4] Editorial Note: Look at the scale on the Y axis in Figure 46.2: it is measured in single millions. It shows the effect of there being population increases which are successively a few million less each year than the year before. Such small changes to the rate of change end up having a huge effect, if the rate continues to stagger downwards as it has done since 1971.

below with the dot again marking where we are *now*.[5] The trends from 1950 to 2011 are identical, but under this alternative median variant scenario births decline just a fraction more rapidly because – between the booms of the past – there were troughs which we currently ignore as we project forward from a time of boom. That potential error has great cumulative effects.

As Figure 46.3 shows, if the change in change repeats the most recent little bit of history we have enjoyed – then a human population maximum is reached in 2060 at 9.295 billion, but by 2100 there would be just 7.362 billion of us, the same number as currently, officially, are projected to be alive in around five years from now.

Figure 46.3: World population estimates, projections and annual population change – alternative median variant scenario.

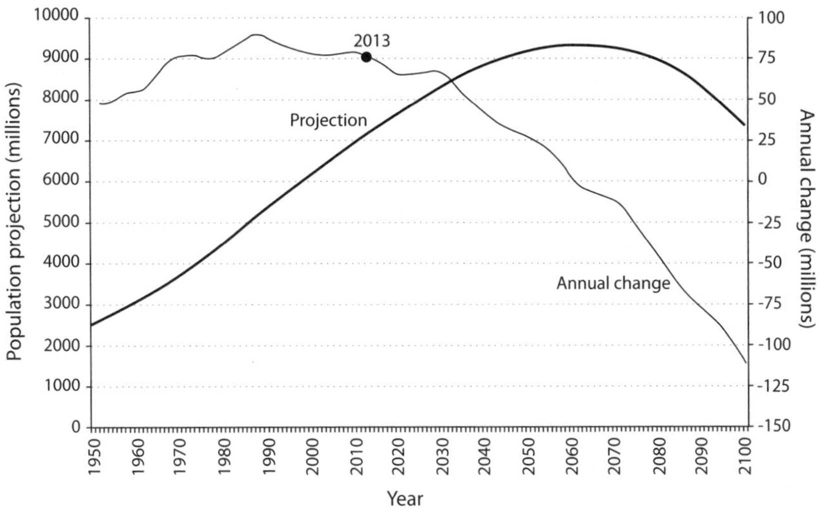

Note: The result of applying the change shown in Figure 46.2.

Many might hope that the falls were not as abrupt as those shown in Figure 46.3. You only have to continue that rate of decline forward another 38 years and we are extinct. As UN statisticians say, in warnings which are routinely ignored, small variations can produce major differences in the long run. Hopefully history will not repeat the last 32 years so exactly and in the long run our offspring's offspring are not all dead.

---

[5] Editorial Note: And 'now' again being 2013 (it is not easy, this 'thinking in different times' business), but as the piece was written using the same most recent data as that which is available as I write in 2012, just the dot needs to be moved on the graphs. When the UN next comes to revise its projections, then the graphs will alter, but you should not take any single year's projections too seriously. The potential errors are so great, the influences of the most subtle of social, economic and political changes so huge.

A fall to less than 7.4 billion humans by the year 2100 may appear rapid but it is slower than the UN Population Division's own low variant projection which is for world population to fall to 6.2 billion by 2100 if fertility were to fall to just half a child per women less than that expected by the medium variant projection. If women in areas where they are expected, on average, to have 2.5 children have 2, and if those expected to have 1.5 (between a group of them) each instead on average have 1, then there will be even fewer of us, and this would occur even sooner than projecting forward an ever-declining baby booms implies. If we had any firm understanding of how our very short-term futures were likely to pan out, then the United Nations would not endorse projections that vary by some 9.6 billion people (15.8 − 6.2) in just 87 years' time from now. But it is worth contemplating the possibility that soon we will begin to see the emergence of new regularities in our numbers.

The United Nations was born out of a World War, with the mission, above all else, to try to prevent its repetition and the harm that would cause in affluent countries. Over the last seven decades the people in it changed the UN's remit to be concerned much more with all humanity and with much more than primarily war. The same forces that have resulted in much better global population statistics becoming available in recent years might also lie behind the apparent medium-term deceleration in our numbers: better health, better contraception, better literacy, maybe even improved numeracy – worldwide. All of that might be more easily realised in future if we saw suggestions in our recent past that our immediate future might be more benign than we had been planning for.

Whether human beings become extinct depends far more on our behaviour than our numbers, and our behaviour depends greatly on what we understand. This is why it matters whether our recent past suggests there are trends in our collective behaviour which we are not yet aware of. As Shirley Bassey so presciently sang in 1997, just as the fourth post-war baby boom was beginning:

and I've seen it before
... and I'll see it again
...yes I've seen it before
... just little bits of history repeating

47

Future people and shifting power[1]

Dorling, D. and Hennig, B.D. (2011) 'In focus: global population shifts', *Political Insight*, vol 2, no 2, p 34.

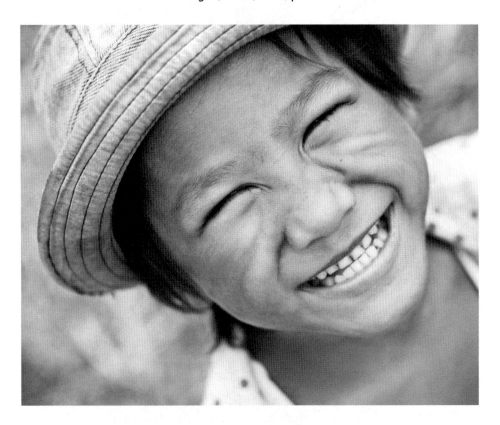

World population is forecast to rise to over 10 billion people by the year 2100 if the future foretold in the most recent United Nations population estimates come to pass. By the end of this year it is thought that the 7 billion mark will have been exceeded. However, the UN itself suggests that it is reasonable to assume a probability range of error for projections for the century's end which includes population possibly falling by then to be lower even than today, or to our numbers more than doubling between now and 2100 if current falls in fertility are not continued.

These three world population cartograms show just the beginnings of that change. The first (Figure 47.1) shows where the extra people assumed to be alive around 2015 will be as compared to those living in each grid cell on the map in 1990. The

---

[1] This article was jointly written in collaboration with Ben Hennig for the back cover of the journal.

Figure 47.1: Population growth 1990–2015 – total change projected on a gridded cartogram.

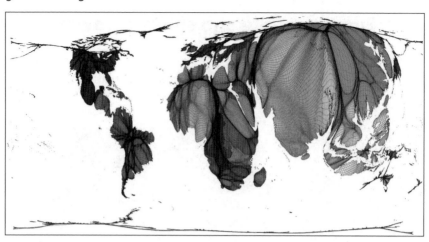

Source: Map drawn by Ben Hennig, using SEDAC data, the GPWv3 gridded population of the world, from Columbia University.

more extra people expected, the larger the areas of each cell in the grid. The second map (Figure 47.2) shows where there are expected to be fewer people in the very near future. Area on it is proportionate to that population loss. On these two world maps each country is coloured differently, but the colours are consistent between the two maps. On the third map (Figure 47.3) each cell is coloured just one of four shades and the area of each cell is drawn in proportion to current population. Areas shaded blue are declining most quickly in terms of people dying or leaving. Areas shaded orange or red are currently areas of the most births and/or in-migrants.

Figure 47.2: Population decline 1990–2015 – total change projected on a gridded cartogram.

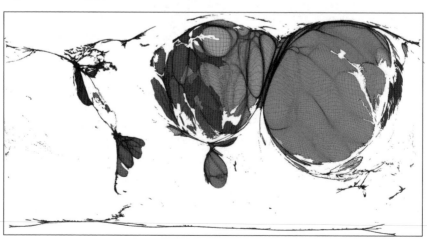

Source: Map drawn by Ben Hennig, using SEDAC data, the GPWv3 gridded population of the world, from Columbia University.

Many countries contain areas where population is currently falling and other areas where it is growing. This is why different parts of China appear on both the first two cartograms. The third world cartogram (Figure 47.3) shows that there is considerable growth in the Pearl River Delta, the factory of the world, where so many of the iDevices and other essentials of our (post)modern lifestyles are made. Elsewhere in China is found a more mixed pattern of growth and decline. Many other countries are expected to soon show the kinds of patterns exhibited already by China and much of Europe, not least the USA.

Figure 47.3: Population growth and decline 1990–2015 – areas of population increase or decrease shaded on an equal population gridded cartogram.

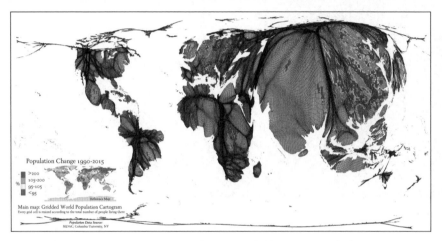

Note: Red areas are experiencing most population growth, blue areas most decline.

Source: Map drawn by Ben Hennig, using SEDAC data, the GPWv3 gridded population of the world, from Columbia University.

48

Looking on the bright side

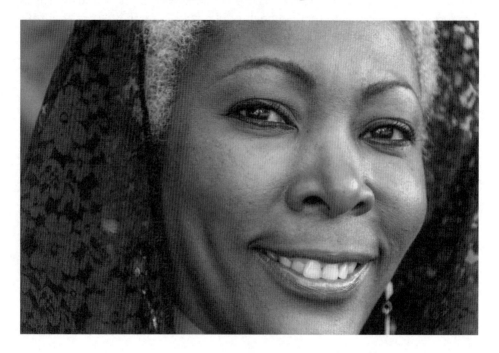

When considering inequalities in health it is all too easy to come to a depressing but incorrect conclusion. This tends to be worded slightly differently depending on the political biases of the proponent, but it mostly comes down to this: misery will always be with us, a great many will always be poor, only a few can be rich, and most will die, on average, much earlier than the best-off. This is not because we cannot control our numbers, invent cures or prevent pain, but because human beings are inherently predisposed to be selfish and, in being selfish, to harm others.

A virtue of selfishness is built up on the political right. The suggestion is that there is no alternative to current levels of selfish behaviour. Some go as far as to say that it is, in fact, essential to ensure we do not prevent a small minority building up huge profits founded on trading across the globe so that the masses can be fed and watered, but not given much more than that. On the political left, capitalism is not seen as curable but only as containable. Most on the left suggest that the very worst effects of unbridled selfish behaviour could be slightly mitigated, so in some rich countries inequalities are lower than in others, but that all rich countries must sustain their affluence at the expense of many others – if not the poor within their own borders, then the poor abroad.

Seeing beyond the theories of selfishness

Selfish intentions can be hidden in what may initially appear as idealistic calls for everyone to take responsibility. When these calls argue that selfishness is a force for good, it is suggested that capitalism is moral, practical and necessary, while government is immoral and unnecessary. This is libertarian anarchy. Its slightly tempered but still savage political near-neighbour is the nightwatchman state. In this state the government's primary role is to have monopoly control over violence, the military, the police and the courts, but it has no right to interfere in financial transactions between people, so that the more selfish are free to exploit those who are less greedy.

The political far-right are calling for either more libertarian anarchy or a nightwatchman state, even as conditions worsen in some of the most unequal of very affluent nations. Ecologically minded anarchy and a much shrunken but less violent state is called for by increasing numbers of younger people on the left, who also suspect that anything which allows too much power to concentrate in the hands of a few will reward selfishness. Other parts of the far-right want an even stronger state and renewed fascism, and similarly other factions of the far-left seek a strong state and new forms of communism. The political centre, meanwhile, appears to be no safe haven for rational debate, but a place where clone politicians can cluster and promote their selfish interests while claiming to do otherwise.

What, however, if most people are not that selfish, but that selfish people are many thousands of times more likely to find themselves holding the levers of power than others? One definition of selfishness is being '... *deficient in consideration for others, concerned chiefly with one's own personal profit or pleasure; actuated by self-interest'* (OED, 1984). This selfishness can be justified by particular ethical positions about the principles of consideration required for cooperating with others. Such justification suggests that people try to fool others into thinking they care about them while remaining chiefly concerned with their own or their own group's interests. They can only do this if they see others or people outside of their group as not being like them.

There is growing evidence that a small proportion of the population is much more likely to engage in unethical behaviour than others and that, as affluent societies are currently constituted, members of this small minority often end up with far more resources and hence more power. The collective ability to control this selfish few has become weakened in recent decades, but there is growing evidence that this is becoming more widely understood, further exposed, and that the malaise is now being acted on. We are becoming better at recognising that some psychopaths are able to rise to the top and we are also beginning to better recognise group psychotic behaviour, where members of an elite and isolated group develop amoral and antisocial behaviour in relation to those outside their group.

Many of those who join this elite lack the ability to love outside the group or to establish meaningful personal relationships; they show extreme egocentricity, fail to learn from experience, and are unable to empathise with people outside their own small group, or even outside of just their immediate family. We are learning that we need to control such an elite. As times are changing, some people in these elite groups are no longer behaving in this way. In many elite academic journals and institutions there is growing evidence of researchers looking outwards, and also getting more evidence from looking inwards too.

During 2012 a study was published in the *Proceedings of the National Academy of Science* (*PNAS*, illustrated by Figure 48.1; see Piff *et al*, 2012). The study reported the results of a series of experiments (conducted by psychologists at the University of California, Berkeley, and the University of Toronto, Canada) on upper-class individuals which found, among other things, that they '*... were more likely to break the law while driving, relative to lower-class individuals. In follow-up laboratory studies, upper-class individuals were more likely to exhibit unethical decision-making tendencies (study 3), take valued goods from others (study 4), lie in a negotiation (study 5), cheat to increase their chances of winning a prize (study 6), and endorse unethical behavior at work (study 7) than were lower-class individuals*' (Piff *et al*, 2012, p 4086). They even found that people could be conditioned to begin to behave like this by being encouraged to feel superior.

Figure 48.1: Upper-class individuals are more likely to engage in unethical behaviour.

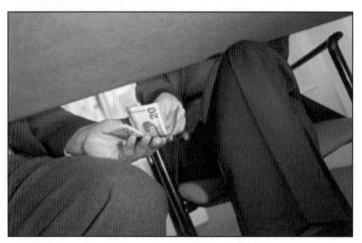

Source: Thinkstockwww.nsf.gov/news/news_summ.jsp?cntn_id=123301.

The results of the *PNAS* study were disseminated worldwide. The National Science Foundation in the US issued a press release (NSF, 2012), and quoted the lead author of the study as explaining: '*The relative privilege and security enjoyed by upper-class individuals give rise to independence from others and a prioritization of the self and one's own welfare over the welfare of others – what we call greed.... This is likely to cause someone to be more inclined to break the rules in his or her favor, or to perceive themselves as, in a sense, being "above the law" ... and therefore become more prone to committing unethical behavior.*'

The most interesting experiment in the study was designed to see whether people would become more likely to behave unethically if they were made to feel superior to others. This was done to check the extent to which it might be possible to alter selfish behaviour. If people could be easily made more selfish then perhaps it would not be naive to believe that a large group could be helped to be far less selfish if they had their eyes and minds opened up to the collective selfishness of their actions.

The results of the study and its nature are so simple that it is hard not to be concerned that it was a spoof, and it may be worth waiting for some replication. I was so suspicious when I read it that I contacted the authors and asked for more details of what they did. I think that says more about myself and the environment I live and work in than any laudable lack of gullibility on my part – living in a more selfish society makes us all less trustworthy and more suspicious. Essentially, what the study reported was that if some adults were made to feel superior to others, then their behaviour became more selfish:

> *Study 4 sought to provide experimental evidence that the experience of higher social class has a causal effect on unethical decision-making and behavior. It was the only study in which researchers manipulated participants into temporarily feeling either higher or lower in social class rank to test whether these feelings actually caused people to behave more or less unethically.... At the end of the study, the experimenter presented participants with a jar of individually wrapped candies, ostensibly for children in a nearby laboratory, but informed them that they could take some if they wanted. This task served as a measure of unethical behavior because taking candy would reduce the amount that would otherwise be given to children.... People in this study, who were made to feel higher in social class rank, took approximately two times as much candy from children than did people who were made to feel lower in social class rank.* (NSF, 2012)

Talking the talk of taxing the rich

When it comes to taking candy out of the mouths of others who have less it is not so much sweets but food that has been the paramount issue in 2012. This was the case even in the most affluent countries of the world such as the US and the UK. In the US 45 million people now rely on food stamps to live, a rise of 70 per cent from four years ago (Martin, 2012). In the UK the numbers having to go to food banks for food has doubled from the much smaller numbers counted 12 months earlier (Butler, 2012). But in other affluent nations, such as Austria, Belgium, Denmark, Finland, France, Germany, Ireland, Japan, the Netherlands, Norway, Sweden and Switzerland (Dorling, 2012), almost all people at the bottom of society have enough money to feed themselves – the decisions to deprive the poorest of so much are political. In the UK, within just two years, the Coalition government had announced measures that would result in the poorest tenth of people in the UK becoming almost 5 per cent worse off (see Figure 48.2). The measures announced in the March 2012 Budget gave most to the sixth, seventh and eighth best-off tenths of the population and, by reducing the top income tax rate from 50 per cent to 45 per cent, reduced taxes for those in the top 1 per cent, so the richest did not all lose out in comparison.

Figure 48.2: Impact of the taxation and benefit changes 2010 to 2014.

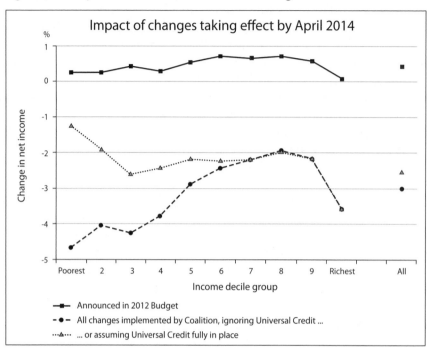

Note: The original graph was produced by the IFS and ignores measures affecting mainly the very rich. These budget measures included changes to taxation law proposed in the budget to prevent very rich people pretending they are giving money to charity, but giving it to something they have set up to look like a charity, to avoid paying tax. That proposal was not implemented, the reason given being that it would apparently affect genuine large charitable donations.

Source: Joyce (2012, Slide 12)

Figure 48.2 shows how a better world is possible. One line in the figure shows what could happen if the government were to introduce the new Universal Credit welfare benefit, a policy that the UK Coalition government says it is committed to. This policy would wrap up all welfare benefits into one single payment, and ensure that it always pays at least a little to be in work. If Universal Credit in this form were implemented, then the worst-off tenth would actually be the least hard-hit by 2014, and the best-off tenth would pay a slightly fairer share towards the common good (Joyce, 2012). To do this the very rich (not shown separately on the graph) would have to experience the largest falls in their net take-home income. That this is the predicted effect of a UK government policy actively being drafted is grounds for optimism. However, given the *PNAS* study reported above, and what we know of the social backgrounds of most UK government Ministers, there are strong grounds to be both suspicious and pessimistic about this particular government achieving anything like the Universal Credit results shown in Figure 48.2. But there are also more and more reasons for a little optimism, albeit tainted with a little scepticism.

In March 2012 the Deputy Prime Minister, Nick Clegg, called for the introduction of a 'tycoon tax' targeting millionaires who employ *'an army of lawyers and accountants'* to reduce their tax bills (Channel 4 News, 2012). And the leader of the Scottish Nationalist Party (SNP), Alex Salmond, committed his party to paying a living wage, saying: *'We have taken the first steps already, with every employee of the Scottish Government, the NHS and our agencies, guaranteed from this year at least the living wage of £7.20 an hour. Two thirds of the thousands who have benefited have been women…. I can announce today that every SNP-led council elected in May will also introduce the living wage'* (STV, 2012).

In April 2012, in the US, President Obama continued to support taxation policies that would reduce income inequality. He stated in his speech on the Republican Budget: *'The income of the top 1 percent has grown by more than 275 percent over the last few decades, to an average of $1.3 million a year. But prosperity sure didn't trickle down. Instead, during the last decade, we had the slowest job growth in half a century. And the typical American family actually saw their incomes fall by about 6 percent, even as the economy was growing'* (*Los Angeles Times*, 2012). He went on to win his second presidential election in the autumn of that year.

During the spring of 2012, Christine Lagarde, then the International Monetary Fund's Managing Director, called on China to reduce inequality, saying *'… more equal societies are able to achieve greater economic stability and lasting growth'*. She will have also known that quintile income inequalities in China and the US are almost identical (IMF, 2012). However, José Angel Gurría, the OECD's (Organisation for Economic Co-operation and Development) Secretary-General, continued the theme, suggesting: *'Inequality should be at the centre of our attention for economic, social and political reasons. Above all, inequality threatens social mobility … countries with high inequality essentially reinforce the vicious cycle of poverty'* (OECD, 2012).

Meanwhile, in Britain, it was announced in the March 2012 Budget that the minimum wage would be increased by just 11p (well below inflation), with the hourly rate for 18- to 20-year-olds frozen at £4.98 and that for 16- to 17-year-olds, frozen at £3.68, while *'Apprentices will enjoy a 5p increase in their minimum wage to £2.65 an hour'* (*The Telegraph*, 2012). If the adult national minimum wage had increased, since it was introduced, by the same rate as the renumeration of the FTSE 100 chief executive officers (CEOs) in the UK, then by April 2012 it would have reached £18.89 an hour (One Society, 2012a). This was followed by the Chancellor, George Osborne, in his 2012 Autumn Statement, announcing real-terms reductions to most welfare benefits, occurring simultaneosly with reductions in corporation tax, so that the very richest individuals would see their wealth rise as the incomes of the poorest fell. What those in power say and what they do is often very different. They may be beginning to say that they recognise growing inequalities are a problem, but if they do not act to reduce them, then their words are hollow.

Walking the walk when following the money

It is always worth doing a little maths. The cost of increasing the minimum wage of UK apprentices to that of 16- and 17-year-old workers, from £2.65 to £3.68 an hour, would be £1.03 an hour. Approximately 457,200 apprentices started work in 2010/11. If they are under the age of 18 they cannot work more than 40 hours a week (legally); £1.03 × 457,200 people × 40 hours is £18.8 million a year. From where could such a huge sum of money be raised?

Barclays' former chief Bob Diamond took home each year £17 million in pay, shares and perks, and Barclays has also paid out £30 million in shares to another eight directors (Treanor, 2012a); GlaxoSmithKline pays its chief executive officer (CEO) £6.7 million (Treanor, 2012b); and in 2011 Pearson's CEO received cash and share awards worth £9.6 million (Bowers, 2012a). Former Reckitt boss Bart Becht is, apparently, in line to receive £45 million in future share awards, which would take his total remuneration to over £200 million for less than six years' 'work' (Bowers, 2012b).

Just one collection of a dozen rich people can easily be identified who were earning or receiving *each* year *on average* £8 million *each*, or in total, £96.6 million a year. If their financial rewards were to be reduced to an average of £6.5 million a year (*each!*), all apprentices across the whole of the UK could receive an extra pound an hour, every hour, every year, for each apprentice. But these dozen rich people do not have the ability to make such a transfer, nor do they know who the apprentices are, or where they live. Such a transfer would have to happen by the government taxing the rich people and redistributing the money to the young apprentices. This is government's job, after all, to do what we are unable to do as individuals. But could the government go further?

Take the next dozen richest people after the nine Barclays bankers and three other CEOs. You could take them from the website that was used to form the list (One Society, 2012b), or from the *Sunday Times* Rich List or, if in government, from income tax records (the fairer way). Then work out who would have to pay a little more tax to achieve other goals: raising everyone's minimum wage to a decent standard, financing more jobs, giving those not working enough money to live on again, and raising the minimum pension income. In countries with so much inequality it is to the rich that we must look to see where the resources that would make these changes possible are being squirrelled away – follow the money!

Health inequalities are worse in those affluent countries where the richest 1 per cent have become the most acquisitive and where their greed is least well controlled by the other 99 per cent. As Figure 1.1 at the very start of this book (page 6) suggested, it is in those countries where overall health is poorer. This is hardly surprising. As Figure 34.1, some two thirds of the way through this book (page 314), illustrates, people become ill when the best-off 1 per cent of the population take up to a fifth of all income, leaving the rest of the population with just four-fifths of the national income to live on.

There is still much debate taking place as to the nature of the mechanisms that lead to more unequal affluent countries having worse health. Some who address this debate suggest that worse is yet to come, as *'income inequality may ... exert its strongest effects on health up to 15 years later'* (Subramanian and Kawachi, 2004, p 86).[1] In studies involving over 60 million subjects in 28 separate trials it was found that the strongest associations between income inequality and ill health existed in the most unequal of countries, since the 1990s, and were strongest when the health effects were measured some time after the rise in inequality (Kondo *et al*, 2009).

A tiny reduction in the income of the very richest 1 per cent, taking their share down by just a percentage point of national income through taxation, would raise much more than adding a penny on income tax for all earners. Taxation on wealth, including on land values, would raise even more, if more were needed.

In contrast to the benefits of the rich having their riches curtailed, having relatively less to live on for those who are poorer makes everybody less likely to share, more frightened and increasingly violent. When the poorest lose the most it is within the rest of the population that inequalities in income grow to be much higher than are found in more equal affluent nations, and people's health and happiness suffer as a result.

But this is an old story. The solutions are well known and there are many different solutions to choose from: greater economic equality brings about more equal health. It is the scandal of our times that inequalities in both health and wealth have been permitted to rise so high with such damaging and potentially long-term effects.

---

[1] See also Subramanian and Kawachi (2003, p 1039) on lag effects. One possibility that their suggestions lead to is that the 'golden generation', people born between 1925 and 1935, have had such good health compared to previous and subsequent cohorts because they have mostly lived through a period of rising equality and then moderately low inequality for the majority of their lives. I am grateful to Madhavi Bajekal for this suggestion. Subramanian and Kawachi (2007, p 597) find that income inequality is more weakly associated with mortality at ages over 64 in the US, and this, too, could be caused by those older generations having spent much of their lives living through periods of much greater income equality than is found today. If lag effects are this important then we may well see far less improvement in health than expected, both in the UK and in the US in years to come, in comparison to far more equitable countries.

References

Bowers, S. (2012a) 'Marjorie Scardino reward package close to £10m last year', *The Guardian*, 23 March (www.guardian.co.uk/media/2012/mar/23/marjorie-scardino-pay-pearson?CMP=twt_gu).

Bowers, S. (2012b) 'Former Reckitt boss Bart Becht in line for £45m in future share awards', *The Guardian*, 30 March (www.guardian.co.uk/business/2012/mar/30/bart-becht-reckitt-45m-pounds-share-awards?CMP=twt_gu).

Butler, P. (2012) 'Foodbank handouts double as more families end up on the breadline', *The Guardian*, 26 April (www.guardian.co.uk/society/2012/apr/26/food-bank-double-families-breadline).

Channel 4 News (2012) 'Nick Clegg's "tycoon tax" plans', 10 March (www.channel4.com/news/nick-cleggs-tycoon-tax-plans).

Dorling, D. (2012) 'Inequality and injustice: some news from Britain', *Urban Studies*, vol 33, no 5, pp 621-9 (http://bellwether.metapress.com/content/m10m3736514222q5/).

IMF (International Monetary Fund) (2012) 'China Development Forum 2012', Luncheon Address by Christine Lagarde, IMF Managing Director, Beijing, 19 March (www.imf.org/external/np/speeches/2012/031812.htm).

Joyce, R. (2012) Institute for Fiscal Studies post-budget PowerPoint: 'Tax and benefit changes, excluding those affecting mainly the very rich', 22 March (www.ifs.org.uk/budgets/budget2012/budget2012robjoyce.pdf).

Kondo, N., Sembajew, G., Kawachi, I., van Dam, R.M., Subramanian, S.V. and Yamagata, Z. (2009) 'Income inequality, mortality, and self rated health: meta-analysis of multilevel studies', *British Medical Journal*, vol 339: 64471.

Los Angeles Times (2012) 'Full text of Obama's speech on the GOP budget', 3 April (http://articles.latimes.com/2012/apr/03/news/la-pn-obama-speech-transcript-20120403/2).

Martin, S.K. (2012) 'Food stamp usage jumps 70 percent – highest it's ever been', *The Christian Post*, 23 April (www.christianpost.com/news/food-stamps-70-percent-increase-highest-its-ever-been-73723/).

NSF (National Science Foundation) (2012) 'New studies determine which social class more likely to behave unethically', Press release 12-038, 27 February (www.nsf.gov/news/news_summ.jsp?cntn_id=123301).

OECD (Organisation for Economic Co-operation and Development) (2012) 'Inequality', Remarks by OECD Secretary-General to the Chinese Academy of Governance, Beijing, People's Republic of China, 19 March (www.oecd.org/document/13/0,3746,en_21571361_44315115_49935501_1_1_1_1,00.html).

OED (Oxford English Dictionary) (1984) *The pocket Oxford dictionary*, Oxford: Clarendon Press.

One Society (2012a) 'How National Minimum Wage is falling behind top pay, and the damage this does to living standards and the economy', Briefing, 1 October (www.onesociety.helencross.co.uk/wp-content/uploads/2012/09/NMW-briefing-27Sept2012.pdf).

One Society (2012b) www.onesociety.org.uk/newsroom/latest-news/

Piff, P.K., Stancato, D.M., Côté, S., Mendoza-Denton, R. and Keltner, D. (2012) 'Higher social class predicts increased unethical behavior', *Proceedings of the National Academy of Science*, vol 109, no 11, pp 4086-91.

STV (2012) 'Alex Salmond's speech to the SNP spring conference', in full, Text of the First Minister's remarks to his Party's gathering in Glasgow, 10 March (http://news.stv.tv/scotland/300287-alex-salmonds-speech-to-snp-spring-conference/).

Subramanian, S.V. and Kawachi, I. (2003) 'Response: In defence of the income inequality hypothesis', *International Journal of Epidemiology*, vol 32, pp 1037-40.

Subramanian, S.V. and Kawachi, I. (2004) 'Income inequality and health: what have we learned so far?', *Epidemiologic Reviews*, vol 26, pp 78-91.

Subramanian, S.V. and Kawachi, I. (2007) 'Commentary: Chasing the elusive null – the story of income inequality and health', *International Journal of Epidemiology*, vol 36, pp 596-9.

The Telegraph (2012) 'Minimum wage frozen for young people', 19 March (www.telegraph.co.uk/news/uknews/9153274/Minimum-wage-frozen-for-young-people.html).

Treanor, J. (2012a) 'Barclays chief Bob Diamond takes home £17m in pay, shares and perks', *The Guardian*, 9 March (www.guardian.co.uk/business/2012/mar/09/barclays-chief-bob-diamond-pay).

Treanor, J. (2012b) 'GlaxoSmithKline chief's pay package more than doubles to £6.7m', *The Guardian*, 12 March (www.guardian.co.uk/business/2012/mar/12/glaxosmithkline-chief-pay-andrew-witty).

Index

Page references for figures and tables are in *italics*; those for notes are followed by n